The Silent Subject

The Silent Subject

Reflections on the Unborn in American Culture

Edited by
Brad Stetson

Foreword by Richard John Neuhaus

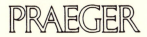

Westport, Connecticut
London

Library of Congress Cataloging-in-Publication Data

The silent subject : reflections on the unborn in American culture /
  edited by Brad Stetson ; foreword by Richard John Neuhaus.
     p. cm.
   Includes bibliographical references and index.
   ISBN 0–275–95032–8 (hc : alk. paper).—ISBN 0–275–95392–0 (pb :
alk. paper)
    1. Abortion—United States—Moral and ethical aspects.
   2. Abortion—Social aspects—United States. 3. Fetus—Moral and
ethical aspects. I. Stetson, Brad.
   HQ767.15.S56   1996
   363.4′6′0973—dc20   95–31397

British Library Cataloguing in Publication Data is available.

Library of Congress Catalog Card Number: 95–31397
ISBN: 0–275–95032–8
     0–275–95392–0 (pbk.)

First published in 1996

Praeger Publishers, 88 Post Road West, Westport, CT 06881
An imprint of Greenwood Publishing Group, Inc.

Printed in the United States of America

The paper used in this book complies with the
Permanent Paper Standard issued by the National
Information Standards Organization (Z39.48–1984).

10 9 8 7 6 5 4 3 2 1

Copyright Acknowledgments

"The Abortion" by Anne Sexton is reprinted by permission of Sterling Lord Literistic, Inc. Copyright
© 1962 by Anne Sexton. Excerpts from HECKEDY PEG, text copyright © 1987 by Audrey Wood,
reprinted by permission of Harcourt Brace & Company.

In Remembrance

Bradley John Stetson
August 15, 1991
II Samuel 12:23

Contents

Acknowledgments   ix

Foreword   xi
Richard John Neuhaus

Preface   xv

Introduction: The Silent Subject
   Brad Stetson   1

Part I: Ethical Perspectives

  1. The Moral Status of Fetuses and Embryos
     John A. Mitchell and Scott B. Rae   19

  2. Ignorance of Fetal Status as a Justification of Abortion:
     A Critical Analysis
     Francis J. Beckwith   33

  3. Moral Duty to the Unborn and Its Significance
     Sidney Callahan   43

  4. The "Medicalizing" of Abortion Decisions
     Thomas Murphy Goodwin   51

Part II: Cultural Perspectives

   5. Feminism and Imaging the Unborn
       Camille S. Williams   61

   6. Sex and Consequences: An Anthropological View
       Olivia Vlahos   91

Part III: Personal Perspectives

   7. Motherhood in the 90's: To Have or Have Not
       Maria McFadden   115

   8. Pregnancy Care Centers: Sisterhood is Powerful
       Frederica Mathewes-Green   123

   9. Women Who Abort: Their Reflections on the Unborn
       David C. Reardon   135

Part IV: Religious Perspectives

  10. When Good Men Do Nothing: Reflections From a Modern-
       Day *Bürgermeister*
       Michael McKenzie   151

  11. The Catholic Debate on the Moral Status of the Embryo
       Tom Poundstone   169

Part V: Legal Perspectives

  12. The Effective Enforcement of Abortion Law Before
       Roe v. Wade
       Clarke D. Forsythe   179

  13. Supreme Court Jurisprudence and Prenatal Life
       Tom Poundstone   229

Selected Bibliography   247

Index   255

About the Editor and Contributors   263

Acknowledgments

I am deeply grateful to each of the contributors to this book for their admirable patience and diligence. Many other people and organizations have contributed to the formation of this book and are due sincere thanks, among them are: William B. Allen, Matthew Berke, Steve Bivens, Lily Bridenbaker, Robert H. Carter, Bob Cheatham, Joseph G. Conti, Carolyn Crawford, Jim Elmore, Brian Finnerty, Marcia Goldstein, Jim Ice, Jeff Johnson, Anne D. Kiefer, Anne Kindt, William W. May, John H. Miller, Frank Montejano, Liz Murphy, Richard John Neuhaus, David Quackenbush, Dennis Rasmussen, John and Carol Stetson, David Stetson, Doug Stetson, Nina Stetson, Ed Trenner, Anthony and Delia Trujillo, Miles Vest, David L. Weeks, The Alan Guttmacher Institute, The Right to Life League of Southern California and The David Institute. These people and groups are not responsible for any errors or omissions contained in this work.

Foreword

Richard John Neuhaus

Nobody would claim that during the last three decades there has been silence about the subject of abortion. Almost no question has been so persistently, heatedly, and often hysterically disputed in our public life. In another sense, however, there has been a most remarkable silence about the subject of abortion — that subject being the human life that is terminated by abortion. That subject, the human life in the womb, is itself silent, and its potential voice silenced by abortion. It (she? he?) is not a participant in our public debates.

Three decades after abortion became a major item on the public agenda, and more than two decades after *Roe v. Wade* made the United States the first democracy in history to effectively abolish abortion law, many readers may be inclined to think that there is nothing new to be said about abortion. That would be a mistake. There is much that is new in *The Silent Subject*, and much that is not new but is explored from perspectives too often neglected. Amidst all the hysteria and sloganeering, we cannot weary of striving for a civil conversation on this most fevered question in our public life. On January 23, 1973, the day after the *Roe* decision, the prestige press and television declared that the Supreme Court had "settled" the abortion question. Of course that turned out to be spectacularly premature, for today there is no more unsettled question in the political arena.

We do not have the civil conversation that is required, indeed it might be argued that we have not even had much of a public debate. A debate requires a measure of honesty, at least the ability to suspend partisan passions enough to allow all relevant considerations to be placed on the table. But it must be admitted that one side in the debate has adamantly insisted upon the exclusion of "the silent subject" from the debate. Surely it is long past time to recognize that we cannot honestly consider the merits of "choice" without considering what is chosen. Many who have gone along with, even championed, the pro-choice position know this, but for whatever reasons have successfully suppressed what they know.

Early on in the controversy, an editorial in *California Medicine* (September 1970) reflected on this phenomenon. "Since the old ethic has not yet been fully displaced it has been necessary to separate the idea of abortion from the idea of killing, which continues to be socially abhorrent. The result has been a curious avoidance of the scientific fact, which everyone really knows, that human life begins at conception and is continuous whether intra- or extra-uterine until death. The very considerable semantic gymnastics which are required to rationalize abortion as anything but taking a human life would be ludicrous if they were not put forth under socially impeccable auspices."

In September, 1994, a National Institutes of Health (NIH) panel on embryo research recommended government funding for the creation of human embryos in the laboratory solely for the purpose of scientific experimentation. The embryos would be discarded when they are no longer useful for research purposes. The panel could not disguise the reality that "everyone really knows," namely, that human life begins at conception. The panelists acknowledged that their recommendation was to produce human lives for research purposes and then destroy them. They spoke about the "profound respect" that is due human life, but then made a critical move by distinguishing a human life from a "person." (For a fuller discussion of the NIH panel and its proposals, see "The Inhuman Use of Human Beings," *First Things*, January 1995.)

The NIH panel differed from the logic of *Roe*, since it candidly asserted what *Roe* suggested we could not know—when a human life begins. Having acknowledged the obvious, the move to the question of "personhood" is perfectly understandable. If we say it is permissible to kill some human beings but not others, it becomes necessary to provide a criterion that distinguishes the protected from the unprotected. The NIH panel, like others who have addressed this question in recent years, seized upon personhood as the needed criterion. The concept of personhood has a complicated history in theology, philosophy, and law, but it is not a scientific concept. It is, rather, an ideological concept, a useful idea that provides a possible justification for doing what we want to do.

In support of its recommendations, the NIH panel cited an article by Professor Ronald Green, himself a member of the panel, "Toward a Copernican Revolution in Our Thinking About Life's Beginning and Life's End." It is indeed a revolution that is proposed by Professor Green and others. The article asserts that there are no "qualities existing *out there*" in any human being requiring us to respect him or her as a person. Whether to grant or deny "personhood" (and hence the right not to be harmed or killed) is, we are told "the outcome of a very active and complex process of decision on our part." In the current language of the academy, personhood is entirely a "social construct." Whether someone is too young or too old, too retarded or too sick, too troublesome or too useless to be entitled to personhood is determined by a "decision on our part." This has a kind of logic to it, but it is obvious that the

American people have not been consulted about, and certainly have not consented to, this "Copernican Revolution" in our understanding of human dignity and human rights.

The proposal that human dignity and human rights are simply social constructs has large ramifications. It has to be squared with our political order's constituting claim that, in the words of the Declaration of Independence, human beings are possessed of "unalienable rights" bestowed by Nature and Nature's God. This is not an esoteric philosophical dispute. If we believe that we bestow standing in the human community—rather than God or some other understanding of ultimate reality bestowing such standing that we are bound to respect—all kinds of possible consequences follow. As much as some people resist the analogy, the question posed is essentially that posed by the *Dred Scott* decision of 1857 which declared that slaves of African descent have no rights that white men are bound to respect. Even more strongly, some people resist the analogy with the Nazi doctrine of *lebensunwertes Leben* —lives that we deem unworthy of life.

The resistance to the drawing of these analogies is perfectly understandable. After all, we are not Nazis and we are not slaveholders. This is the United States in the 1990s, not America in the 1850s or Germany in the 1930s. The differences between our circumstance and those other circumstances are very important, but so also are the similarities important, and deeply troubling. The stakes for how we think about humanity and the human future could not be higher. Also at stake is our understanding of democracy. More than twenty years later, it is obvious to all but the willfully blind that the American people have not ratified the logic and decision of *Roe*. Today the defenders of the unlimited abortion license created by *Roe* have only the Supreme Court to rely upon. In a democracy, this is an extremely dangerous isolation of the judicial power from the democratic process. In addition, it became evident in the 1992 *Casey v. Planned Parenthood* decision that only two justices on the Court are prepared to say that *Roe* was rightly decided, even though another three go along with the abortion license that it established.

Significant change in the law now seems probable. The goal of the pro-life forces, as I understand it, is quite unequivocal: That every unborn child be protected in law and welcomed in life. Given the limits of law and public policy, as well as the fallen condition of humanity, that goal will never be perfectly achieved. It is precisely that, a goal to strive toward. The goal of the pro-choice forces, at least until now, is unmistakably clear: To maintain the status quo of *Roe*, which is the legal availability of abortion for any reason during the entire nine months of pregnancy. Those of us who have followed the survey research data over the years know that at no time have more than 20 percent of the American people supported that goal, and even that support seems now to be declining. The overwhelming majority of Americans desire some kind of accommodation, which would include laws more protective of the unborn and policies more responsive to the needs of women with crisis pregnancies. There is reason to believe that that desire will grow and achieve greater political effect in the years ahead.

Essays in this volume make the compelling case that women, too, are often "the silent subject" in abortion. As this controversy has developed it has become increasingly obvious that the dispute is not between men and women. We must also hope that it will become more evident that the dispute is not simply between those who call themselves pro-life and those who call themselves pro-choice. Nor is it a dispute between the religious and the secular. All those divides are pertinent to the dispute, but finally the questions facing all of us have to do with the definition of humanity, the criteria for membership in the political community, the basis of our civilization's claims about human rights, and our responsibility to those who cannot protect themselves. When, God willing, the abortion controversy is behind us, partisans of the pro-life and pro-choice positions are going to have to live together in this society. That is why, while sloganeering and passionate polemics are inevitable, civil conversation is essential. And that is why *The Silent Subject* is such a gift to all of us at this point in the controversy.

Preface

This eclectic collection of essays pondering the significances of human fetal life and analyzing the social and cultural forces which shape public understandings of it speak to questions which have long needed answers. But because of the unique and highly contentious nature of the abortion debate, answers have been slow in coming.

This social silence on the manifold meanings of nascent human life is indeed ironic, given the political prominence of abortion debates. This book exposes that irony, opening venues of reflection seldom entered in the public square, thereby bringing before the public mind a subject that is tremendously underconsidered in proportion to its value and significance.

Together the essays in this work constitute a sensitive, public argument for a reconstruction of the confused—yet dominant—popular attitudes toward nascent human life and its value. Unlike virtually all arguments from this viewpoint, it offers no strictly religious or exclusively sectarian warrants for its assertions—instead bearing a more secular cast, it speaks to a generalized and pluralistic audience. As a whole *The Silent Subject* embraces no specific, particular political ideology. Its contributors represent a broad spectrum of professional interests, political perspectives and social philosophies—all of which indicates the fundamentally humanistic and apolitical nature of concern for the unborn and the degree to which they are esteemed.

The essays in this collection are idiosyncratic, being a product of each author's special personal concerns and perspective on the contemporary cultural devaluation of human fetal life. But while each reflection is unique, they all thematically dwell on a subject which is at the core of the most urgent and intractable moral issue of our time (abortion)—a core paradoxically shrouded in silence by the intimidating force of political correctness and the controlling authority of social custom.

The book is divided into five perspectival sections: Ethical, Cultural,

Personal, Religious and Legal. In each discrete section the authors address seminal issues and questions relevant to that particular sphere of inquiry. Each author speaks in his or her own voice, and on behalf of only themselves. Thus, the reader may find points at which different writers hold distinctly separate views on the same topic. This variety of opinion indicates the vitality, tolerance and intellectual diversity of pro-life sentiment in America. As well, it serves as an invitation to the reader to further consider the assertions and implications of these articles, writings which stand as a challenging testament to the objective and socially transcendent value of every human life—wherever it is, and however silent.

The Silent Subject

Introduction: The Silent Subject

Brad Stetson

[T]here has been virtually no reporting at all on the debate over the moral status of the fetus. What is being aborted, after all?

—James Davison Hunter, sociologist, 1994[1]

[W]e at NPR [National Public Radio] just do not cover this issue [abortion] because we think it has been decided

—NPR reporter[2]

So much has been written and said over the last three decades about the complex of issues surrounding abortion and abortion politics that one would think it difficult, if not impossible, to say something new about them. But it is not. Indeed, it is very easy, if one is willing to set aside the rigid conventions of public debate that reign in this country, and if one is willing to resist the culturally embedded understandings of what today constitutes "tolerant," "fair" and "compassionate" comment on the topic. For the truth is that the subject of every abortion—the unborn human being whose life is being ended—has received little genuinely comprehensive and sustained conversational attention in the American public square. Yes, the unborn might be the subject of a bumper sticker slogan, or pasted onto a protest sign, or perhaps vaguely referred to in legal papers as something the government might be interested in, *but as a central topic of widespread and probing public contemplation, nascent human life is verböten.*

In abortion and public policy discussions, to broach the topic of the beauty and awesome nature of nascent human life, details of fetal development or personal obligations implicated by the value of the unborn is to be derided as "carrying on a love affair with the fetus," as former surgeon general Joycelyn Elders once said abortion opponents did—to their great shame, in her eyes. For Dr. Elders and those of her ilk—as her remarks imply—the human fetus is not a legitimate object of love. Deep concern for it is misplaced, and fetal life is not worthy of the sort of close, sustained attention and reflection one associates with an affection as intense as "love." This is an extremely significant understanding rooted in much of American culture. Of course, the irony of Dr. Elders, formerly the leading national health officer—*and a pediatrician*—holding such a view is substantial. It is a testimony to the depth to which unborn human life has been denigrated and dehumanized. Thirty years after the advent of institutionalized abortion practice, the human fetus is not to be regarded as an appropriate object of love. This disquieting reality is only underlined by the fact that the perspective Dr. Elders' remarks reflect is one that holds ascendance among bureaucratic, political and media elites. It is the norm among many opinion makers.

Without question the regnant conversational and attitudinal restrictions about the unborn are a direct consequence of the unborn's legal and moral disenfranchisement. But to point that out is only to underline the extent to which our cultural discourse has eclipsed the significance of nascent human life. This is a silence that is uncomfortable for us as a nation. It does not coincide with our national history of protecting the vulnerable, or with what we have traditionally known to be the unique value of human life and the beauty of new birth. Nor does it coincide with the plain facts of biology as we apodictically know them to be. Yet it is a silence that persists, and has been diffused in American culture to the point of a matter of protocol in public debate and political discussions. Civilized and thoughtful people are expected to step around the violent death of the unborn accomplished by every abortion. To mention it in dialogue or debate is to solicit angry glares, impatient sighs and apparently learned expressions of skepticism about knowing when "human life begins."

All of which helps incline the body politic to the fiction that "compassion" requires us as a nation to embrace liberal abortion laws.[3] This is an extremely powerful moral judgment in American life. It has ascended to the level of "public truth"—that is, a generally accepted, unquestioned feature of the social and cultural landscape. There is no such thing, in the agora of public opinion, as being compassionate to the unborn. Not only are they not accorded the legal status of persons, but they are not even admitted into public discourse as legitimate objects of concern. Thus, the devaluation of their lives is not just a legal and moral reality, it is largely a patterned response and presupposition of reflection which has been installed within the public consciousness itself. To realize the power of this settledness, we only need note that opinion polls consistently show that most Americans oppose the morality and legality of most abortions performed and that most Americans are stunningly ignorant of current abortion law.[4] The result: abortions—throughout the three trimesters of pregnancy—continue at the rate of about 1.5 million annually.[5]

So, there has unquestionably been an unnatural cleaving in American society between moral sentiment and social practice. This lacuna is enforced and perpetuated by a social silence—a palpable social pressure strongly shaping public discussions—about information and new understandings that would threaten to expose the absurdity of this gap.[6] Consider, for example, the following instances of censorship and suppression:

- A college newspaper is forbidden by its editor in chief from running an ad placed by a pro-life group, which includes photos of fetuses in the womb and a simple description of common abortion procedures. The editor says its readership is pro-choice, and will be "greatly offended" by the ad.[7]
- A planned speaker at a high school honor society induction dinner is disinvited because the vice-president of the society fears the speaker's opposition to abortion might be "offensive" to some of the honor students.[8]
- A billboard in upstate New York reading "Abortion has two victims—one dead, one wounded," is repeatedly defaced, with special attention given to obliterating a phone number advertising access to eight different agencies providing abortion alternatives, including free prenatal care, housing, parenting classes and adoption counseling.[9]
- A fifth grade child in Alaska is ordered by a public school superintendent to disassemble and remove from classroom display her science project "Is abortion murder?—Yes," which presents photographs of aborted human fetuses. The superintendent says the student has not selected an "appropriate topic" for study.[10]
- Democratic governor Robert Casey of Pennsylvania is forbidden from speaking at the 1992 Democratic National Convention, because his pro-life position is at odds with the official position of the party. Later, when invited by *The Village Voice* to speak on the possibility of being a pro-life liberal, he is shouted down by audience members who disagree with his views.[11]

And the examples could be multiplied many times. The hegemony of the spirit of "choice" and its assorted baleful consequences are clearly the result of the contemporary *zeitgeist* with which the apotheosis of personal liberty—understood as the minimization of self-responsibility and constraint on individual desire—is thoroughly consonant. In postmodern America, where all things normative bear a heavy burden of suspicion, if not outright revilement, the public mind is inclined away from consideration of the intrinsic value of unborn human life and the personal and social obligations individuals bear toward it.

Importantly, it is the turn to the subject in American philosophy, the antitraditionalistic moralism of political-correctness, the general relativism and solipsism in American society along with the popular focus on self and unfettered "self-expression" which all converge to provide fertile intellectual and social contexts for the insinuation and legitimation of this ethos of "choice." But the "expressive-individualism" which results reflects a distorted view of the human person, void of the community ties and intimate relationships which decisively contribute to our self-formation and moral life. Thus, one's participation in it inevitably leads to frustration, alienation and an unrealistic self-understanding.

We are not the unencumbered, shorn selves autonomously choosing perceived goods and exercising rights that is the picture of the American individual featured by the culture of "choice."

But apart from the anthropological inaccuracies and psychological confusion generated by the existential enthroning of "choice," choice itself is bankrupt as an ethically ordering concept. Many people today believe that merely because they have made a behavioral choice or selected a position on a given topic or issue, their decision is therefore morally right and impervious to critical evaluation. But the act of making a choice cannot by itself serve as an ethically right-making consideration. "Choice" is not itself a moral value. It is only a faculty of the will, a formal category. Choice itself is a morally empty process without any intrinsic moral qualities. It is neither good nor bad in itself, but rather depends upon the antecedently established moral quality of its subject for its own moral warrant. Choice—the act of making a decision—alone, without any ethical and social context, is simply a mechanical mental operation, like adding two and two.

But does the mere fact that a decision has been made automatically render that decision morally justified? Obviously not. The worth of our decisions and expressions of autonomy is not independent of the courses decided or the expressive ends chosen. The moral quality of our choices is wholly determined by what it is we have chosen to do and why we have chosen it. The absolutizing of freedom in contemporary American life and the *prima facie* rightness accorded actions done by individual "choice" obscures this, and insulates the work of "choice" and "self-expression" from moral criticisms of even the simplest sort.

The truth is in other areas of life, free from the confusing fog of political correctness enshrouding consideration of nascent human life and abortion, we routinely—as individuals and as a public—approve or disapprove of individual and social choices based on the content and substance of those choices. The recent national *mea culpa* over interning Japanese Americans during World War II, and the current cultural vigilance regarding racism and hate crimes, all attest to our felt need to evaluate morally the substance of our choices.

But to point this out is only to affirm the fact that the manifold impoverishment of public discourse and moral aphasia infecting this country is rightly a matter of rather comprehensive record.[12] The stunted nature of public moral consideration is, of course, in no small part the result of a reified and practiced manipulation of language, seen most clearly in the way we as a public talk about unborn human life and abortion. Through the anodyne of "appropriate" words, we have learned how to dull our conscience and protect ourselves from the jarring reality of our cultural practice of abortion. As Michael Bauman frankly comments:

> We hide the fetal holocaust that surrounds us every day just as effectively as
> the Nazis hid their extermination of the Jews. And we do it the same way. We

cannot bring ourselves to utter the "M" word, though we commit the "M" act. That is, we do not murder unborn children, we "abort fetuses". . . . Some of the more squeamish among us are unable even to say the "A" word. Though by aborting fetuses rather than murdering babies our linguistic sleight of hand has hidden the real nature of our action (murder) and the real identity of our victim (baby), some people require a still heavier dose of verbal opium. We must tell them they are merely "terminating a pregnancy," which eliminates overt reference to any living thing. . . . If "terminating pregnancies" is still too overt a verbal description because the word *pregnant* tends to evoke unfortunate images of happy women large with child, we can hide the crime behind an even more impersonal wall of words. We can say that the murdering of unborn children is nothing more than the voluntary extraction of the "product of conception," or, as nearly all abortion clinics have it, "removing the POC." What could be more innocent.[13]

An important effect of this sanitized language is that it lends to our remarks about the abortion of the unborn the *appearance of reasonableness*. It allows us to believe that we have seriously and forthrightly engaged the full moral meaning of abortion, that we have acted as responsible and mature moral agents. But in fact all we have done is take our place in the long procession of people who have participated in a rhetorical dance of obfuscation and self-justification regarding the human target destroyed by the violence of every abortion committed. This participation only works to strengthen the intellectual atmosphere and ambient sociocultural forces which superintend the culture of "choice" and our talk of abortion.

This noosphere pervades the dens of elites as well as the warrens of popular culture. In both arenas, one questions the acceptability of abortion on demand only at risk to one's reputation and trustworthiness. As a matter of course, assorted *ad hominems* such as "misogynist" and "extremist" await any expression of doubt about the social and moral wisdom of abortion. In many schools of medicine, for example, students are tacitly taught not to consider and openly debate the ethical question posed by abortion. In the polite and learned setting of medical school, one doesn't bring that up. While ethics courses for physicians in training are proliferating, it is still uncommon for them to comprehensively broach this topic of *sui generis* significance. Remarks one medical school professor, "The majority of people going into medicine are trained not to make a judgment as to whether abortion is right or wrong, they are trained to avoid such moral judgments. This assists in dehumanizing the unborn, because people have never been expected to make a rigorous moral evaluation about them. Most people who go through medical school have not had their moral learning and capacity for ethical reflection keep pace with their medical and scientific training."[14]

Such cultural drifts are part of the larger shift in American society from a pre-1960s general commitment to the bourgeois, middle-class values of thrift, diligence, self-discipline and delayed gratification to the postmodern 1990s ethos of atomistic individualism and liberal social engineering.[15] A cardinal result of this change, and one which has played no small role in mediating to us the culture of "choice," is the rise in American society of a backward distinction between the public and private. This has the curious and perverse result of taking things that should always be private and making them very public, such as peoples' sex lives and sexual preferences. Conversely, things that ought to be public—for example, the way one conducts oneself in society, raises one's family and deals with one's neighbors—are regarded as though they were merely private questions. This is a perversity that strongly contributes to our moral tenor where a developing human being, simply because of its temporary (and natural) location inside a woman, can be degraded to the point of chattel—ironically, just as women once were and still are in many non-Western cultures.

With specific reference to the abortion of the unborn, we can get a feeling for the magnitude of America's cultural shift if we realize that Planned Parenthood, today among the most vociferous pro-choice lobby groups, recognized in one of its 1964 pamphlets that "Abortion kills the life of a baby, once it has begun," and in 1947 one of its officers referred to the being produced by conception as "the new baby which is created at [that] exact moment."[16] Today, the clinics of Planned Parenthood systematically accomplish tens of thousands of abortions every year, bringing in millions of dollars of revenue.

This societal inclination marginalizes the substantial interests of unborn human beings in public debate and deliberation. The resulting routinized closing of the American mind to the unborn is so inveterate that people who say they are "pro-choice" actually tend to disapprove of the legality and morality of many abortions, when particular circumstances are identified.[17] This indicates the rehearsed, politically correct and sterile quality of peoples' attitudes toward the unborn. Unless the usual tracks of public discussion are broken and they are reminded of the life and humanity of the unborn, many people simply manifest the opinions cued to them by their social milieu.

In the same vein, the experience of one pro-life attorney who has debated the topic of abortion before pro-choice gatherings indicates a presumption operating in peoples' minds against according favor and full moral standing to nascent human life. She says she no longer relies on oral argumentation and rational persuasion—based on biological and philosophical realities—to make her case. Such an approach has proved ineffective. "I've really lost a lot of respect for people's ability to think clearly," she says.

> People generally aren't persuaded by sound argument anymore, now you've got to punch them with an image, you've got to grab their heart and shake them up. I've found that only when I actually show people physical evidence, photos of babies killed by abortion, do they respond with a realization of the violence of abortion. I often hear, 'Oh, I didn't know that is what an aborted baby looks like. I thought it was only a blob of tissue. It's legal so how could

it be this horrible, its head separated from its arms and legs?'[18]

But even though the contemporary flavor of American culture and society devalues unborn human life and inhibits open, comprehensive public reflection on it, there is no question that Americans are becoming less comfortable with the regime of abortion on demand. People are growing more cognizant of the use of abortion as *ex post facto* contraception, and of the rhetoric of choice as an asylum from personal moral responsibility, for both women and men.[19] Recent proof of this is to be found in the 1994 elections, in which no pro-life incumbent lost and pro-life challengers defeated more than thirty clear abortion advocates. *New York Post* columnist Ray Kerrison comments that the election shows that the "U. S. is rapidly, astonishingly, and mercifully revolting against abortion."[20] Furthermore, most voters in the election who were polled by Richard Wirthlin said that they preferred a pro-life Republican to a pro-choice Democrat for the 1996 presidential election, 48 to 35 percent.[21]

All of which would seem to indicate that Americans are decisively growing in their unease over the chasm between their moral expectations and the shape of current abortion law and practice. Those who are able to unhitch their thinking from the dominant paradigms of the day or become aware of the simple biological realities of fetal development and abortion practice are often not willing to consent to the sweeping reduction of abortion to "a woman's right to choose," no matter how persistent the elite establishment or abortion lobby is in incanting that slogan.

And for good reason, for the presence of a separate living human being is undeniable, as indicated by these widely recognized facts of fetology: a unique and permanent independent genetic identity (since conception); a beating heart (since three and a half weeks postconception); detectable brain activity (since six weeks postconception); fully formed fingers and toes, and all internal organs (since eight weeks postconception). By three months, this human being is autonomously active, forming fists, bending arms, curling toes, and growing rapidly.[22]

Awareness of these realities, coupled with recognition of the very real violence of abortion, bears the potential of overcoming the ethical complacency and conversational controls to which we as a social body have become accustomed. And certainly this habituation is powerful, as it is able to stunt the reporting of even the most morally perverse and ethically repelling transgressions of the abortion culture. For example:

- Recently a woman shot herself in the stomach in order to kill the 20-week fetus inside of her. The baby survived the attack, was born alive, but later died after efforts to save it. The woman, nineteen years of age, was charged with third-degree murder and manslaughter.[23] Of course, had she aborted in an abortion clinic, killing the child—at the same stage of development and even later—would have been perfectly legal.

- Recently a 24 week old fetus received life saving surgery while still in-utero.[24] But had the mother wished to have this fetus killed through abortion, in every state of the nation it would have been legal for her to do so.

- In California the state Supreme Court has held that someone who causes the death of a fetus as early as seven weeks can be charged with fetal murder.[25] This does not apply to doctors who, with the mothers' consent, cause the death of fetuses sometimes much later in pregnancy.

- The ACLU argued that a 1970 California law against fetal murder could not be used against a pregnant woman who caused the stillbirth of her full-term unborn baby by going on a two-day drug spree just before the child's birth, because the law violated the woman's right to privacy by intruding on her freedom to make decisions about childbearing and health care.[26]

- Under the category of the bizarre, the mother of Ana Rodriguez expressed relief that Dr. Abu Hyatt—with whom she had contracted to kill via abortion her eight-month preborn child—had been convicted of assault. Hyatt sliced off the arm of the now 16-month-old Ana Rodriguez during a failed abortion attempt. The maimed young girl's mother said she hoped Hyatt received a long prison term.[27]

- In Dr. George Tiller's place of business—an abortion clinic in Wichita, Kansas—where ten to twenty late second- and third-trimester abortions are performed each week, it is routine for several women at a time to lie on cots in a central room in the clinic basement, in labor to deliver their nearly full-term—but dead—babies. Tiller charges from $1,850 to $3,000, cash only, for each abortion, and incinerates the aborted babies in his own basement crematorium on the premises.[28]

- A pioneering new method for late second- and third-trimester abortions—the D & X (Dilation and Extraction)—calls for the doctor to pull all of the baby except the head down into the vagina. The doctor then takes a pair of blunt scissors and forces the scissors into the base of the baby's skull, spreading it to enlarge the opening. Using a suction catheter, he then sucks out the brain of the human being, killing it. One Dr. Martin Haskell, who teaches the procedure to other doctors at National Abortion Federation seminars, has done this more than seven hundred times to unborn babies 20 to 26 weeks developed.[29]

- A Los Angeles doctor who operates two abortion clinics is called "an unselfish and committed provider" by a judge who sentenced him to one year probation for the deaths of two women to whom he was administering abortions.[30] Later, following review by the Medical Board of California, the doctor, who has performed approximately 100,000 abortions, had his medical license revoked.[31]

- Fully one out of ten fetuses in the United States is exposed to cocaine in the womb, affecting three hundred thousand babies a year.[32]

- In the New York State Legislature, efforts at requiring doctors to notify parents if their newborn children are HIV positive have repeatedly failed, since to do so allegedly violates the parents' right to privacy.[33]

Given the media-saturated time in which we live, and the popular obsession with violence and horror, one might think that these lurid tales would cadge the lenses and pens of the press. But they rarely do, and when they do it is certainly not an attention that is commensurate with the awfulness of the events. Again, we see the effect of the rules of discourse controlling public discussion. The victim status of women in the regime of political correctness, the political power of the women's rights establishment and the left-liberal sympathies of most print and electronic journalists render sustained attention to the suffering of the unborn and the moral perversities of the abortion culture out of bounds.[34]

Yet, certainly moral responsibility requires that we move beyond the politically safe media constructions of reality and vie for the objective truth about the nature of nascent human life. In an insightful yet simple attempt to make plain the logically and biologically obligatory conclusion that every human life begins at conception, bioethicist Sidney Callahan writes, "If we took a movie of everyone alive and ran it backward, we would see that we are continuous with our embryonic beginnings . . . we can rationally infer that the child and the infant—and before that the fetus and the embryo—are continuously us."[35] This thought experiment was tellingly borne out by the experience of one Los Angeles obstetrician, who wrote of why he no longer does abortions. After the onset of depression and self-loathing following years of abortion practice, Dr. George Flesh explained how his change of heart came about:

Early in my practice, a married couple came to me and requested an abortion. Because the patient's cervix was rigid, I was unable to dilate it to perform the procedure. I asked her to return in a week, when the cervix would be softer.

The couple returned and told me that they had changed their minds and wanted to "keep the baby." I delivered the baby seven months later. Years later, I played with little Jeffrey in the pool at the tennis club where his parents and I were members. He was happy and beautiful. I was horrified to think that only a technical obstacle had prevented me from terminating Jeffrey's potential life.[36]

So Jeffrey's is one life spared from the altar of "choice." He will go on to realize a life of possibilities, but such a future is denied to millions of other unborn human beings who are put to death by abortion for reasons that are usually unremarkable. This is a truth full of pain, and so it is a truth the voice of which we as a society seek to deny in myriad ways. In no small part, this denial is accomplished by the *de facto* codes of public debate which sustain silence, codes whose force holds at bay understandings that might shatter the dominant plausibility structures of the reasonableness of "choice."

Before he was overcome by liberal political ambition, Jesse Jackson spoke out against the rationality of the abortion culture, and on behalf of the unborn. He once asked: "What happens to the mind of a person, and the moral fabric of a nation that accepts the abortion of the life of a baby without a pang of conscience? What kind of a person, and what kind of a society, will we have 20 years hence if life can be taken so casually?"[37]

The sorry answer to that question is on the front page of newspapers every day and leads off the six o'clock news every night. We have a society which has become coarsened and brutalized, one that has radically devalued human life.[38] But since we have legally, morally and culturally given credence to the idea that an unborn human life has the same value as ex-utero human lives only if its mother wants it to have such value, can we really expect anything more? We have fostered many definitions of moral reality, and we now endure the pervasive chaos and social convulsion such relativism insinuates within a society.

Those who would see our prodigal nation return to an understanding it once held to be self-evident—that the right to life is inalienable—are obliged to continue to speak out in a voice however dissonant with the spirit of our age. Ferment over abortion, the most intractable of battles in the culture war, will continue, apparently without any cessation of hostilities or armistice of wills. And perhaps no such peace should be soon expected, for, as a variety of authors have suggested, arguments about abortion are really assertions about much more than the issue itself.[39] Yet amid the prolonged cultural sound and fury, there remains the silent unborn human being that we all once were, and in whose innocence there reposes the best of each of us. It is a dignity and value we did not earn, but is unrivaled by any living thing on earth. Perhaps it is our greatest and most far-reaching social pathology that we have cheapened it to the profound depths we have.

NOTES

1. James Davison Hunter, *Before the Shooting Begins: Searching for Democracy in America's Culture Wars* (New York: Free Press, 1994), p. 163.

2. Ibid., p. 165.

3. See Mary Ann Glendon, *Abortion and Divorce in Western Law* (Cambridge, Mass.: Harvard University Press, 1987) for an explanation of the development and permissiveness of American abortion law, especially with regard to the positions of other developed nations on this subject.

4. Some recent polls documenting this are to be found in *The Boston Globe*, 31 March 1989, pp. 1, 12; "Poll: Abortion Key for Voters," *USA Today*, 2 January 1990, pp. 1A, 2A; "Abortion Legislation Poll," *Newsweek*, 17 July 1991, p. 17; and "Gallup Poll: America is Pro-Life," *The Washington Times*, 28 February 1991, p. 1. For a clear and concise description of the current scope of abortion law, including the

often denied fact that abortion in the United States is legal throughout the nine months of pregnancy, see Hunter, *Before the Shooting Begins*, pp. 247–249.

5. The most stringently conservative recent reporting puts the abortion total, for 1991, at 1.3 million, having steadily risen from 193,000 in 1970, with 45 percent of all abortions in 1991 having been performed on women who've already received at least one abortion. See "Abortion Surveillance—United States, 1991," Centers for Disease Control and Prevention, CDC Surveillance Summaries, 5 May 1995, MMWR 1995; 44 (No. SS-2), pp. 27–29, 49. It should be noted though, that such numbers are undoubtedly low, since not all states collect and report all their abortion data, and individual abortion providers within the states are not subject to having their own data checked or verified by any independent government, health, or law enforcement body. Indeed, even the Alan Guttmacher Institute (Planned Parenthood) cites the 1991 and 1992 abortion totals at more than 1.5 million each. See their report "Abortion Services in the United States, 1991 and 1992," by Stanley K. Henshaw and Jennifer Van Vort, published in *Family Planning Perspectives* 26, no. 3 (May/June 1994): 100–106, 112.

6. All of which is simply to say that there is great pressure in this society to be pro-choice. This force directs people to those attitudes which are laudable and popularly reasonable. In this way this force of political correctness—a sort of peer pressure writ large—conditions public sentiment, since the accepted norms of opinion in a given social context significantly affect the opinions people choose to hold. For full explanations of the psychological and sociological dynamics of this effect, called by Elizabeth Noelle-Neumann the "spiral of silence," see her work "The Spiral of Silence: A Theory of Public Opinion," *Journal of Communication* 24 (Spring 1974): 43–51; and *The Spiral of Silence* (Chicago: University of Chicago Press, 1984). For representative discussion of this phenomenon at work in public considerations of other controversial issues, such as affirmative action and racial politics, see Frederick R. Lynch, *Invisible Victims: White Males and Crisis of Affirmative Action* (New York: Praeger Publishers, 1991) and Joseph G. Conti and Brad Stetson, *Challenging the Civil Rights Establishment* (Westport, Conn.: Praeger Publishers, 1993), respectively.

7. "Pro-Choice, Anti-Speech," *The Wall Street Journal* 30 November 1992, p. A14.

8. Nat Hentoff, "The War Against Offensiveness," *Orange County Register* 5 December 1994, Metro p. 7.

9. Ibid.

10. Reported on "CNN Headline News" with Judy Fortin, 4 March 1995, 1:30p.m. Pacific Standard Time broadcast.

11. See Nat Hentoff, "Pro-Choice Bigots," *The New Republic* 30 November 1992. Reprinted in the *Human Life Review* 19, no.1 (Winter 1993): 21.

12. See, for example, William Bennett, *The De-Valuing of America* (New York: Summit Books, 1992); William Donohue, *The New Freedom* (New Brunswick, N.J.: Transaction Publishers, 1990); Alisdair Macintyre, *After Virtue* (Notre Dame, Ind.: University of Notre Dame Press, 1984) and *Whose Justice? Which Rationality* (Notre Dame, Ind.: University of Notre Dame Press, 1988); Richard John Neuhaus, *The Na-*

ked Public Square (Grand Rapids, Mich.: William B. Eerdmans Publishing Co., 1984)
and *America Against Itself* (Notre Dame, Ind: University of Notre Dame Press, 1992);
Os Guiness, *The American Hour* (New York: Free Press, 1993); William Sullivan, *Reconstructing Public Philosophy* (Berkeley: University of California Press, 1986),
and Robert Bellah et al., *Habits of the Heart: Individualism and Commitment in American Life* (Berkeley: University of California Press, 1985).

13. Michael Bauman, "The Euphemisms of Abortion Hide the Crime," *Orange County Register* 9 January 1989, reprinted in Francis J. Beckwith, *Politically Correct Death: Answering the Arguments for Abortion Rights* (Grand Rapids: Baker Book House, 1993), p. 181.

14. Brad Stetson, Interview with Jeffrey L. Johnson, M.D., assistant professor of Clinical Pediatrics, University of Southern California School of Medicine, 20 October 1994. Perhaps emblematic of this ethical myopia is the founding of the student group, "Medical Students for Choice" at several medical colleges across the country.

A concrete example of the lack of moral rigor Dr. Johnson is citing is to be seen in the reactions of doctors to the case of a woman, 22 weeks pregnant, who sought an abortion. The abortion was to be administered by two injections. First, an abortifacient was to be injected, followed by a drug to stimulate contractions. The resident doing the procedure inadvertently administered the injections in reverse order, causing the baby to be delivered alive. By law, efforts to resuscitate the baby had to be made. The mother, however, did not support such efforts, describing her newborn as "the doctor's problem." Two days later the baby died. Ironically, most of the physicians with whom Dr. Johnson spoke regarding this episode did not find it ethically troubling, or even worthy of careful reflection. It was legally correct, and that was all that mattered.

15. For discussion of the effects of this shift, particularly on the underclass, see Myron Magnet, *The Dream and the Nightmare: The 60's Legacy to the Underclass* (New York: William Morrow, 1993).

16. George Will, "The Case of the Unborn Patient," *Newsweek* 22 June 1981.

17. See chapter 4, "The Anatomy of Ambivalence," in Hunter, *Before the Shooting Begins*, particularly pp. 86–99, for a detailed discussion of the many nuances of public opinion on abortion.

18. Brad Stetson, interview with Anne Kindt, 16 September 1994.

19. As many writers have argued, *Roe v. Wade* and the common practice of abortion benefits men not women, by freeing them from the consequences of their sexual behavior. Indeed, a significant percentage of women who abort report that they did so under pressure from a man. For discussion of males pressuring females to abort and the various psychological sequelae suffered by women as a result of abortion, see the comprehensive survey work of David C. Reardon, *Aborted Women, Silent No More* (Chicago: Loyola University Press, 1987), especially pp. 27–40; 45–47; 328–337. Of course this is a great and tragic paradox, since it is women's rights groups who championed the legalization of abortion, who defend it today with little regard for the harm it causes women, and who hold it out as *the precondition* for women's social and economic equality with men. For a sensitive statement on how and why the interests

of women should not be seen as mutually exclusive with a pro-life ethic, see "A New American Compact: Caring about Women, Caring for the Unborn." *First Things*, No. 27, November 1992, pp. 43–46; and Frederica Mathewes-Green, *Real Choices: Offering Practical, Life-Affirming Alternatives to Abortion* (Sisters, Oreg.: Questar Publications, 1994).

20. Quoted in "For the Record," *National Review*, 19 December 1994, p. 10.

21. Ibid.

22. These developmental markers are noted in standard texts, including F. Beck, D. B Moffat, and D. P. Davies, *Human Embryology* 2nd ed. (Oxford: Blackwell, 1985); Keith L. Moore, *The Developing Human: Clinically Oriented Embryology* 2nd ed. (Philadelphia: W. B. Saunders, 1977); Andre E. Hellegers, "Fetal Development," in Thomas A. Mappes and Jane S. Zembaty, eds., *Biomedical Ethics* (New York: Macmillan 1981), pp. 405–409; Landrum Shettles and David Rorvik, *Rites of Life: The Scientific Evidence of Life Before Birth* (Grand Rapids: Zondervan Publishing, 1983).

23. "Woman Who Shot Herself Is Charged in Fetus' Death," *Los Angeles Times*, 10 September 1994, p. A34.

24. "Fetus to Get Surgery for Birth Defect," *Santa Barbara News Press*, 9 September 1993, p. A1.

25. Susan Carpenter McMillan, "...While in California, a Court Affirms the Humanity of a Fetus," *Los Angeles Times*, 20 May 1994, p. B11.

26. "Murder Charge Is Rejected in Drug-Related Stillbirth," *Los Angeles Times*, 22 August 1992, p. A13.

27. "Botched Abortion," *Orange County Register*, 25 February 1993, p. A12.

28. These facts are documented in Jessica Shaver's article, "Attack on Doctor Shifts Focus from the Violence of Abortion," *Orange County Register*, 29 August 1993, Commentary p. 3. Regarding the ethical issues surrounding violent attacks on doctors who perform abortions—attacks which have rightly been condemned by virtually all opponents of abortion—see Richard John Neuhaus, "Bloody-Minded Compassion," *First Things*, No. 40, February 1994, pp. 48–50; and "Killing Abortionists: A Symposium," *First Things*, No. 48, December 1994, pp. 24–31.

29. Nat Hentoff, "No Limit on 'Choice?' Here's the Ugly Result," *Los Angeles Times*, 26 July 1993.

30. See *National Right to Life News*, 7 September 1994, p. 20.

31. See "Abortion Deaths Cost Doctor License," *Los Angeles Times*, 25 May 1995, pp. A3, A40.

32. "In the Name of the Children," *Los Angeles Times Magazine*, 7 August 1994, p. 14.

33. "AIDS: Civil Liberties vs. Lives," *The Wall Street Journal*, 13 September 1994, p. A16. See also Peter Hellman, "Suffer the Little Children," *New York*, 21 February 1994 and John Leo, "Babies Have Rights, Too," *U. S. News and World Report*, 1 May 1995, p. 23.

34. See Los Angeles Times reporter David Shaw's seminal study of pro-choice media bias in his series, "Abortion Bias Sweeps into News," *Los Angeles Times*, 1 July 1990, p. 10f. See Hunter, *Before the Shooting Begins*, pp. 154–168 for a thor-

ough discussion of the topic. Of late, the carefully shaded nature of reporting has again been seen in the way many pundits and the press were duly skeptical of research findings showing that an induced abortion raises a woman's risk of contracting breast cancer by at least 50 percent, and by 300 percent if the abortion occurs before she is eighteen years old. (See "Induced Abortion Hikes Breast Cancer Risk, Study Says," *Los Angeles Times*, 27 October 1994, p. A3; and "Linking Abortion and Breast Cancer," *U. S. News and World Report*, 7 November 1994, p. 70). For discussion of the studied silence of the media on the abortion—breast cancer link, see David Rothbard and Craig Rucker, "No 'Buts' About It: Bias in Science-Reporting," *Orange County Register*, 25 November 1994, Metro p. 23 and Mona Charen, "Breast Cancer: The Hidden Link to Abortion," *Orange County Register*, 19 October 1994, Metro p. 9.

35. Sidney Callahan, "The First Stage of Life Is Life," *Los Angeles Times*, 19 June 1991, p. B.7. Of course one common way some commentators attempt to avoid Callahan's conclusions is by importing gradations of human life into consideration of the ontological status of the unborn. But any and all talk of "partial human-ness" is inevitably arbitrary and subjective, since it must appeal to a particular religious or otherwise ideological touchstone of "complete human-ness," the warrant for which is itself going to be private and parochial—and in strong need of comprehensive justification. Some writers who appeal to gradations of humanity often reserve "partial human-ness" for the earliest stages of pregnancy (e.g., one day, three weeks), where they presumably see abortion as unproblematic. It is important to point out, however, that the earliest abortions are not performed before six weeks postconception, so that the doctor performing the procedure is able to reassemble ex utero the dismembered body, in order to verify the completion of the procedure, and reduce the risk of infection. Thus, the appeal to embryonic "partial human-ness"—even if wrongly accepted as legitimate—is irrelevant to the abortion debate, since no abortions are performed at that stage of pregnancy. The specter of RU-486, the so-called "abortion pill," being employed as an abortifacient at this early stage of pregnancy is problematic as well, since (1) it is still a means of abortion and susceptible to all the arguments against abortion; and (2) it is simply untrue that RU-486 is safe and clinically unproblematic. For two brief discussions of some of the dangers of RU-486, see Janice G. Raymond, "RU-486: Miracle Drug Turns Nasty," *Los Angeles Times*, 11 April 1993, p. M5 and Callahan, "The First Stage of Life Is Life."

36. George Flesh, "Why I No Longer Do Abortions," *Los Angeles Times*, 12 September 1991. I should point out that Dr. Flesh was not prevented from terminating Jeffrey's "potential life," as he says, but Jeffrey's actual life, along with the future realization of Jeffrey's potential.

It is instructive to note that Dr. Flesh's experience underlines the plain yet often overlooked biological and linguistic reality that words like "embryo" and "fetus" have *developmental* not *ontological* significance. That is, they refer to a definite and established type of being at a certain stage of its existence, not a being which at its present stage is ontologically different from what it will later become. In this general regard see the essay by John A. Mitchell and Scott B. Rae below.

37. Quoted in Patrick Buchanan, "Christians, Nazis and Jesse Jackson," *Los An-*

geles Times, 13 December 1994, p. B7.

38. For example: In 1991 a resident of Los Angeles had a greater chance of dying from a bullet wound than from a car accident; over the last three decades violent crime in America has increased 560 percent; since 1960 the teen suicide rate has more than tripled, and it is now the second leading cause of death among American adolescents; in 1960, 5 percent of all births were out of wedlock, by 1991 the number had risen to 30 percent; the United States has the highest divorce rate in the world, presently approximately half of all American marriages end in divorce. For full documentation of these and other troubling social trends, see William Bennett, *The Index of Leading Cultural Indicators* (New York: Simon and Schuster, 1994).

39. They are claims about concepts and values as broad as family, motherhood, independence, identity, and meaning in life. Most notably in this regard, see Kristen Luker, *Abortion and the Politics of Motherhood* (Berkeley and Los Angeles: University of California Press, 1984), and Hunter, *Before the Shooting Begins*, part I.

Part I

Ethical Perspectives

Chapter 1

The Moral Status of Fetuses and Embryos

John A. Mitchell and Scott B. Rae

It is a genetic fact that a fertilized human ovum is 100 percent human. . . . All that is added between conception and death is food, water and oxygen.
— J. P. Moreland and Norman L. Geisler[1]

We have raised a whole generation that believes we have more in common with an opossum than with a human fetus.
— Dennis Prager[2]

At the root of all discussion regarding human rights is the fundamental question, "Who counts as a human person?" And, more specifically, "When does human personhood begin and end?" The answer to the question at both ends of the spectrum requires metaphysical reflection in three areas: (1) What is a substance and what is a property-thing?; (2) What does it mean to be a human being?; and (3) What does it mean to be a human person? In this chapter, we address these questions and attempt to lay a metaphysical foundation for ethical decision making concerning human rights at the edges of life. While the implications of this analysis extend to a variety of ethical issues, we limit our application to the ontological status of the unborn, and argue that zygotes, embryos and fetuses (hereafter referred to synonymously) are fully and equally human beings and, consequently, human persons.

SUBSTANCES VERSUS PROPERTY-THINGS

Developing an ontology of unborn human beings first requires drawing a distinction between substances and property-things. In the tradition of Aristotle and Aquinas, acorns, dogs and human beings are examples of substances. Every substance is an individuated essence that bears accidental properties (i.e., nonessential properties, like the arrangement of spots on a dog or the I.Q. of a human being) and exists as a deeply unified whole that is ontologically prior to its parts. That is, a substance is more than the aggregate or emergent sum of its parts and properties. Most importantly, a substance possesses a defining, internal principle within its essence that informs its law-like change and behavior. Conversely, an artifact is a property-thing or an ordered aggregate. A Ford Aerostar is an example of such an entity, existing as a loosely unified aggregate of externally related parts. There is no underlying bearer of properties existing ontologically prior to the whole, and no internal, defining essence that diffuses, informs and unifies its parts and properties. It is merely a collection of parts, standing in external, spatial-temporal relations that, in turn, give rise to a bundle of externally related properties that are determined by those parts.

The same is not true with a substance, say a dog. The properties of a dog adhere differently than the properties of an automobile. The properties of the dog are grounded in, unified by, and emerge from the capacities that constitute the internal structure of the dog's essence. Thus, a dog is more than the external organization of its parts functioning in a given way. Its properties are deeply unified and related *internally* as part of the essential nature of "dogness." A dog is what it is apart from convention, and its properties exist only in the context of a coherent, ontological whole. Conversely, a Ford has no ontology beyond its additive or emergent properties, bundled together to form a loosely unified whole. Lacking an internal essence or nature, an ordering principle is externally imposed upon a set of parts to form a bundle of properties by human convention. To possess an internal nature, then, is possible only for substances, all of which belong to a natural kind and exist in a manner essentially unique to a particular class of beings. Their essential nature informs their being and affords the essential properties peculiar to their natural kind. All members of a given species instantiate the same essential nature. Thus, it is unintelligible to assert that a substance can exemplify its nature to a greater or lesser degree, since the essential nature underlying a given member of a species is nondegreed. That nature either is or is not exemplified by some particular.

So, while substances possess an internal nature, property-things do not. There is no internal, ordering principle to ground a Ford's unity, govern its law-like change, or guide its movement toward an ontological *telos* (end). Instead, there are only modifications caused by external forces. Specifically, human minds designed and built the automobile by configuring its materials into a functional pattern. These materials had no proclivity to be so structured and are externally related in an artificial manner. The shape, location and function of the materials could have been radically different, and each component could have been used for an entirely different purpose than constructing an automobile. By contrast, that which moves a puppy to maturity or an acorn to an oak tree is an internal, defining essence or nature. This nature directs the developmental process of the individual substance and establishes limits on the variations each substance may undergo and still exist. The acorn will not grow into a dog, and the dog will not become an oak tree. Consequently, a substance functions in light of what it is and maintains its essence regardless of the degree to which its ultimate capacities are realized. Thus, while morphology and the degree of functional expression may vary among members (individual substances) of a natural kind, such variance does not affect the essential nature of their being. For it is the underlying essence of a thing, not its contingent state of development at a given point, that constitutes what it is. We would not, for example, say that an oak sapling is of a different kind than an adult oak tree. As a substance grows, it does not become more *of* its kind, but rather, it matures according *to* its kind. The actualization of its potentialities or capacities is both controlled by and a reflection of the substance's essential structure. The capacities for the acorn one day to develop a trunk, branches and leaves are already embedded within the acorn, prior to their realization. This is true whether or not the acorn actually grows into a tree, since such development is dependent on accidental (nonessential) conditions that are wholly independent of the acorn's essential nature. When such conditions are met, however, including the proper soil, environment, and so on, the acorn will express its latent capacities in the fullest sense. The absence of such conditions is irrelevant to the essential nature of the acorn.

This principle of potentiality and actuality is best explained in terms of a hierarchical structure of capacities. Consider human beings. Smith has the first-order capacity to speak and write in English. He also has the second-order capacity to develop the first-order capacity, currently lacking, to speak and write in French. Smith's capacities proceed in a structural hierarchy until ultimate (foundational) capacities are reached. Smith's set of ultimate capacities constitute his human nature, and they exist in Smith as long as he has being.

A further distinction between substances and property-things follows from the above discussion. Specifically, substances maintain their ontological identity through change, while property-things do not. An individual substance endures through change because it is more than the aggregate set of its parts, formed according to an external ordering principle. The accidental parts or properties of a substance can change without altering the thing itself. This is true because it exists as a deeply unified, ontological whole that *possesses* these parts and properties. A dog, for example, can lose a tooth or shed its fur, but remain the same dog throughout these processes of change; for the dog is not an aggregate sum of its parts, nor an emergent whole whose parts are prior to the whole. Instead, the whole is prior to the parts, and these parts exist in virtue of their internal relations to each other, grounded in the enduring essence of the dog. By contrast, a property-thing is an ordered aggregate—that is, a whole that is constituted *by* its parts. Thus, it cannot sustain literal identity when it gains or loses parts. No single entity endures through change, but, instead, a successive series of ontologically distinct, though perhaps similar, entities begin and cease to exist over time. Since property-things are identical to the sum of their bundled properties and ordered parts, a change in any property or part necessarily causes one "entity-stage" to end and another to begin. Thus, property-things have no enduring essences to ground their sameness through change.

THE HUMAN BEING AS A SUBSTANCE

Regarding the theme of this chapter, it is arguably the case that a human being is not a property-thing but a substance. While space does not permit an exhaustive defense of this view beyond what has already been said, it will be helpful to briefly sketch four lines of argument in its favor.[3] This will at least formally establish the metaphysical issues one must consider when arguing for or against the position. First, every human organism is an ontological whole whose parts, properties and capacities are related internally. The "human" identity of bodily organs and structures of consciousness presupposes their participation in the whole of which they are parts and structures. Second, every human being exhibits species specific behavior, betraying an essential nature that is common to all members of the human species. All growth and development is governed by and restricted to the law-like process informed by the essential human nature. Third, absolute personal identity through change implies a substance ontology. Introspective awareness, as well as the problems with ancestral chain models (i.e., the counterintuitive notion of "person-stages") lends support to the claim that human persons are substances that endure through change. Finally, a necessary condition for libertarian free will is the existence of an agent (e.g., agent-causation or noncausal agent theory); and a substance ontology of the agent is arguably a necessary condition for agency theory.

Although we acknowledge that each of these metaphysical claims has been disputed, we cannot defend them here. The crucial point that we want to make is that if these theses regarding human beings are true (i.e., they are organic, nonemergent wholes that exhibit law-like stages and limits to development, absolute personal identity through change and [arguably] libertarian freedom), then human beings are substances, not property-things. Before we apply the preceding discussion to the question of the ontological status of the unborn, we need to consider briefly three objections to the view that humans are substances. These criticisms focus primarily on problems with the notion of essential natures. First, some claim that the traditional doctrine of substance and essence is too restrictive and lacks the explanatory power of views that emphasize external relations. This position is expressed and held to varying degrees.[4] Charles Curran summarizes a form of this objection: ". . . . Reality does not consist of separate substances completely independent of each other. Reality can be understood only in terms of the relations that exist among the individual beings.".[5] Speaking specifically of human persons, he writes, "The individual person has no intrinsic orientation (a nature) necessarily bringing about personal perfection; rather, according to Aristotle, one depends more on the contingent and the accidental.".[6]

Curran is correct that reality, taken as a whole, reflects relations among substances and not merely substances in isolation. Indeed, the human experience includes contingency and accident, and Aristotle's "good life" demands these elements. However, by acknowledging the role of accident and contingency, we must not deny or unnecessarily minimize the restrictive role of essential natures. The simple fact is that there are limits to the kind of change a human can undergo and remain human, as well as to the kinds of relations a human can sustain to other things. These facts are most consistent with and best explained by the doctrine of natures. Furthermore, what sense can be given to the notion of the contingent or accidental if there is no enduring essence to serve as a contrast with these notions? One can assert that a thing is what it is and not another thing without ignoring its contingent relations to other existents, since the members of a given species possess a deeply unified and law-like structure that remains unaffected by contingency and accident. An essential nature, then, plays an irreducibly crucial role in defining what a thing is. Moreover, it sets limits and serves as the final cause for the growth and development of the being.

A second objection centers on the entrenched metaphysical debate over realism and nominalism. Roughly, the former view asserts that immutable natures or essences exist and are exemplified fully in particular instances of their kind. Conversely, the latter view asserts that only particulars exist, and no two particulars exemplify a literally identical essence (not even two members within the same species). Against the typological (realist) view defended in this chapter, some argue that "essence" is a mere chimera, lacking empirical defense. J. M. Thoday suggests that genetic variations are so significant among members of any given population that regarding human beings, "there are as many human natures as there are men."[7] The obvious question for Thoday is why he refers to all men as having *human natures*. What is it that unifies this group of existents under the classification, "human?" He may respond that each human being has an *individually distinct* human nature, and thus may be grouped into the set we *refer* to as "humans" (e.g., {Human Nature$_1$, Human Nature$_2$, Human Nature$_3$ . . . Human Nature$_n$}).[8] But this clearly does not solve the problem. For now the question is, What unifies the members of this set to warrant calling it the set of individual *human* natures? To avoid an infinite regress of individualized natures within natures, we must eventually point to a universal human nature that allows us to refer ostensibly to the unified group of existents we call humans.[9] For " . . . unless there is some tacit, generalizable understanding of what the word 'human' means, some universal signification, then it could not be used to describe more than one organic entity."[10]

A third argument against the essentialist view suggests that entering a species is a process. Speaking of the human species, Lawrence Becker asserts,

Human fetal development is a process analogous to metamorphosis, and just as it makes good sense to speak of butterfly eggs, larvae, and pupae as distinct from the butterflies they become (to say that they are not butterflies) so too it makes sense to say that human eggs, embryos, and fetuses are distinct from the human beings they become—that they are not human beings, only human becomings. When can we say that the fetus is a human being rather than a human becoming? Surely only when its metamorphic-like process is complete— that is, when the relatively undifferentiated mass of the fertilized human ovum has developed into the pattern of differentiated characteristic of the organism it is genetically programmed to become.[11]

Becker's view is riddled with problems. First, he fails to distinguish between epistemic convention (the way we describe what we see) and essential natures (what a thing actually is). From the fact that we draw an epistemological distinction between "pupae," "larvae," and "butterfly," it does not follow that each is its own species. Becker himself acknowledges that "caterpillars and butterflies are both stages in the same insect."[12] Although the former is modified morphologically into the latter, the *essential nature* of the *one* insect is identical in both cases. This is what justifies the belief that these are different stages in a single organism. Similarly, although we distinguish between human newborns and adults, it does not follow that they are of different species. Nor does it follow that because we distinguish between human fetuses and two-year old children, they belong to different species. Thus, Becker's distinction between human beings and human becomings, though epistemologically useful, is metaphysically unhelpful.

To illustrate this problem with Becker's view, consider a man entering a room.[13] One can enter a room gradually, be halfway in, three quarters of the way in and then fully in the room. During all stages of entrance, the man must exist fully to do the entering. Likewise, to be in the process of entering the human species, I must first be, in toto. I cannot be in the process of coming into being, since I must first exist to enter any process. Although it might be an open question as to exactly what I am, to be a mere "human becoming" is an incoherent notion.

A second problem with Becker's view is the suggestion that the fetus becomes a human being only after "its metamorphic-like process is complete . . . [when] . . . the relatively undifferentiated mass of the fertilized human ovum has developed into the pattern of differentiated characteristic of the organism." This judgment is highly arbitrary, especially when applied to human beings, since the development process continues for decades after birth. Thus, it is difficult to see when Becker's "metamorphic-like" process is complete. Size and shape, as well as physical and mental capacities, continue unfolding well into the teenage years and beyond. Certainly, the eighteen year old is no more human than the five year old; but since the older person is further along in the (metamorphic) process, Becker's distinction implies this conclusion. It seems apparent that both the child and the adult are equally human. Moreover, the most obvious explanation for this equality is that they both possess a common human nature that informs and directs the "metamorphic-like" process throughout the stages of human growth and development. Arguably, the same essential nature directs the process before birth. Nothing in Becker's argument dissuades this suggestion.

Finally, Becker equivocates between "human-becomings" and "human beings." All organisms, he claims, are "genetically programmed to become" specifically differentiated entities. Presumably, this genetic program allows the being to develop into its adult form. But what is this genetic program if not a manifest essential nature? Moreover, how can this nature continually direct an entity's becoming without continuing to be present in that entity? Both the embryonic and adult stages of the organism possess the *same* genetic program (nature). This unity of being allows Becker to refer to the fetus as the "it" whose metamorphic process will one day be complete, affording "it" the status of human being. On what basis, then, can Becker draw a metaphysical distinction between so-called human-becomings and human beings? It seems that there is none. Thus, he gives us no reason to doubt that the human embryo, possessing an identical genetic program as the adult she will become, is a bona fide member of the human species.

HUMAN PERSONHOOD AND THE UNBORN

The following argument defends the humanity of the unborn.

P1. An adult human being is the end result of the continuous growth of the organism from conception.
P2. From conception to adulthood, there is no break in this development which is relevant to the ontological status of the organism.
P3. Therefore, one is a human being from the point of conception onward.[14]

Although few would deny premise P1, and Premise P3 clearly follows from P1 and P2, the success of this argument rests on the truth of P2. In defense of P2, the fetus certainly seems to be a substance; an ontologically distinct organism, instantiating an essential nature. As such, the fetus can and does undergo dramatic development and change, though remaining identical to itself as an individuated substance throughout the process. Furthermore, since the fetus belongs to the human species (instantiates an essentially human nature) at some point during the process, it must belong to the human species from the point of conception, since there is no ontologically significant break in the process (i.e., the same essential nature governs a single process from conception to adulthood). To deny that the fetus is fully human from conception, one must point to an ontologically significant (substantial) modification that occurs between conception and birth. So far as we can tell, there is no good reason to believe that such a modification occurs at any point in the process (as opposed to important but normal developments within the life of one organism). Some disagree with this claim, however, and point to either "criteria for humanness" or "decisive moments" at which the fetus first acquires the status of human personhood.

The most common decisive moment, and the one currently endorsed by the Supreme Court is *viability*—that is, the point at which the fetus is able to live on its own outside the womb. Currently , the average fetus is viable at roughly 24–26 weeks of gestation. Once this point is reached, some argue, the fetus acquires the status of personhood, by virtue of its ability to live on its own, though still dependent on medical technology, but not dependent on a uterine environment.

"Viability" as a determinant of personhood is unhelpful, if for no other reason that viability cannot be measured precisely. It varies from fetus to fetus, and medical technology is continually pushing viability back to earlier stages of pregnancy. Moreover, since viability continues to change, this raises questions about its reliability as an indicator of personhood. But proponents of viability argue that it is possible, at least in principle, that medicine will reach a lower limit, say at 20 weeks gestation, and at this point, there may be no reasonable prospect of pushing it back any earlier. Given this scenario, viability will be a more stable concept, and thus it is argued that it is more reliable as a determinant of personhood.

But what does viability actually measure about a fetus? The concept of viability is a commentary, not on the essence of the fetus but on the ability of medical technology to sustain life outside the womb. Viability relates only to the fetus's location and dependency, not to its essence or personhood. There is no inherent connection between the fetus's ability to survive outside the womb and its essential nature as a human being. Thus, while viability is a helpful measure of the progress in medical technology, it has no bearing on what kind of a thing the fetus is or is not.

Perhaps the next most commonly proposed decisive moment is *brain development*, or the point at which the brain of the fetus begins to function, at roughly 45 days of pregnancy. The appeal of this decisive moment is the parallel with the definition of death, which is the cessation of all brain activity. Since brain activity is what measures death, or the loss of personhood, some argue, it is reasonable to take the beginning of brain activity as an indication that personhood has begun. This decisive moment, however, is unhelpful as well. The problem with the analogy to brain death is that the dead brain has no capacity to revive itself again. It is in an irreversible condition, but the fetus only temporarily lacks first-order brain function. Its electroencephalogram (EEG) is only temporarily flat, whereas the dead person has a permanently flat EEG. In addition, the embryo from the point of conception has all the necessary capacities to develop full brain activity. Until around 45 days gestation, those capacities are not yet realized but are latent in the embryo. However, that a capacity is not instantiated in the first order has no bearing on the essence of the fetus, since that capacity is only temporarily latent, not irreversibly lost. Thus, there are significant differences between the fetus who lacks the first-order capacity for brain activity in the first four to five weeks of pregnancy, and the dead person who lacks both the potentiality and the actuality for any brain activity whatsoever. Pointing to brain activity as the decisive moment for personhood, then, is a nonstarter.

A third suggested decisive moment is *sentience*, or the point at which the fetus is capable of experiencing sensations, particularly pain. The appeal of this point for the determination of personhood is that if the fetus cannot feel pain, then there is less of a problem with abortion, and it disarms many of the pro-life arguments that abortion is cruel to the fetus. As is the case with the other decisive moments, however, sentience has little inherent connection to the personhood of the fetus, since it confuses the experience of harm with the reality of harm. Simply because the fetus cannot feel pain or otherwise experience harm, it does not follow that it cannot be harmed. If I am paralyzed from the waist down and cannot feel pain in my legs, I am still harmed if someone amputates my leg. In addition, to take sentience as the determinant of personhood, one would also have to admit that the reversibly comatose, the person in a persistent vegetative state (a person who has sustained a very serious head injury leaving only the brain stem functioning), the momentarily unconscious and even the sleeping person are not persons. One might object that these people once did function with sentience and that the loss of sentience is only temporary. But once that objection is made, the objector is admitting that something else besides sentience is determinant of personhood, and thus sentience as a decisive moment cannot be sustained.

Another suggested decisive moment is *quickening*, or the first time that the mother feels the fetus move inside her womb. Historically, this has been the first evidence of life to be detected clearly. This was obviously before the use of sophisticated medical technology such as ultrasound that can see the fetus from the early stages of pregnancy. Upon close examination, it becomes clear that quickening as a determinant of personhood is unacceptable because the essence of the fetus cannot be dependent on someone's awareness of it. This criterion confuses the nature of the fetus with what one can know about the fetus. In other words, this decisive moment confuses epistemology (knowledge/awareness of the fetus) with ontology (the nature or essence of the fetus). A similar confusion is involved in the use of the appearance of humanness of the fetus as the decisive moment for personhood. The appeal of this view is primarily emotional in that, as the fetus comes to resemble a baby, one begins to associate it with the kind of being that they would normally consider a full human being (e.g., a newborn). But what the fetus looks like has no inherent relationship to what it is, and from the point of conception, the fetus has all the capacities necessary to one day exemplify the physical characteristics of a normal human being. The appearance of the fetus, then, is an unhelpful criterion for human personhood.

A few assert that *birth* is the decisive moment at which the fetus acquires personhood. But this assumption is deeply problematic. It seems intuitively obvious that there is no essential difference between the fetus on the day prior to its birth and the fetus on the day after its birth. The only difference between the prebirth and postbirth fetus/newborn is her location. But as is the case with viability as the determinant of personhood, birth says nothing about what kind of thing the fetus is; it merely offers a commentary on her location. But just because I change venues, it does not follow that there is any essential change in my nature as a person. Likewise, just because the unborn human substance changes its location, this does not change its essential nature as a fully human being.

A final suggested decisive moment is *implantation*, and proponents of this view offer at least three reasons in its defense. First, it is at implantation when the embryo establishes its presence in the womb by the "signals" or the hormones it produces. Second, since anywhere from 20 to 50 percent of the embryos spontaneously miscarry prior to implantation, some suggest that implantation is critical not only to the development of the embryo, but also to its essence. Proponents also suggest that if we claim that a full human person exists before implantation, then we are morally obligated to save all the embryos (something that very few people hold). Third, twinning, or the production of twins, normally occurs prior to implantation, and, according to some, this suggests that individual human personhood does not begin until after implantation.

Although placing personhood at implantation would have little effect on the abortion question (since most induced abortions occur well after implantation), the ethical implications of this decisive moment are significant. First, if correct, it would make any birth control methods that prevent implantation, such as many forms of the birth control pill and the "abortion pill," RU-486, morally allowable, since an embryo that has yet to implant itself is not considered a person. Furthermore, leftover embryos that are kept in storage in in vitro fertilization could be discarded or used in experiments without any moral problem, since those embryos do not possess personhood.

Several things can be said against the arguments for implantation as a decisive moment. First, just because the embryo establishes its presence by the hormonal signals it produces, it does not follow that personhood is established at this point. The essence of the fetus is independent of another's awareness of its existence, whether that awareness includes physical awareness, as in quickening, or chemical awareness as in the production of specific hormones. Second, just because up to 50 percent of conceived embryos spontaneously miscarry, it does not follow that personhood comes at implantation, since the essential nature of the fetus is not dependent on the number of embryos that do or do not survive to implant. Moreover, even if the pre-implantation embryo is a full human person, as we contend, we are not morally obligated to save them all since there is no moral obligation to interfere in the embryo's natural death. Not interfering to prevent a spontaneous miscarriage is not the same thing as killing an embryo any more than removing life support on a terminally ill patient and allowing him or her to die is not the same thing as actively killing such a patient.[15] Third, just because twinning occurs prior to implantation, it does not follow that the original embryo was not a full human person before the split. In fact, it is equally possible that two persons existed prior to implantation and only individualized after that point. Thus, implantation fails to serve as an ontologically decisive moment for personhood.

Given the apparent inadequacies of the above decisive moments, ethicists like Mary Ann Warren draw a more sophisticated demarcation between so-called "genetic humanity" and "moral humanity," claiming only those in the latter group are persons. Persons, she claims, must meet one of five criteria: (1) Consciousness, especially the ability to feel pain; (2) reasoning, the developed capacity; (3) self-motivated activity; (4) the capacity to communicate; (5) the presence of self-concepts.[16] To this list, Joseph Fletcher adds (1) self-control; (2) a sense of the future and the past; (3) the ability to relate to others; and (4) curiosity.[17] Similar to Mary Ann Warren's "genetic/moral" distinction, James Rachels draws a distinction between "biographical" and "biological" life,[18] placing the emphasis on the possession of low-order capacities of persons. In our view, the entire project of defining personhood in functional terms fails, since, as argued above, a thing is what it is, not what it does. Moreover, as J. P. Moreland argues, the absence of lower order (expressed) functional capacities does not mean that the individual's ultimate capacities to express those abilities are absent. Instead, "Higher order capacities are realized by the development of lower order capacities under [them]. . . . When a substance has a defect, (e.g., a child is born color blind), it does not lose its ultimate capacities. Rather, it lacks some lower order capacity it needs for the ultimate capacity to be developed."[19] Thus, applied to the unborn, from the assertion that the unborn, defective or otherwise, may[20] be incapable of first-order human person skills like reasoning, communication, willing, desiring, self-reflection, aspiring, and so on, it does not follow that they are not human persons. For these capacities still exist within the individual human substance as ultimate capacities constituting its essence. Therefore, even if these criteria were among the legitimate epistemological identifiers of personhood, every human substance, born and unborn, would qualify as a human person, since a human being is a substance with all the *ultimate* capacities for fully expressed personhood, including those listed by Warren, Fletcher and Rachels.

The ontological inadequacies of functional definitions are clearly evident if we try to practice them consistently. Applying any of the above criteria, counterintuitive and ethically troubling results abound. Consider the person under general anesthesia. He is clearly not conscious, has no expressed capacity for reason, is incapable of self-motivated activity, cannot possibly communicate, has no concept of himself, and cannot remember the past or aspire for the future. According to the functionalist view expressed by Warren, Fletcher and Rachels, he is not a full person—but this is absurd. In response, it may be argued that the adult lacks the first-order capacity to respond but still has the capacity to exercise the first-order capacity when free from anesthesia, and is therefore a person who is *temporarily dysfunctional*. But this *ad hoc* claim is not available without appealing to something outside of first-order functional criteria. Appealing to *unexpressed*, higher order capacities as evidence of personhood smacks of essentialism; that is, defending the personhood of the anesthetized human seems to require pointing to higher order or even ultimate capacities that are embedded in his human nature. To argue that the person before anesthesia remains a person while under anesthesia, we must point to what that person *is*, irrespective of his first-order functional capacities. To insist that he remains a person because he had once expressed first-order capacities of consciousness begs the question, since this merely re-asserts the functional premise as a defense against the essentialist counterargument.

Finally, if essential personhood is determined by function, it follows that essential personhood is a degreed property. After all, some will realize more of their capacities to reason, feel pain, self-reflect, and so on, than others. Moreover, it is undeniable that the first several years of normal life outside the womb include an increasing expression of human capacities. Likewise, the last several years of life may include a decreasing expression of human capacities. Consequently, if the functionalist view is correct, the possession of personhood could be expressed by a bell curve, in which a human being moves toward full personhood in her first years of life, reaches full personhood at a given point, and then gradually loses her personhood until the end of her life. Presumably, the commensurate rights of persons would increase, stabilize and decrease in the process. Without appealing to something other than function, it is difficult to resist this counterintuitive conclusion. Indeed, intellectual honesty has driven many to embrace this conclusion , and the slope is ever so slippery. Helga Kuhse and Peter Singer comment on the ontological status of newborns:

> . . . . When we kill a newborn, there is no person whose life has begun. When
> I think of myself as the person I am now, I realize that I did not come into existence until sometime after my birth. . . . It is the beginning of the life of the
> person, rather than of the physical organism, that is crucial so far as the right
> to life is concerned.[21]

While we applaud their intellectual consistency in applying their notion of personhood evenly in ethical issues, their chilling consistency reveals, at least to us, the danger of defining human personhood in functional terms. Not only are the unborn and newborns less than persons, but apparently all of us are subject to graded personhood and the commensurate rights therein.

In this essay we have argued that to be a human person is to possess an essential human nature. The unborn are individual human substances, possessing an essentially human nature; therefore, they are human persons. Functional definitions of personhood are arbitrary, metaphysically inadequate and ethically problematic. Metaphysical insight prompts us to remember that a thing is what is, not what it does. Essence precedes function—to possess an essential human nature is to be a human person, regardless of whether or not first-order functional capacities are instanced.

NOTES

1. J. P. Moreland and Norman L. Geisler, *The Life and Death Debate: Moral Issues of Our Time* (Westport, Conn.: Greenwood Press, 1990), p. 34.

2. "The Dennis Prager Show," KABC Talkradio, Los Angeles, 9 June 1994.

3. We express our thanks to Dr. J. P. Moreland for his insights regarding this issue.

4. See W. V. Quine, *Ontological Relativity and Other Essays* (New York: Columbia University Press, 1969) for the most radical explication of this view. Others embrace ontological relativity in widely varying degrees.

5. Charles E. Curran, "Natural Law in Moral Theology," *Readings in Moral Theology No. 7: Natural Law and Theology* (New York: Paulist Press, 1991), p. 276.

6. Ibid., p. 277.

7. J. M. Thoday, "Geneticism and Environmentalism," in J. E. Meade and A.S. Parker eds., *Biological Aspects of Social Problems* (Edinburgh: Oliver Boyd, 1965), p. 101, as quoted by Daniel Callahan, "The 'Beginning' of Human Life," Michael F. Goodman, ed., *What Is a Person* (Clifton, N. J.: Humana Press, 1988), p. 41.

8. For a detailed defense of metaphysical realism, see Reinhardt Grossman, *The Existence of The World: An Introduction to Ontology* (New York: Routledge, 1992), pp. 14–45.

9. The Nominalist may respond that the exact similarity relation among human beings is simply a primitive fact, and may insist that no further explanation is necessary. But this response is unsatisfying, since merely asserting that two human beings happen to be exactly similar lacks any explanatory power whatsoever. The realist view, however, offers a more satisfying explanation for this similarity by accounting for both *what* a thing is and for the fact that *it* is an individualized member of that kind. Those who assert that individual human beings just happen to be similar, then, stop their analysis too early and fall short of an irreducible explanation. Conversely, the realist analysis provides a more thorough explanatory account for the sameness that individual humans share, by arguing that their similarity is a function of their possession of an identical property (i.e., human-ness).

10. Daniel Callahan, "The 'Beginning' of Human Life," in Goodman, ed., *What is a Person,* p. 41.

11. Lawrence Becker, "Human Being: The Boundaries of the Concept," in Goodman, ed., *What Is a Person,* p. 60.

12. Ibid., p. 60.

13. Roderick M. Chisholm, *On Metaphysics* (Minneapolis: University of Minne-

sota Press, 1989), p. 58.

14. Cf. Richard Werner, "Abortion: The Moral Status of the Unborn," *Social Theory and Practice* 4 (Spring 1975): 201–222.

15. There is some debate on the parallel between killing and allowing to die through euthanasia. See for example, James Rachels, *The End of Life* (New York: Oxford University Press, 1987).

16. Mary Ann Warren, "On the Moral and Legal Status of Abortion," in James A, Sterba, ed., *Morality In Practice* (Hartford, Conn.: Wadsworth), pp. 144–145, as quoted by W.F. Cooney, "The Fallacy of All Person-Denying Arguments for Abortion," *Journal of Applied Philosophy* 8, no.2 (1991): 163.

17. Joseph Fletcher, "Indicators of Humanhood: A Tentative Profile," *Hastings Center Report* vol. 2 (1972). Cited by Scott B. Rae, "Views of Human Nature at the Edges of Life," in J. P. Moreland and David Ciocchi, eds., *Christian Perspectives on Being Human: An Integrative Approach* (Grand Rapids:Baker, 1993), p. 239.

18. Rachels, *The End of Life*, p. 5.

19. J. P. Moreland, "Wennberg, Personhood, and the Right to Die," *Faith and Philosophy* 12 (January 1995): 6,7.

20. Much of this argument boils down to epistemological, not metaphysical issues. Our ability to reliably ascertain the functional abilities of the unborn is hardly exhaustive. The budding field of prenatal psychology, experimental though it may be, indicates that much of the cognitive/self-awareness capabilities of the unborn remain unexplored.

21. Helga Kuhse and Peter Singer, *Should the Baby Live* (New York: Oxford University Press, 1985), p. 133. It is quickly apparent that Kuhse and Singer equivocate on the question of personal identity. After all, if *I* do not exist until sometime after *my* birth, in what sense is the birth *mine?* The only way for "*my* birth" to be more than a linguistic convention is to admit that "I" existed before I was born, or at least at the time of my birth. But if this is the case, Kuhse and Singer's attempt to define personhood in terms of function fails.

Chapter 2

Ignorance of Fetal Status as a Justification of Abortion: A Critical Analysis

Francis J. Beckwith

[T]o accept the fact that after fertilization has taken place a new human has come into being is no longer a matter of taste or opinion. . . . [T]he human nature of the human being from conception to old age is not a metaphysical contention, it is plain experimental evidence.

—Jerome Lejeune, Genetecist, 1981[1]

In what is arguably the most quoted passage from *Roe v. Wade*, Justice Harry Blackmun, author of the majority opinion, writes: "We need not resolve the difficult question of when life begins. When those trained in the respective disciplines of medicine, philosophy, and theology are unable to arrive at any consensus, the judiciary, at this point in the development of man's knowledge, is not in a position to speculate."[2]

Justice Blackmun is arguing that since experts disagree as to when life begins, the Court should not come down on any side. That is, since experts disagree about when and if the fetus becomes a human life, then abortion should remain legal.

In popular debate, Justice Blackmun's claim is often put forth by abortion-rights advocates when they affirm that "no one knows when life begins," and from that affirmation conclude that abortion is morally justified. There is a difference, however, between claiming that "no one knows when life begins" and "experts disagree as to when life begins." My guess is that when people use the former in popular debate, they are in fact arguing that it is justified by the latter:

(1) Experts disagree as to when life begins.

Therefore,

(2) No one knows when life begins.

Of course (2) does not necessarily follow from (1). It may be that experts disagree as to when human life begins, but some of them are wrong while others in fact know when human life begins. This would not be surprising, since historically some faction of experts usually turns out to be correct about a disputed issue, such as in the cases of slavery, women's suffrage, and the position of the earth in the solar system. In some cases, expert disagreement can be accounted for by some factions ignoring contrary evidence or alternative theories. In other cases, it may result from holding an irrational belief, clinging to a religious or secular dogma, or wanting not to appear politically incorrect. By treating all expert disagreement over fetal personhood as philosophically and scientifically indistinguishable; by giving the impression that all the arguments of all the factions in the abortion debate are equally compelling; and by simply appealing to expert disagreement rather than wrestling with the actual arguments proposed by these experts and evaluating these arguments for their logical soundness, the Court was able simply to discard the issue of fetal personhood while pretending to actually take it into consideration.

The Court turned this evasion into a virtue in the 1992 case which upheld *Roe* as precedent, *Planned Parenthood v. Casey*. In that case the Court asserted the following about the meaning of the Fourteenth Amendment:

> Our law affords constitutional protection to personal—decisions relating to marriage, procreation, family relationships, child rearing, and education. . . .
> At the heart of liberty is the right to define one's own concept of existence, of meaning, of the universe, and of the mystery of human life. Beliefs about these matters could not define the attributes of personhood were they formed under compulsion by the State.[3]

Evidently, the Supreme Court has chosen to abandon a rigorous defense of philosophical argument in the free marketplace of ideas only to replace it with a New Age *mantra* in the convenience store of slogans.

The claim, however, that "no one knows when life begins" is a misnomer, since no one seriously doubts that individual biological human life is present from conception. Thus, what the abortion-rights advocates probably mean when they say that "no one knows when life begins" is that no one knows when personhood or full humanness is attained in the process of human development by the individual in the womb.

It is interesting to note that the U.S. Senate Subcommittee, which interviewed numerous scientific and bioethical authorities in conjunction with its study and analysis of the 1981 Human Life Bill, came to a similar conclusion. It concluded that "no witness [who testified before the subcommittee] raised any evidence to refute the biological fact that from the moment of conception there exists a distinct individual being who is alive and is of the human species. No witness challenged the scientific consensus that unborn children are 'human beings,' insofar as the term is used to mean living beings of the human species." On the other hand, "those witnesses who testified that science cannot say whether unborn children are human beings were speaking in every instance to the value question rather than the scientific question. . . . [T]hese witnesses invoked their value preferences to redefine the term 'human being.'" The committee report explains that these witnesses "took the view that each person may define as 'human' only those beings whose lives that person wants to value. Because they did not wish to accord intrinsic worth to the lives of unborn children, they refused to call them 'human beings,' regardless of the scientific evidence."[4]

Consequently, from a legal perspective Justice Blackmun and other abortion-rights advocates are arguing in the following way:

(1) Experts disagree about when human life becomes valuable (or a person or fully human, as some ethicists have put it).

Therefore,

(2) No one knows when human life becomes valuable (or "begins").

Therefore,

(3) Abortion should remain legal.

I will call this the agnostic argument for abortion rights (or AA). I believe that this argument is flawed in at least four ways.

CRITIQUE OF THE AGNOSTIC ARGUMENT

1. *The AA is in principle difficult if not impossible to maintain in practice.* Recall what Justice Blackmun said in *Roe v. Wade*: "We need not resolve the difficult question of when life begins. When those trained in the respective disciplines of medicine, philosophy, and theology are unable to arrive at any consensus, the judiciary, at this point in the development of man's knowledge, is not in a position to speculate."[5] Hence, the state should not take one theory of life and force those who do not agree with that theory to subscribe to it, which is the reason why Blackmun writes in *Roe*, "In view of all this, we do not agree that, by adopting one theory of life, Texas may override the rights of the pregnant woman that are at stake."[6] Thus, for the pro-life advocate to propose that non-pro-life women should be forbidden from having abortions, on the basis that individual human personhood begins at conception or at least sometime before birth, is a violation of the right to privacy of non-pro-life women.

But the problem with this reasoning is that it is self-refuting and question-begging. For to claim, as Justice Blackmun does, that the Court should not propose one theory of life over another and that the decision should be left up to each individual pregnant woman as to when protectable human life begins, is to propose a theory of life which hardly has a clear consensus in this country.[7] For once one claims that certain individuals (pregnant women) have the right to bestow personhood and/or value on unborn humans, one affirms a theory of humanity which in practice excludes unborn humans from constitutional protection.

Thus, the Court actually did take sides on when life begins. It concluded that the fetus is not a human person, since the procedure permitted in *Roe*, abortion, is something that evidently would have been permitted if it were conclusively proven that the fetus is not a person. In fact, according to Justice Blackmun, the constitutionality of *Roe* hinges on that very question: "If the suggestion of personhood [of the unborn] is established, the appellant's case, of course, collapses, for the fetus' right to life is then guaranteed specifically by the [Fourteenth Amendment]."[8] Although verbally the Court denied taking sides, the practical effect of its opinion is that the fetus in this society is not a human person worthy of protection.

Imagine that the Court, if confronted with the issue of enslaving African Americans, delivered the opinion: "We need not resolve the difficult question if blacks are human persons. When those trained in the respective disciplines of medicine, philosophy, and theology are unable to arrive at any consensus, the judiciary, at this point in the development of man's knowledge, is not in a position to speculate." Suppose that the Court on that basis *allowed* white Americans to own blacks as property. It would appear that, although the Court would be making a verbal denial of taking any position on this issue, the allowance of slavery would for all intents and purposes be morally equivalent to taking a side on the issue, namely, that blacks are not human persons. Likewise, the Court's verbal denial of taking a position on fetal personhood is contradicted by its conclusion that abortion is a fundamental constitutional right and that fetuses are not persons under the Constitution.

By permitting abortion for virtually any reason during the entire nine months of pregnancy, abortion rights advocates have decided, for all practical purposes, when full humanness is attained. They have decided that this moment occurs at birth. Despite their claim that "no one knows when life begins," abortion-rights advocates act as if protectable human life begins at birth.

2. *The AA is contrary to the benefit of the doubt argument.* If it is true that we don't know when full humanness begins, this is an excellent reason not to kill the unborn, since we may be killing a human entity who has a full right to life. If one killed without knowing whether the being killed (in this case, the unborn) is fully human with a full right to life, it would be negligent to proceed with the killing. To use an example, if game hunters shot at rustling bushes

with this same philosophical mind-set, the National Rifle Association's membership would become severely depleted. Ignorance of a being's status is certainly not justification to kill it. This is called the benefit of the doubt argument, since we are giving the unborn the benefit of the doubt.

Professor Robert Wennberg of Westmont College, however, does not agree with this. He asks us to consider the following case:

A thirty six-year-old woman with four children, worn down and exhausted by poverty and terrible living conditions, married to an alcoholic husband finds herself pregnant. Although not the sole source of income for her family, the woman does work and her income is desperately needed. After wrestling with her predicament, the woman decides that an abortion would be in the interests of herself and her family. . . . Concerned about whether abortion might be the killing of a being with a right to life, she consults two moralists, both of whom appeal to the Benefit of the Doubt Argument. One is a "conservative" who warns her to avoid the possibility of a great moral evil terminating the life of what might be a holder of a right to life. The other is a "liberal" who encourages her to secure what she *knows* to be good—avoiding considerable suffering for herself and her family. It seems to me that both pieces of advice are reasonable and that neither is clearly superior to the other.[9]

The point of this story is that the benefit of the doubt argument can be used by either the conservative or the liberal. For the liberal, the benefit of doubt should be given to eliminating the woman's predicament, since we know that she is a real person in a real predicament, whereas we are unsure of the fetus's right to life and/or full humanness. On the other hand, for the conservative, the benefit of the doubt should be given to the unborn, since the magnitude of the evil one may be committing (i.e., killing an innocent person for the sake of relieving one's own suffering) is so great that it should be avoided at all costs.

Wennberg's response, however, fails to appreciate the pro-lifer's use of the benefit of the doubt argument. Wennberg's account does not seem to grasp the magnitude of killing an innocent human person. Consider the following revised version of the above story:

A thirty six-year-old woman with four children, worn down and exhausted by poverty and terrible living conditions, married to an alcoholic husband, finds herself pregnant. Although not the sole source of income for her family, the woman does work and her income is desperately needed. After wrestling with her predicament, the woman is approached by a wealthy benefactor who presents to her the following proposition which would get her out of her predicament: "If you detonate the building across the street, which I own, I will pay you $25,000 a year for the next 20 years, adjusting the sum every year in accordance with inflation and the cost of living, and provide you a housekeeper free of charge. (This will, of course, more than make up for the burden another child places on the family.) However, there is one catch: there is a 1 in 10 chance that in the basement of this building there is a perfectly healthy and innocent eight-year-old child. Thus you run the risk of killing another human being. Is your personal well-being worth the risk?"

If the woman decides to blow up the building, I believe that few, if any, would judge her actions as morally justified. Even if the odds were 1 in 100, it would seem incredible that anyone would even consider the risk of killing another human being so insignificant that she would take the chance. But keep in mind that the AA implies a nonprobabilistic ignorance. It is different from the agnosticism one finds concerning the existence of extraterrestrials or the faked death of Elvis. That is to say, the use of the AA by Justice Blackmun and other abortion-rights advocates seems to imply that the different positions on fetal personhood all have able defenders, persuasive arguments, and passionate advocates, but none really wins the day. To put it another way, the issue of fetal personhood is up for grabs; all positions are in some sense equal, and none is better than any other. But if this is the case, then it is safe to say that the odds of the fetus being a human person are 50/50. These odds, of course, make Wennberg's fictional scenario all the more perplexing.

To better understand the flaw in Wennberg's story, let us revise the story even further and suppose that the thirty six-year-old woman is independently wealthy, childless, lives in a beautiful home, and has a wonderful caring husband. Would Wennberg argue that the risk of homicide would be justified in this case? If not, then his position is tantamount to saying that risking homicide is morally acceptable for poor people but not for the wealthy, which means that relief of personal economic and familial burdens is sufficient justification for risking homicide, even when the odds are 50/50. This seems to be morally counterintuitive. If his answer is yes—that the risk of homicide when the chances are 50/50 is justified in the case of the well-off thirty six-year-old—then the relieving of personal economic and familial burdens is not relevant in the justification for risking homicide, and Wennberg's support of a liberal use of the benefit of the doubt argument collapses.

3. *Proponents of the AA mistakenly assume that questions of the beginning of life are "religious."* Some abortion-rights literature, which I am certain is quite embarrassing to the more sophisticated proponents of this cause, claims that "personhood at conception is a religious belief, not a provable biological fact."[10] What could this assertion possibly mean? Is it claiming that religious claims are in principle unprovable scientifically? If it is, it is incorrect, for many religions, such as Christianity and Islam, maintain that the physical world literally exists, which is a major assumption of contemporary science. On the other hand, some religions, such as Christian Science and certain forms of Hinduism,[11] deny the literal existence of the physical world. Moreover, the arguments used to support the view that life begins at conception, or any other view on abortion for that matter, are not even remotely religious, since they involve the citing of

scientific evidence and the use of philosophical reasoning.

But maybe this assertion is claiming that biology can tell us nothing about values? If this is the case, it is right in one sense and wrong in another. It is right if it means that the brute facts of science, without any moral reflection, cannot tell us what is right and wrong. But it is wrong if it means that the brute facts of science cannot tell us to whom we should apply the values of which we are aware. For example, if I don't know whether the object I am driving toward in my car is a living woman or a mannequin, biology is important in helping me to avoid committing an act of homicide. Running over mannequins is not homicide, but running over a woman is.

Maybe this assertion is saying that when human life should be valued is a philosophical belief which cannot be proven scientifically? Maybe, but this cuts both ways. For isn't the belief that a woman has abortion rights a philosophical belief which cannot be proven scientifically and over which people obviously disagree? But if the pro-life position cannot be enacted into law because it is philosophical (or religious), then neither can the abortion-rights position. The abortion-rights advocate may respond to this by saying that this fact alone is a good reason to leave it up to each individual woman to choose whether she should have an abortion. But this begs the question, for this is precisely the abortion-rights position. Furthermore, the pro-lifer could reply to this abortion-rights response by employing the abortion-rights advocate's own logic. The pro-lifer could argue that since the abortion-rights position is a philosophical position over which many people disagree, we should permit each individual unborn human being to be born and make up her own mind as to whether she should or should not die.

4. *Proponents of the AA avoid the question of the beginning of human life by inadequate appeals to "tolerance" and "pluralism."* This fourth objection to the AA is a variation on the third. Some people, at least as the abortion debate is framed in popular discourse, apparently assume the correctness of the AA and then bypass the issue of fetal personhood by appealing to "tolerance" and "pluralism." They argue in the following way: since people disagree about abortion, we ought simply to permit each person to decide for himself or herself whether the fetus is a human person and/or whether abortion is immoral. Consequently, if abortion opponents believe that abortion is homicide, that is fine. They need not fear state coercion to have an abortion or to participate in the procedure. On the other hand, if some people believe that abortion is not homicide and/or it is morally permissible, then they need not fear state coercion to remain pregnant. This, according to conventional wisdom, is the tolerant position one ought to take in our pluralistic society.

The problem with this reasoning is that its proponents seem to fail to grasp why people oppose elective abortion. Consider the following. During the 1984 presidential campaign when questions of vice-presidential candidate Geraldine Ferraro's Catholicism and its seeming conflict with her support of abortion-rights were conspicuous in the media, then New York Governor Mario Cuomo, in a speech given at the University of Notre Dame, undertook to give the tolerance argument intellectual respectability. He tried to furnish a philosophical foundation for Ferraro's stance. Cuomo failed miserably. For one cannot appeal to the fact that we live in a pluralistic society, as Cuomo maintained, when the very question of who is part of that society (that is, whether or not it includes fetuses) is itself the point under dispute. Cuomo lost the argument because he begged the question.

The failure of the tolerance argument can also be illustrated by the actions of the radical anti-abortion group, Operation Rescue (OR), which disobeys trespassing laws by blocking the entrances of abortion clinics in order to prevent fetuses from being aborted. Regardless of what one thinks about the moral justification of the group's tactics,[12] the members of OR do bring home the undeniable fact that if one believes that fetuses are fully human persons, then the fetuses carried in the wombs of abortion-rights proponents are just as human as those carried in the wombs of abortion opponents. To the member of OR, a fetus carried inside the womb of Whoopi Goldberg, Cybil Shepherd, or Kate Michelman is just as much a person as the fetus carried inside the womb of Phyllis Schlafley, Beverly LaHaye, or Shirley Dobson.

Although many of us may not agree with either the mainstream or the radical opponents of abortion, let us use our imagination and try to understand their position. To tell these people, as many defenders of the tolerance argument do, that "pro-lifers have a right to believe what they want to believe about the fetus" and that "they don't have to get abortions if they don't want to" is to unwittingly promote the tactics of OR. Think about it. If you believed, as abortion opponents do, that a class of persons were being killed by methods which include dismemberment, suffocation, and burning, wouldn't you be perplexed if someone tried to ease your outrage by telling you that you didn't have to participate in the killings if you didn't want to? That's exactly what abortion opponents hear when abortion-rights supporters tell them, "Don't like abortion, don't have one" or "I'm pro-choice, but personally opposed." In the mind of the abortion opponent, this is like telling an abolitionist, "Don't like slavery, don't own one," or telling Dietrich Bonhoeffer, "Don't like the holocaust, don't work in a concentration camp." Certainly, abortion opponents may be totally wrong, absolutely misguided, or terribly misled in their view of the fetus and the moral status of abortion. But the tolerance argument does not address this. Consequently, for the defender of the tolerance argument to request that pro-lifers "should not force their pro-life belief on others," while claiming that "they have a right to believe what they want to believe," is to miss the central point of why most abortion opponents oppose elective abortion.

It seems, then, that the tolerance argument is not as neutral as its proponents believe, and neither does it provide a sufficient reason to ignore fetal status as central to the morality of abortion. For to say that women should have the "right to choose" to kill their fetuses, as abortion-rights proponents proclaim, is tantamount to denying the pro-life position that fetuses are human persons worthy of protection. And to affirm that fetuses are human persons with a "right to life," as abortion opponents proclaim, is tantamount to denying the abortion-rights position that women have a fundamental right to terminate their pregnancies, since such a termination would result in a homicide. It seems, then, that the tolerance argument is inadequate in resolving the current debate.

NOTES

1. In expert testimony before United States Congress, 23 April 1981, as quoted in J. P. Moreland and Norman Geisler, *The Life and Death Debate: Moral Issues of Our Time* (Westport, Conn.: Greenwood Press, 1990), p. 34.

2. Justice Harry Blackmun, "Excerpts from Opinion in *Roe V. Wade*," in Joel Feinberg, ed., *The Problem of Abortion* 2nd ed. (Belmont, Calif.: Wadsworth Publishers, 1984), p. 195.

3. Justice O'Connor, Justice Kennedy, and Justice Souter in "*Planned Parenthood v. Casey* (1992)," in Louis P. Pojman and Francis J. Beckwith, eds., *The Abortion Controversy: A Reader* (Boston: Jones and Bartlett, 1994), p. 54.

4. *The Human Life Bill—S. 158*, Report together with Additional and Minority Views to the Committee on the Judiciary, United States Senate, made by its Subcommittee on Separation of Powers, 97th Congress, 1st Session (1981):11. For a detailed presentation of the biological facts of human development as well as a philosophical defense of fetal personhood, see Francis J. Beckwith, *Politically Correct Death: Answering the Arguments for Abortion Rights* (Grand Rapids: Baker Book House, 1993), Chapters 3 and 6; and Dianne Nutwell Irving, "Philosophical and Scientific Analysis of the Nature of the Early Human Embryo," Ph.D. diss., Georgetown University, Washington D. C. (8 April 1991).

5. Blackmun, "Excerpts from Opinion in *Roe V. Wade*," p. 195.

6. Ibid., p. 196.

7. See the results of *The Boston Globe/WBZ-TV* nationwide poll recently published in *The Boston Globe*, which concluded that "Most Americans would ban the vast majority of abortions performed in this country...While 78 percent of the nation would keep abortion legal in limited circumstances, according to the poll, these circumstances account for a tiny percentage of the reasons cited by women having abortions" (Ethan Bronner, "Most in US Favor Ban on Majority of Abortions, Poll Finds," in *The Boston Globe* 31 March 1989), pp. 1, 12.

8. Blackmun, "Excerpts from Opinions in *Roe V. Wade*," p. 195.

9. Robert Wennberg, *Life in the Balance: Exploring the Abortion Controversy* (Grand Rapids: William B. Eerdmans Publishing Co., 1985), p. 59.

10. This is from a pamphlet distributed by the National Abortion Rights Action League, "Choice—Legal Abortion: Abortion Pro and Con," prepared by Polly Rothstein and Marian Williams (White Plains, N.Y.: Westchester Coalition for Legal Abortion, 1983), n. p.

11. On Christian Science, see Walter R. Martin, *Kingdom of the Cults*, 3rd ed. (Minneapolis: Bethany House, 1985), pp. 126–165. On Hinduism and New Age thinking, see Elliot Miller, *A Crash Course on the New Age Movement* (Grand Rapids: Baker Book House, 1989), pp. 16–18, 22.

12. It is clear that among pro-lifers there is serious disagreement about the moral justification of employing civil disobedience in their fight against abortion. See, for example, Randy Alcorn, *Is Rescuing Right?* (Downers Grove, Ill.: InterVarsity Press, 1990); Beckwith, *Politically Correct Death*, pp. 155–165; John S. Feinberg and Paul D. Feinberg, *Ethics for a Brave New World* (Wheaton, Ill.: Crossway Books, 1993), pp. 91–98; Norman L. Geisler, *Operation Unbiblical: Should Christians Ever Break the Law?* (Lynchburg, Va.: Quest Publications, 1989); Donald P. Shoemaker, *Operation Rescue: A Critical Analysis* (Seal Beach, Calif.: Grace Community Church, n.d.); and Randall Terry, *Operation Rescue* (Springdale, Pa.: Whitaker House, 1988).

Chapter 3

Moral Duty to the Unborn and Its Significance

Sidney Callahan

Although we invent medical and legal definitions to devalue and dehumanize prenatal life, although we declare it non-living, non-viable, non-human, or a non-person, from the moment of our conception we are never anything less than human life with a human face that will manifest itself in due time.

How can we teach our children to value and respect human life while through the example of hundreds of thousands of abortions each year we show them that human life has value only if wanted, planned and not inconvenient?

—Nathaniel Davis[1]

There is much more to abortion than abortion. It has numbed, as if with Novocain, a respect for life in American society. . . . [O]nce killing of any kind is legal, it becomes easier, with time, for the harvest of death to increase. And once anything is legal, most people believe that it is moral. . . .My reason for opposing abortion—in addition to a desire to stop the mass killing—is that it is anesthetizing the society.

—Nat Hentoff[2]

The unborn are not without influence. Our society is shaped by the story we tell ourselves about life before birth. Conflicts and questions mar present accounts. What kind of entity is a developing human organism? Do we have any moral obligations to it?

Beliefs about embryonic and fetal life will necessarily apply to one's personal prenatal history as well as form general attitudes toward having children. Every image, schema, concept, or idea we hold about the unborn subtly but powerfully affects our perspectives on the nature and worth of a human being.

As we envision the relationships of the unborn with mother, father, grandparents, extended families and larger communities, we create prototypical patterns of human connections—or lack of them.

PERSPECTIVES ON THE UNBORN

Today science and technology have allowed us to see that famous series of photographs, or the even more amazing movie, detailing the incredible journey from conception to birth. A new human life can be observed as it progresses from a zygote to a fully developed nine-month-old fetus barely indistinguishable from a newborn. Once seen, these images can arouse the same kind of awe and expanded perspectives as did the first pictures of earth taken from the moon's surface.

Of course, reactions of wonder can always be muted. The dynamic development from conception to birth can be dismissed as "merely" another biological process which has little importance compared to the intelligent decision making and self-conscious rationality characteristic of normal adults. For some observers of the human condition, only the possession of fully rational capacities counts as an adequate criterion for human status; only self-governing persons should be accorded moral equality or human rights.

By contrast, all forms of human life that are "immature," "unformed" or "prerational" will be seen as being embedded in a natural world that is subject to human dominion and constructive interpretation. For many, the meaning and value of natural processes depend solely upon the meaning and value given them by the deliberations of rational human beings. *Ergo*, if the legal community and polity decide that an embryo is to be valued as a human being only if it receives its mother's emotional investment and affirmation of its existence, then so be it.

Such a view of the contingent value of fetal development assails the foundational moral belief that certain values and realities exist whether or not humans recognize them. Reality can be defined as that which exists despite what humans might or might not wish to be so. Dynamic growth, development and irreversible one-way trajectories through time characterize all of reality and human life as we know it.

Each human embryo possesses its own eon worth of evolutionary genetic heritage, with its own incredibly complex program for dynamic development. This potentiality of the individual springs from its membership in the human species, which itself emerged from the evolutionary developmental processes of selection taking millions of years. The dynamics of embryonic development are still not fully understood. But consider, in one telling example, the fact that at one point in human development brain cells in the fetus are created and migrate to their positions at the rate of 250,000 cells a minute.

Even after birth each human being is still shaped by processes of its unique genetic program. Innate fixed patterns of ordered development interact with novel environmental influences. An adult body maintains its pattern through time because the information in the genetic program regulates the continual replacements of matter and energy from the environment. When the genetic program runs its course, then adult bodies die and disintegrate. The fetal body and an adult body share genetic continuity in maintenance operations.

If we could rerun a moving picture taken of every person now alive, we could go back day by day, minute by minute, to that moment when a particular sperm meets and joins with a specific egg. This is true despite the fact that no one can remember either encounter or all those stages of infancy and childhood that are experienced before the development of self-consciousness and continuous memory. The rational decision-making self emerges too late and functions too sporadically to be the marker and criterion of human value. Besides, as we now understand the brain's operations, we can see that many of the adult human being's most vital operations operate without conscious awareness.

In the end, it is impossible to deny that fetal life needs only time and nurture to develop its future potential. If we protect helpless immature newborns then why not the fetus? Indeed, the journey from conceptus to newborn does not seem nearly as immense as the change that takes place between a 6 pound newborn and a 6 foot, 180 pound adult male in the peak of his powers.

When the embryo's developmental processes through time and its future potential are denied as an independent objective reality with intrinsic value,then other kinds of human potential lose their moral claim. If only the present achieved status of a human life is taken into moral account, then society is going to suffer. Permitting the destruction of fetal life because of its immature dependent status and lack of development sets a chilling precedent.

Once future potential no longer counts then those who have power, strength, health and achieved status need no longer be committed to the future potential of newborns, children, women, the ill or oppressed minorities. After all, schooling, healing professions, reform movements like feminism and altruistic parental caretaking are based on the moral injunction to fulfill human potential and keep faith with the future.

But, some say, doesn't the minuscule size of the human embryo make a difference in our evaluation of it? Embryos would be invisible without sophisticated ultrasound technologies and other like marvels which allow us to be aware of their functioning. But why should size be seen as a relevant guide to importance once we have learned that the whole universe right after the Big Bang was smaller than a zygote? Power and vast potentialities are released in microevents as we know from the effects of splitting the atom and epidemics caused by infectious viruses. As we become more scientifically educated, we realize that what is visible to the naked eye is not the measure of objective reality. It takes almost eight weeks before a fetus looks like a baby in miniature, but the programmed information which informs the dynamic developmental process is present after the initial microevent. Something real happens, a human life begins.

Perceived size, in any case, depends upon the framework that exists. If one thinks of the expanded universe with its vast reaches of space and billions of stars, then even a fully grown adult person on our small planet resembles but a speck of dust. In the same way, a long life of ninety plus years would seem but a nanosecond compared to the life and death of stars.

Numbers and scale need not numb our powers of appreciation. The number of human embryos of Homo sapiens who have ever been conceived or been born would seem minute compared to the millions upon millions of existing stars. When people worry over the proportion of (probably) normal embryos which are lost before birth, the so-called wastage problem, they are not fully cognizant of the vast numbers of entities that emerge and then die in the known universe.

If we decided that the survival rate of embryos must mean that they could not have value, what do we make of the thousands of infants and children who die before reaching maturity? Earth has always been a place of death and extinction arising from plagues, floods, fires and other natural and manmade disasters. Human beings have always died before their time, but this does not mean that they have no value and can just as well be destroyed. Indeed, in the midst of so much death every instance of human life can be seen as being even more meaningful and valuable.

Once we withdraw value from the human embryo because of its size or immaturity or the fact that so many human embryos die before birth, we are logically drawn on to diminishing the value of all humankind. Within the framework of the universe, every finite human life exists as but a microevent for a moment. Are we to despair and conclude that human life is meaningless? Is it really the case that "We are to the gods as flies to wanton boys, they kill us for their sport." Never.

Happily, a new ecological consciousness of the value and interdependence of all forms of life is emerging. Human beings not only depend on the environment for sustenance but also, through their common genetic heritage, are biologically connected with other species. Instead of praising humanity's dominion and sovereignty over the world, we now are given new models to emulate, such as befriending the world and cooperating with its ecosystem. Many ecofeminists have held up the image of mothering the earth and nurturing the environment. At the very least, careless persons and policies must desist from selfishly exploiting natural resources and arrogantly destroying other forms of life.

RELATIONSHIPS AND MORAL OBLIGATIONS TO FETAL LIFE

As the newly dawning ecological consciousness of caretaking begins to affirm that all life is interdependent in a larger ecosystem, will we not have to reconsider human responses to fetal life? If we are to mother the earth and nurture life, we will have to give up modes of unilateral control. Our civilization must heed Erik Erikson's urging to carefully reflect on the relationship between the will to master totally, in any form, and the will to destroy.

In the interests of survival, cooperation, and human flourishing, a new ecological consciousness encourages us to have a sense of solidarity with all the members of the human family, as well as with other species sharing the environment. This new view of caretaking makes us concerned about our responsibilities to the future potential of those now alive as well as for those future generations of our kind who will inherit the earth. We're forced into asking new questions about what is private and what is public; where does individual liberty end and justice for all begin?

At this point we find disturbing inconsistencies in American polity. Certain species, such as eagles and their nesteggs, are protected from destruction while fetal life can be aborted and killed on demand. In some towns, such as my own, a tree cannot be cut down without permission from a local commission, while a nearby abortion clinic freely extinguishes fetal life by the thousands year after year. The killing of a developing fetal life is supposedly justified in order to grant a woman her autonomy, privacy and right to totally control her reproductive capacity.

Here two kinds of power can be discerned. One kind of power follows the logic of domination and insists on unilateral control by repression, coercion and destruction to achieve a willed outcome. Another type of power is actualizing power or the power to create, engender and bring existing potential to fruition and fulfillment.

Both of these forms of power spring from the evolved capacities of the human species for using foresight, planning, and taking the role of another. Human beings are able either to nurture or destroy in unique ways because of their intense rational and emotional capacities. The human capacity for empathic understanding of the needs of others can be used either to lovingly care for them or to manipulate and even torture others for one's own ends.

In exercises of actualizing power, persons who identify with their own prenatal past can empathize with fetal life; in solidarity they will act to protect immature but potential development and well-being. Following the logic of domination, however, adult persons will feel free to kill or selectively destroy a fetus which is not wanted, planned for, or does not measure up to some acceptable criteria, including gender.

Women have been enjoined to think of abortion as a sacrament or a rite of passage. In this message exalting the autonomous will, a woman must be courageous enough to destroy a fetus which threatens her own individual development of self. To grow strong, the individual must choose self before others and break free from any bonds which may entrap. Fetal life may be recognized as a necessary human sacrifice or be discounted by being labeled a "parasite" or "tissue."

Such a permissive view of abortion affirms that an individual may define reality (I decide whether a truly human life has begun) as well as determine morality (only my emotional investment and choice create any moral claim upon me). If a society takes this route of absolutizing individual autonomy and choice, even to the point of self-definitions of reality and moral obligations, then other moral claims must fall.

Can it be that only freely willed and consciously contracted relationships can create moral obligations? If so, then all moral responsibilities in relationships which we have not entered into with informed consent will be endangered. Our parents, siblings, neighbors and compatriots would have no claim upon us.

Such a constricted view of moral responsibility appears both unconvincing and unworthy of human life. Indeed, no one has ever given informed consent to be born into earth's ecosystem, yet we can have obligations to care for the earth and the environment out of gratitude for sustaining our life. Surely we have other bonds and moral obligations that we have not chosen. Life is full of unexpected encounters and unplanned events that demand a moral response. Think of the obligations we would have to rescue someone with whom we had been in an automobile accident. So, too, obligations to care for an unborn life may exist even if we did not plan the conception. Of course, the obligation to a woman's unborn fetus would be strengthened by the sharing of kinship ties and the complete, if temporary, dependence upon the mother for the preservation of life.

If we as a human community abandon the completely helpless powerless unborn life, then actualizing nurturing power once more gives way to the logic of domination. Already under the rule of the marketplace and the jungle's law of survival of the fittest, there are calls for selective infanticide as a parent's right. Infanticide, we should remember, was approved of as a respectable practice in ancient Roman society, for any reason whatsoever, even to increase the family fortune. Modern abortion can be seen as a resurgence of one of the oldest of human customs, selectively killing unwanted offspring.

Once human life has been deemed expendable and it is exploited at will, it becomes difficult to stop the process. Suicide rates have climbed at the same alarming rates in the decades since abortion has become a routine way of solving the stressful problems of unwanted pregnancy. Everywhere in our society we see violence and abuse of the powerless by the more powerful and dominant.

It seems puzzling that so many advocates of abortion as a tragic necessity still believe that a destructive and violent solution permitted in one stage of the human life cycle will not generalize to other stressful situations in life. If a child only exists on its parent's sufferance and by choice, its claim to inalienable rights and dignity are more fragile. The commandment against killing has always supported the moral rule against using another person as a means to an end. Breaking both of these cultural taboos by allowing the killing of the unborn pollutes our moral ecosystem. Women, children, the aged, the ill and the impaired will suffer the consequences.

CONCLUSION

The unborn human being has value because it is a member of the human family and shares in the heritage of the human species. The human status and human potential of the dependent embryo deserve respect and protection.

Current struggles over the treatment of the unborn exemplify a larger cultural conflict between the logic of domination and the exercise of nurturing actualizing power. This moral strife will hardly remain confined to the abortion controversy, but will spread to other domains and other human relationships.

Is human life a gift which we accept gratefully? Do we have moral obligations to mother the earth, nurture the immature and protect dependent lives? A vision of human bonding and the value of all the living urges us to answer yes. A yes to the unborn is both an assertion of justice and an affirmation of hope for humankind.

NOTES

1. Nathaniel Davis, Letters to the Editor, *Los Angeles Times*, 12 May 1994.

2. Nat Hentoff, Introduction to David Mall, ed., *When Life and Choice Collide: Essays on Rhetoric and Abortion* Vol. 1 in *To Set the Dawn Free*, David Mall, ed., (Libertyville, Ill.: Kairos Books, Inc., 1994), pp. 2, 3, 5.

Chapter 4

The "Medicalizing" of Abortion Decisions

Thomas Murphy Goodwin

I will neither give a deadly drug to anybody if asked for it, nor will I make a suggestion to this effect. Similarly I will not give to a woman an abortive remedy. In purity and holiness I will guard my life and my art.

—The Hippocratic Oath

The paradigm of all peace and security should be the peace of the unborn child in the womb.

—Dr. Alan Keyes[1]

Moral decisions related to medical matters require, fundamentally, the unbiased representations of competent medical authority.[2] Information may come from the scientific literature, from individual physicians who are involved directly in a given case, or from physicians who are acting as consultants. In each case, suitable moral analysis requires the firm base of unbiased scientific data.

Despite a common perception to the contrary, the medical-scientific domain is no less subject to bias than any other. Indeed, much of the emphasis in clinical research in recent years has been directed toward standardizing study design in order to remove bias in clinical investigation. But there are certain sources of systematic bias in the medical community which influence the ability to pose moral questions fairly and have far-reaching consequences for all who come in contact with the medical establishment. I would like to discuss one of these sources of bias in particular. It is that which arises from the merging of the legal and political dimension of the abortion debate into medical judgment and decision making. I would like to develop this idea just as it presented itself in practice, through the case histories of individual patients. The cases which I will present provide a vantage point for viewing the politicized landscape surrounding the pregnant woman today.

My practice and clinical research are in one of the sub-specialties of obstetrics and gynecology, maternal fetal medicine, which is concerned with the whole spectrum of pregnancy complicated by maternal or fetal disease. There are few situations more daunting to those who advocate a consistent ethic of life than the circumstance in which the life of the mother is threatened by the continuation of the pregnancy itself. Although I do not acknowledge this conflict as justifying abortion, even the most dedicated of advocates for the life of the unborn are awed by this dilemma. Indeed, the power of this image has been one of the principal wedges moving forward the advocacy of abortion in general in the United States and elsewhere. What do we know about it objectively?

In Table 1 are listed the conditions that can be diagnosed in advance which are known to be associated with the greatest risk of maternal mortality. Taken altogether, abortions performed for these conditions make up a barely calculable fraction of the total abortions performed in the United States, but they are extremely important to the extent that they have been used to validate the idea of abortion as a whole. They stand as a sign that the idea of abortion is in some sense unavoidable—that it can be the fulfillment of the good and natural desire of the human person (in this case the mother) to live.

Table 1
Conditions   Associated   with   a   Greater   Than   20%   Risk   of Maternal   Mortality

Pulmonary hypertension
Primary
Eisenmenger's syndrome
Marfan's syndrome with aortic root involvement
Complicated coarctation of the aorta
Peripartum cardiomyopathy with residual dysfunction

The first point I would like to emphasize is how rare these conditions associated with the high risk of maternal mortality are. Our obstetric service has been the largest in the United States for most of the last fifteen years, averaging 15,000 to 16,000 births per year. Our institution serves a catchment area for all high-risk deliveries among 30,000 per year. Excluding cases that have been diagnosed late in pregnancy, we do not see more than one to two of these cases per year; these are exceedingly rare conditions. This does not diminish the tragic dimension of these difficult cases but they are seen in perspective when their numbers are compared to the total number of abortions performed.

If we examine other conditions which have been associated with significant, though lesser, risk of maternal mortality for which abortion is often recommended (Table 2), we find that in many cases the prognoses are changing, both because of a better understanding of the natural history of disease processes and because of advances in therapy. Some examples of this are seen in the cases which follow.

Table 2
Other Conditions Associated with Significant Risk of Maternal Mortality

Severe aortic or mitral stenosis
Prior myocardial infarction (especially in diabetic)
Marfan's syndrome
Uncorrected tetrology of Fallot
Coarctation of the aorta

Here is the paradox: as the actual risks to the mother are diminishing because of medical advances, concern about maternal and fetal risks from complications of pregnancy is still offered as a justification for many abortions. From the case histories that follow, taken from just this last year in our clinic, I will attempt to illustrate the distorted milieu of medical practice into which most pregnant women now enter.

CASE 1

A twenty one-year-old woman in her nineteenth week of pregnancy was referred for "immediate abortion." She had complained of shortness of breath, and a full evaluation revealed a complex maternal congenital heart lesion, tetrology of Fallot. This is a lesion that is frequently listed as a contradiction to pregnancy because of the increased risk of maternal mortality. The senior house office who was coordinating the abortion asked for a second opinion from our high-risk clinic because the patient was distraught over the recommendation. Despite having been told that she had a significantly increased chance of dying if she remained pregnant, she had not reconciled herself to the abortion.

Repeat evaluation confirmed the diagnosis but showed that the particular manifestations of the condition in this patient were such that she could be expected to tolerate pregnancy without difficulty. She was a so-called "pink tet," tetrology of Fallot in which the patient is still receiving adequate oxygen. This fact could have been determined by the referring physician. As it was, the patient very nearly underwent an abortion for nonindication. The patient delivered without significant complications following induction of labor in her thirty-eighth week of pregnancy.

CASE 2

A twenty five-year-old woman in the twelfth week of her first pregnancy had shortness of breath and was found to have severe narrowing of one of the valves of the heart, mitral stenosis. Her physician recommended abortion and asked our opinion for confirmation. We suggested that the patient be offered the opportunity to discuss balloon valve repair during pregnancy with a cardiologist skilled in that technique. We provided references showing that this could be accomplished safely in pregnancy. Her physician expressed his concern about his liability if there were any abnormality of maternal or fetal outcome. "She's young," he opined. "She can have the valve repaired and try again."

CASE 3

A thirty eight-year-old woman was referred by her pastor. She was 11 weeks pregnant and was found to have breast cancer with spread to the regional lymph nodes. She was told that, for the best chance of long-tern survival, she should undergo chemotherapy, but that the pregnancy should be terminated first. She was told that her prognosis would be worse if she remained pregnant and that the chemotherapy would definitely harm her baby. Her abortion had been scheduled.

We discussed with her the published experience showing that breast cancer is not affected by pregnancy and that the chemotherapy regimen required for her condition is apparently well tolerated by the fetus. Of course, the experience with any given chemotherapy regimen is limited, and we were frank with the patient that there were open questions about long-term sequelae. When her physician was informed of the patient's desire to undergo chemotherapy and continue the pregnancy, he suggested that we take over her care and accept the liability.

The patient underwent chemotherapy (Adriamycin and Cytoxan) and delivered a baby boy who appeared entirely normal at birth. That many chemotherapy regimens can be continued without apparent ill-effect in pregnancy is information readily available to any interested physician. Why was the patient not informed?

CASE 4

A twenty-year-old woman in the eighteenth week of her first pregnancy presented with severe renal disease which appeared to be due to new-onset systemic lupus erythematosus. The first consultant who saw her recommended abortion in anticipation of favorably affecting the course of the disease and out of concern that the medication required to control her disease might injure her fetus. The patient was anxious not to abort. We were able to tell her that, although the chance of successful pregnancy outcome was low, abortion would not predictably affect the course of the disease. We discussed the considerable experience available with the medications that she would require (principally steroids) and the fact that there were no apparent serious fetal affects related to this type of treatment. The patient elected to continue her pregnancy.

Subsequently, a kidney consultant recommended kidney biopsy as part of efforts to confirm the diagnosis—but not until the patient was aborted. We presented data showing that renal biopsy can be accomplished safely in pregnancy and that the need for this test should not be considered an indication for abortion.

Finally, the patient required a lengthy procedure under X-ray fluoroscopy. The radiologist recommended abortion because of significant X-ray exposure. After consultation with the radiation physicist, however, it was clear that the actual X-ray exposure to the fetus in this case posed no significant risk. The patient ultimately delivered a premature infant at 27 weeks gestation. The child did well for one week until dying, suddenly, of an overwhelming infection.

All the recommendations for abortion in these cases were partly the result of ignorance of the data, but also of something else—a belief that it is better to err on the side of abortion if there are doubts about the effect of the pregnancy on maternal or fetal outcome.

We have discussed some cases in which the risk is entirely maternal and others in which both fetal and maternal risks have factored into a recommendation for abortion. In many cases, the risk is entirely fetal.

CASE 5

A thirty two-year-old nurse had herself tested for cytomegalovirus at 7 weeks gestation. This is a type of virus known to be capable of crossing the placenta and infecting the fetus, sometimes resulting in retardation and multi-organ system disease, especially if the infection has occurred for the first time in pregnancy. The results of her testing profile suggested a recent infection indicating the possibility that her baby could be infected. She was advised to terminate the pregnancy and she had made plans to do so, although with great regret. Her doctor stated that he had confirmed his recommendations with a "high-risk pregnancy specialist."

She was referred to us by a physician colleague who was her neighbor. On initial review of the tests, it did appear that there had been an acute infection during the pregnancy. We presented to the patient the data on the likelihood of her child being seriously affected—4 in 100, one-half of these represented by isolated hearing loss. She was stunned and relieved to learn that the risk was no greater than that. As it turned out, a more specific indicator of infection which we recommended be checked before any decision was made revealed that there had been no infection at all. She delivered a healthy boy at term. She frequently referred to her "miracle baby," a pathetic reflection of the circumstances which nearly took that baby from her.

All this patient received was an accurate assessment of the risk to her child. That was enough for her, even before she learned that there had been no infection. It might not have been for the next woman. In fact, the same woman could have had an abortion for no reason at all the next day. *But it would not have been under the pretense of a medical indication.*

The purpose of exposing this pretense is simply to restore a rational medical assessment to these issues. Personally, we may be required to do much more. But in our professional lives, this role of strictly focusing the issue of medically justified abortion draws attention to the way in which medical judgement has been vitiated in this area.

These cases are just some of those we have seen in the last year. They include only women who, usually because of their own convictions, could not easily accept the recommendation for abortion and sought more information. There is no doubt that many others have received such recommendations and have proceeded to abort simply on the basis of the doctor's authority.

But the significance of these cases lies not in the individual stories themselves, however disturbing they may be. Such cases are an insignificant number compared to the total number of abortions. In addition, the ethical dilemma in such cases is commonly understood in a context which accepts the notion that abortion would indeed be appropriate if there were a significant risk to the mother or if the fetus were seriously malformed. The real significance of these cases though, lies in what they reveal about the attitudes of the physicians these women first encountered.

Why are physicians not providing readily available information that could affect their patients' judgement regarding termination of pregnancy? I believe that there are two related reasons for this phenomenon, and that they go much deeper than simple ignorance of the facts. One is the transference of the ambivalent attitude toward the developing human, virtually codified in *Roe v. Wade*, into the medical arena. Since the fetus can be aborted for any reason, the physician may see fit to suggest, if not recommend, the alternative of abortion for almost any reason. The basis for such an attitude is closely linked to a second concern: the unbalanced legal burden of informed consent.

When a mother presents with a major medical problem in pregnancy (or indeed any medical problem), the medical record must reflect, in practical terms, the patient's informed consent to continue with the pregnancy despite the risk. By failing to disclose these risks, the doctor is negligent because the patient could have chose a different course of treatment (abortion). To compound the problem for the physician, there are no clear legal guidelines to determine which risks are so small as not to warrant communication to the patient. A fact is considered to be material if a reasonable, prudent person in the position of the patient would attach significance to it in deciding whether or not to submit to the proposed treatment.[3] The accurate assessment of the risks in a given case can be a tedious process. Should any untoward outcome result from the pregnancy (always a possibility), the record may well be scrutinized intensely. Yet, no method of documentation is watertight.

The doctor's alternative, to suggest or recommend that abortion is the safest route, carries no such legal liability. There does not appear to be a legal precedent for a physician's liability in a case where abortion was recommended on supposed medical grounds that were subsequently found to be baseless or misrepresented.

With regard to fetal abnormalities, the burden is equally one-sided and even more clearly delineated in law. Physicians have legal and, some would say, ethical duties to inform pregnant women of prenatal tests that would affect their willingness to continue the pregnancy. The concept of "wrongful birth" in law establishes that failure to inform of tests that are widely accepted in the medical community as part of the standard of care could lead to legal liability for the physician.[4] The related concept of "wrongful life," though less commonly invoked legally, is instructive for distilling the idea behind the law. In such cases, the child sues, claiming that it would be better not to have been born than to have been born with defects.[5]

The concept of informed consent, then, although simple in theory, is almost impossible in practice. For many physicians, it translates into simply recommending every possible test and erring on the side of suggesting abortion whenever there is a question of risk to the mother or fetus. There is a tremendous imbalance between the liability involved in not informing of risks compared to the liability of suggesting the alternative of abortion. All pregnant women, no matter what their personal convictions, are subjected to the effects of this imbalance.

The circumstances where this dilemma arises because of real or even perceived increased risk to the mother or fetus, as I have presented above, are actually relatively infrequent. Much more common in practice is the situation in which a presumably healthy mother (and healthy fetus) are offered screening tests in the hopes of identifying various congenital anomalies of the fetus. Maternal serum alphafetoprotien (MSAFP) screening, which is capable of identifying fetuses with neural tube defects or Down's syndrome, was introduced into this country in the early 1980s. Its place in practice was virtually mandated by the 1985 liability alert from the American College of Obstetricians and Gynecologists, which itself was a direct response to the perceived liability under the concept of wrongful birth.[6] Every physician must inform patients about these tests or make himself liable for the results. The patient may refuse the test but is usually required to make a positive statement refusing the test. The inescapable implication is that the woman who refuses the test is outside of the norm.

More recently, various tests of maternal blood designed to identify fetal Down's syndrome have been introduced into clinical practice. The number of tests on the horizon which will allow identification of other fetal abnormalities appears limitless. The ineluctable logic of these legal precedents affects every pregnant woman and her child. No matter what the personal convictions of the mother, she must receive her care in a system in which every possible problem of maternal or fetal well-being is a test of whether the pregnancy will be allowed to continue. In that balance, the developing human has little or no value. There is no counterweight to "wrongful birth." There is no "wrongful abortion."

Although few women may actually abort because of this bias, many will learn the lesson: that a new human being is accepted conditionally, one test at a time.

NOTES

1. Alan Keyes, in press release announcing candidacy for the United States presidency, 22 March 1995.

2. This essay is an expanded and revised version of a speech delivered by the author to the 1994 North American Catholic Bishops' winter symposium at the Pope John XXIII Center in Braintree, Massachussetts.

3. R.R. Lenke and J. M. Nemes, "Wrongful Birth, Wrongful Life: The Doctor Between a Rock and a Hard Place," *Obstetrics and Gynecology* 66 (1985): 719–722.

4. J. A. Robertson, "Legal and Ethical Issues Arising from the New Genetics," *Journal of Reproductive Medicine* 37 (1992): 521–524.

5. M. Z. Pelias, "Torts of Wrongful Birth and Wrongful Life: A Review," *American Journal of Medical Genetics* 25 (1986): 71–80.

6. American College of Obstetricians and Gynecologists professional liability alert, 1985.

Part II

Cultural Perspectives

Chapter 5

Feminism and Imaging the Unborn

Camille S. Williams

We have to remind people that abortion is the guarantor of a woman's . . . right to participate fully in the social and political life of society.
—Kate Michelman, abortion rights activist[1]

A people who perceive needs and seek to satisfy their needs without giving thought to the means they are using will often find themselves drinking poison rather than helpful medicine. This is a testimony to the power of a teaching droned in over a long period of time—even when it's inaccurate—to alter a peoples' view of their universe, of their reality.
—William B. Allen, political scientist[2]

To understand contemporary views of the unborn, we must survey briefly our conceptions of maternity and the ways in which mothers and their unborn are known. This is a question not of materiality but of maternal desire. We see the unborn through their mothers, if we see them at all, and we see mothers rather differently than our mothers saw themselves. Coincidentally, perhaps, the 1.4 million women who seek fertility services yearly[3] is a near mirror of the number of abortions recorded each year in the United States. Some women who have postponed childbearing for the sake of a career are desperate now for conception.[4] Intuitively, it might be assumed that these groups of women have vastly different images of the unborn. Their views are remarkably similar: many women who abort view the unborn as their own living child of possibilities. It is true that those searching for conception see the unborn as a gift just beyond their reach, whereas those who abort see their unborn as a threat to their autonomous lives; the factor distinguishing between women reaching for the unborn and women aborting the unborn—apart from their relative levels of fertility—appears to be how those women view themselves as potential mothers.[5]

As poststructuralistically impaired as it may appear, I offer in this chapter a partial reading of some textual images of mothers and their interactions with the unborn. I assert that the desire for children, though sometimes masked, may be as deeply held by contemporary women as it was by women in the past. Efforts to re-educate women's desires away from childbearing and childrearing may have caused at least as much sorrow as would shaping women *only* for motherhood, if indeed such error ever occurred.

FEMINISM, MOTHERING AND THE UNBORN

During the past thirty years, the women's movement in the United States has interrogated, problematized, displaced, deconstructed and reconstituted the image of mothering. The simultaneous expansion of the theory and practice of legalized elective abortion has been central to that effort.[6] In order to re-establish mothering as a respectable-when-voluntary option—and to distinguish *our mothering* from that of earlier generations (who, it is alleged, were mothers because they had or perceived no other choice)—feminist writings have worked to separate women's sexual activity from procreation, and childrearing from childbearing.[7]

As though it were news, feminist theorists explain that "we have come to re-alize that women's reproductive capacities are not brute phenomena isolated from their social context."[8] As might have been anticipated,

> Feminist criticism has recently joined forces with advanced technology to throw many of our settled beliefs about motherhood into disarray.

> Feminists have debunked traditional expectations about women's reproductive role and have called for a radical reconfiguring of that role. Many feminists, Simone de Beauvoir among them, have argued that women should regard motherhood as an option, not as a biological imperative, and that women must cease to expect their main fulfillment to come from procreation.[9]

The unavoidable result of this effort has been one species of privatization of motherhood. Pregnant women no longer automatically join the ranks of honorable motherhood across the ages: if you want to give birth, proceed at your own risk; decide what the unborn means to you personally, and negotiate your own place in society. To turn Orania Papazoglou's phrase, in despising our mothers, we learned to despise mothering.[10] As the status of ordinary mothering (as opposed to mothering with a raised consciousness) was explored, so was the status of those we mother, especially the unborn child.

Feminist legal scholar Deborah L. Rhode links technological change to changing attitudes toward mothering, the unborn and abortion:

> During the 1960s, many of the same forces underlying liberalized contraception policy also encouraged abortion law reform. Women's increasing sexual activity and labor force participation increased the number of unwanted [*sic*]

pregnancies. As improvements in medical technology reduced the circumstances in which abortion was necessary to preserve a mother's life, the rigidity of existing statutes became more apparent.[11]

Actually, what became apparent was that abortion was seldom necessary for physical health, but was much in demand for other reasons.

Once it was clear that there were truly few situations in which a pregnancy would endanger a woman's life or good health, defenses of abortion rights worked to deny the moral status of the unborn. Philosopher Bonnie Steinbock's discussion of abortion rehearses a pedigreed ethical argument.[12] A commonplace of philosophical justifications for elective abortion is that we can confidently label the previable unborn as *presentients* who cannot be harmed, and thus, are not entitled to our moral concern.

Should we be surprised that the cognitively able select *their strength* as the determinant of moral status? I confess to a sense of unease with such cognicentric assertions. Whether listing the requirements for personhood or dividing up the living into "conventional persons," "potential persons," "future persons," and "actual persons," each with a specific "moral status,"[13] such defenses evince the prejudice[14] that unless an entity can prove itself in some manner *we* can recognize, we do no harm in destroying it. I recognize that *ad hominem* is unseemly, but perhaps we think too much of ourselves: because we have formal training, we think we are wise.

Steinbock refutes various pro-life arguments on behalf of the unborn. The "happiness of the potential child is not determinative—indeed, not even relevant to the decision to abort," she claims.[15]

> A pregnant woman who wishes to be responsible and conscientious in making a decision about abortion is not required to consider the child who might have been born. In order to justify having an abortion, she does not have to claim that her child would be miserable. She can acknowledge that, if she does not abort, the resulting child might well have a very happy life. . . . There is no obligation to bring happy people into the world, only an obligation to try to give the children one decides to bring into the world a decent chance at happiness.[16]

The unborn in the womb *is* within the world of her parents; her presence in their world is the cause of their felt obligation, be it an obligation to give life or an obligation to abort. While it may not be relevant to the logic of an argument for abortion, for actual women making the decision to continue to carry or abort a child, the potential happiness of the child is salient. The assertion that "only future actual people . . . can be harmed, not merely possible people"[17] sounds very much like a general rule that is applicable in no specific case—ideology dressed up like analysis.

"Your sentience or your life!" seems a crude motto for a gang of cognoscenti;

the judgment is occasionally softened. "A human fetus," Steinbock acknowledges,"even a preconscious one, is a potential person and a powerful symbol of humanity, and, as such, should be treated with respect."[18] The respectful treatment is due more developed fetuses, if for no other reason than public sensibilities. "By 12 to 14 weeks of gestation, a fetus *looks human. It evokes in most people the same instinctive responses of protection that newborn babies do.*"[19]

In addition to making fine distinctions among categories of human life, abortion advocates have depicted the psychological burden of an unwanted pregnancy—keeping the focus on the image of the suffering woman. The fetus's dependence on her or his mother's body was likened to the use a rapist would make of a woman's body,[20] or the use a dying violinist, sharing the woman's vital organs, would make of her body for an extended period of time.[21] Pregnancy was also analyzed as "an illness for which [American women] regard the appropriate treatment to be abortion,"[22] or the unborn characterized as a parasitic, invasive growth.[23] Images of the unborn are, to a large extent, shaped by whether the woman wants a child, whether she wants to be a mother:

> A woman who wants a child lives in compliance with her biological condition if she becomes pregnant; a woman who is pregnant against her wish lives at war with her body. The fetus is a foreign body whose growth consummates inside her without her being able to do anything about it on her own strength and from her own will. Her biological function produces in her ego a disastrous defeat. No man is subject to this stress situation between body and consciousness.[24]

Both women and men may feel at war with the body. The apostle Paul and Stephen Hawking might relate to the plight of the woman struggling with her body—except, of course, their afflictions did not have a nine—or ten—month cap.

The image of ourselves as aborters keeps getting in the way of seeing the unborn at all. The liberty to abort has been with us in this country for only two decades. The *Casey* Court's covenant to preserve abortion for future generations is a reflection of the double-mindedness of our society as a whole: we want the best for our children, and to achieve it we destroy a full third of them before birth.

Rhode assesses the *Roe* Court's trimester scheme, in light of technological development since 1973, acknowledging that the state's interest in maternal health "surely exists prior to the point at which abortion is riskier than childbirth. Yet now abortion is safer than childbirth until the third trimester of pregnancy, the original health justification for distinguishing first and second trimester procedures has disappeared."[25] She concedes that "Society's interest in affirming the value of human life and minimizing physical and psychological complications argues for ensuring that abortions occur before the point of fetal survival, except under limited extenuating circumstances."[26] Technological advances, it seems, have made it both easier to know our preborn children and safer to destroy them without physically harming the mother—a mixed triumph over nature. *Casey* gave legal sanction to the notion that with contraception and abortion today's women can and must shape their own spiritual imperatives.[27] The Court alluded to the "fact that for two decades of economic and social developments, people have organized intimate relationships and made choices that define their views of themselves and their places in society, in reliance on the availability of abortion in the event that contraception should fail."[28] We have developed merely at the cost of the unborn.

Some consider abortion a necessary evil, a temporary solution that will be little used once women are fully integrated into public institutions. Others see abortion as no evil, a merely regrettable episode that will fade from personal and collective memory once contraceptive technology makes unplanned pregnancies a risk of the past.

THE UNBORN AS THREAT

Since philosophy, feminism, and medical technology have changed the image of *mother*, it should not startle us that the image of the unborn has changed. There is a good deal of irritation among some feminists about the contemporary tendency, fueled by technology, that allows study of the fetus, to view the unborn as subjects to whom we have obligations. "Science has inspired doctors to view the fetus as a second and interesting patient, separate from the mother. But fetal rights [derivable from the fetus as subject] may lead us to treat women simply as fetal containers."[29] This horrifying projection seems unlikely to anyone who is or has had a mother.

Some pro-choice advocates consider the emphasis on the humanity of the unborn misleading or deceptive, betraying "ignorance and contemptuous attitudes to women" by diverting attention from the woman carrying the child to representations of the unborn in "tearjerking pictures of the sweet little pink embryo with its sad eyes staring out of its plastic bag, pleading: let me live!"[30] Cultural studies scholar E. Ann Kaplan contends that images of the fetus as "cosmic entity," "perfected being," "full-blown subject," and "safe haven" are "imbued within an ideological discourse" which marginalizes the mother's body and subjectivity."[31] This reasoning is quite backward. Social and legal pressure to encourage women to save prenatal life or health does not demonstrate that women are considered lacking in legal capacity. On the contrary, when women have been charged, for example, with prenatal abuse of their unborn children, the charge itself is a recognition of the agency, power and subjectivity of the woman. Like a trustee, the mother is viewed as having special power over the unborn child. As one standing in a position of trust relative to one vulnerable or without legal capacity, the woman is, intuitively at least, held to a high standard of care *because* she has both legal capacity and power.

Considering the unborn as subjects in their own right is hardly a new idea. Whereas generations past learned about gestational development from a study of fetuses that miscarried, today fetal monitors, ultrasound and surgery *in utero* have yielded detailed knowledge about life between conception and birth. Legal abortion has provided some researchers with numerous "subjects" for study. This new technology has been used by partisans on both sides of the abortion debate.

Despite a virtual revolution in the knowledge of the physical, psychological and behavioral development of the child *in utero* and its link to the traits of newborns, a view that is "often defended by scientists and medical professionals" describes

> the fetus as a passive agent that grows in an unchanging world buffered from environmental stimuli. The fetus sleeps during most of its existence before birth, exhibits only sporadic, reflexive movements, and is influenced only as a receiving object in an environment regulated by the mother. Only at the time of birth is the fetus transformed into an active and interactive organism.[32]

That view of the unborn as passive during most of gestation is a mainstay for many who seek to protect women's access to legal abortion. It is a necessary fiction for those who fear that recognizing the humanity of the unborn will in some sense decrease the humanity of the women who carry those children. Ultrasound and other "prenatal procedures gives the fetus social recognition as an individual separate from the mother . . . producing a context in which women's procreative rights achieved only recently after decades of struggle are threatened."[33]

It is becoming more difficult to think of the unborn as only potential human beings.[34] Robert H. Blank notes that

> until the recent decade the fetus in utero could not take on the social recognition of a human except conceptually. . . . One of the most critical elements of recognition is visualization. Only in the last ten years has it been possible to visualize the fetus in utero through sophisticated electronic equipment. As ultrasound technology has advanced to produce more explicit real time images of the fetal limbs and movement, it is reasonable to expect a tendency to perceive the fetus as a small baby instead of an unseen organism residing in the womb.[35]

The aggravating propensity of the general public (as distinguished from trained philosophers, demographers, and feminists) to think of the unborn as like us is regarded as dangerous ignorance that not only damages women, but also places cutting-edge research in jeopardy. Dr. Steven Muller, chair of a federal ad-

visory panel on fetal research, regards the public outcry over fetal experimentation as ignorance exploited by those in opposition to such experimentation.
Most Americans, he contends, "know little about the intricate details of human
reproduction" and are needlessly alarmed, since very young embryos do not have
the same moral status as infants and children, though they do merit significant
respect.[36] This is, of course, a premise stated as a conclusion.

The fear is that as the unborn gain a reputation for humanness, the woman
carrying the child will disappear as a subject in her own right. "Earlier the fetus
was merely an object, or a part of the mother's body. Where before there was one
subject, and one body (the woman's, in pregnancy, carrying a developing extra
part), suddenly there are two subjects, two bodies, from the moment of conception."[37]

It is arguable that the unborn have long been subjects apart from their mothers; furthermore, there is no logical necessity that the mother as subject disappears if the unborn attain subject status. In fact, making subject status a zero-
sum proposition bears an uncanny resemblance to the charges that men have
viewed women's increased status as a threat to male power and dominance.

Some feminists worry that "late-twentieth-century displacement of the
mother reworks" either the "Catholic" doctrine that personhood begins at conception or the "medieval concept of the homunculus in the man's sperm," reducing
the mother to incubator rather than giver of life. The incubator image would be
more accurate if the fetus were considered part of the woman's body. The view
that the unborn have social and moral status elevates human gestation and maternity to a meaningful, charitable, purposeful act. These analysts have no desire
to go back to a cult of domesticity, where "the mother was overinstalled in the
symbolic."[38] There is an admission, however, that prior to our generation
"motherhood at least gave women an opportunity to gain attention, to fulfill an
important function for the aristocracy and then the bourgeoisie (that is, reproduction of the class), and, at times, to gain a certain amount of power within the
home, despite its constraints."[39] Now, it is posited, these "benefits" are displaced
onto the fetus, and "the mother *herself* is no longer important . . . the mother's
own body, and along with it, her subjectivity, are sidelined to make the fetus
central."[40]

Alternatively, it could be argued that the fetus as a subject was cut loose
from the mother by feminist theorizing itself. Since *Casey* gave each individual
woman the liberty to define her "own concept of existence, of meaning, of the
universe, and of the mystery of human life,"[41] we cannot make any assumptions
about the woman whose body encases the developing being. Were we to emphasize her noble sacrifices, her "intimate and personal" suffering,[42] we would be
likely to collapse into essentialism, stereotyping all women or all mothers on
the basis of reproductive capacity. However, if we explore the growth of the unborn while simultaneously reminding ourselves that at any and every minute the
woman carrying the unborn has no special obligation to continue life support,

we risk eliciting sympathy for those unborn who *are* aborted, and concomitantly, may encourage people to think that "'fetus' equals "baby," and may promote automatic anti-choice sentiments."[43] We of the anti-choice persuasion find that result both logical and unproblematic.

Surely, there are aspects of parenting that are socially constructed; perhaps there are also some experiences that are common, if not universal, to the human condition. That experience is tied neither to an innate ability to nurture nor to reproductive capacity as "hardwired," or as socially constituted. It is tied to the human—not exclusively female—capacity to feel pity, to have compassion on our children in their weakness. We see our own weaknesses, too, but are sometimes moved to behave better than we might otherwise. While an appeal to the milk of human kindness may seem insufficiently postmodernist, reading human impulses as tending to mercy is no greater leap of logic than the facile assertion that generations of women were either hopelessly oppressed, or relentlessly brainwashed, into nurturing roles.[44]

VIEWS OF THE UNBORN

Both as individuals and as a group, the unborn have been a felt presence for many people throughout the ages. Their presence and promise have sometimes motivated their parents to act in their behalf. "Everything in our life happens as though we entered upon it with a load of obligations contracted in a previous existence . . . obligations whose sanction is not of this present life, [which] seems to belong to a different world, founded on kindness, scruples, sacrifice, a world entirely different from this one, a world whence we emerge to be born on this earth, before returning thither."[45] According to Erik Erikson in *Gandhi's Truth*, "deep down nobody in his right mind can visualize his own existence without assuming that he has always lived and will live hereafter; and the religious world-views of old only endowed this psychological instinct with images which could be shared, transmitted, and ritualized."[46]

An awareness of and a concern for the unborn are seen in texts both ancient and contemporary, ranging from Wordsworth's familiar: "Our birth is but a sleep and a forgetting: /The Soul that rises with us, our life's Star, /Hath had elsewhere its setting, / And cometh from afar," to traditional tales of the Osage Elders of The First Race: The First of the race/ Was saying, "Ho, younger brother! the children have no bodies./ "We shall seek bodies for our children."[47]

Whatever it may have been called in the past, parents were tied to their children before birth. Current technologies which allow us to see the unborn early on help "parents bond with their babies very early in the pregnancy. The result is a parent-infant bond that can be strong and intense, even in its earliest stages."[48] This may account for the chagrin one California women felt after a first-trimester prenatal exam that included an ultrasound. "They let me listen to the heartbeat, then they showed me my baby moving inside me, *then* they asked me whether I wanted to terminate the pregnancy—how could they do that?" she wondered. Maybe to those of us who grew up with TV, the ultrasound image on screen can seem unreal. It is surprising what can be believed despite ocular proof. One abortion activist I've had the pleasure of associating with in public spectacles was insistent before an audience that most abortions occur so early in fetal development that all you're dealing with is a "tiny, tiny, tiny little spot of blood." Images of the nearly intact aborted child have proven too controversial for pro-choice proprieties. *Some abortion advocates refuse to participate in debates with pro-life representatives unless the pro-life side is prohibited from showing any pictures either of fetal development or of the results of abortions.*

Showing pictures of aborted fetuses is considered inflammatory or too gauche for words. "*Hard Truth*," a video which for the most part presents against a musical backdrop the portrait of the unborn aborted in the second or third trimesters of life, has been blamed in the popular press for Michael Griffin's attack on abortionists.[49] Maryland artist Mary Cate Carroll's reliquary for an aborted five-month-old fetus was banned from exhibit at Mary Washington College because the art director judged its showing a "flagrant and crass exploitation of [that] pathetic form," which, in her judgment, demonstrated a lack of respect for human life by the artist.[50] How is respect for unborn life to be promoted when such respect has been reduced to personal preference rather than moral obligation?

In *Life Before Birth* Sarah Hinze recounts the experiences of thirty nine parents or families who were given knowledge about or who communicated with their unborn children. One, a woman reluctant to be pregnant, dreamed of a beautiful young girl in a place as serene as heaven. "Who is that little girl?" she asked; "She's a spirit child waiting for her turn on earth," a voice answered her. Why isn't she happy then? the woman asked. The distant voice replied "She sees how sad you are that she is coming." The woman felt that she had hurt her unborn child and despite a series of health problems elected to give birth to a healthy daughter.[51]

Parents and siblings share their "visions" and dreams of unborn children, some of whom play the role of guardian angels. One woman, after being assaulted in her own home by a stranger, felt the presence of a young woman beside her as she listened to the rapist ransack her home. "Who are you?" she asked aloud, feeling that the "spirit essence was a blood relative . . . ,"a guardian angel" who would take her to "the other side" should she be killed. She felt that the spirit beside her, not the intruder, was in charge, although the criminal was still in her home. Shortly after she heard the intruder leave, her "spiritual friend" departed, too. Ten months later—after six and a half years of wanting another child—she found that she was pregnant. She knew she was to have a daughter. She described the birth of her child as a "great miracle" taking place; it seemed that the child had an aura about her head. When her mother held her for the first time she reported, "I looked into her eyes and her focus caught mine. Her little eyes became transfixed on me and we had an immediate bond. I said, 'It was you.' No one else knew what I meant, but I knew she did." Her mother felt "the strength and power of her spirit. It was as though she had been watching me for a long time. I felt that this child had been my protector before her birth . . . this day was the reason my life was spared: so that I could bring her to earth."[52]

Several of the unborn who communicated with their parents were initially unwanted by women who felt that they had neither the physical nor the emotional strength to care for another child; many of the parents were struggling financially. The message of the unborn child was, for most of them, a strengthening, comforting experience that allowed the parents to accept the conception and birth of children they had not sought to bring into the world.

"Janet M." tells of caring for her fourth son shortly after returning home from the hospital and "hearing the cry of babies." She would rush to her infant's room "thinking it was him only to find him sleeping peacefully." This continued for three months; Janet began to wonder whether she was "crazy." When she told her husband, he remarked that maybe they were "supposed to have more kids." Feeling already overwhelmed with child care and a part-time job, she prayed that "the crying would go away. Within days it stopped," and she felt relieved. Six months later the crying resumed. As she nursed her baby late at night, she listened again to "the sound of a crying baby." One day as she worked in the kitchen while the older children played outside and the baby slept she heard a child's voice cry "Mommy, Mommy!" When she turned around, she saw a "little girl about five years old." She knew immediately that the child was to be her daughter. The child did not speak again, but they "communicated spirit to spirit." The visit was to let her mother know she was anxious to join the family: "I had not hearkened to the message in the baby's crying. She told me she loved me, and as she grew dimmer, I knew I loved her too. Then she was gone."[53] Janet and her husband discussed what her "vision" meant; because her other pregnancies had been difficult, they were reluctant to attempt another pregnancy unless both felt a sense of peace with the decision. After her daughter's presence followed her for two days straight, they felt they should try to have the child and made arrangements for hospitals and doctors. This fifth pregnancy was more difficult than all the others; at times Janet worried that they hadn't made the right decision. Despite significant health risks, a healthy girl was safely delivered. The life Janet "thought was so full before, would be empty without this choice little person" in the family.[54]

Hinze also interviewed a number of infertile couples who were assured by the unborn that they would have children of their own bodies, or would adopt the unborn who communicated with them. One baby "spoke these words as one adult speaks to another, 'I have been waiting a long time and I have your name on me.'"[55]

Anne Taylor Fleming's *Motherhood Deferred* elucidates the lives of women such as herself who, "armed with [their] contraceptives and [their] fledgling feminism," went to college as "the golden girls of the brave new world, ready, willing and able to lay our contraceptively endowed bodies across the chasm between the feminine mystique and the world the feminists envisioned."[56] She and the women of her generation would not be restricted to the "comfortable concentration camp" of home, they would not be "buried alive" in the traditional roles of wife and mother.[57] With self-fulfillment as moral imperative, some pursued sexual experiences as part of their education. Many now infertile women came by their "infirmity" through sexually transmitted diseases, which marred their reproductive organs and made "life-giving difficult if not impossible."[58]

Now, no longer so inspired by de Beauvoir's argument that the oppression of women is directly linked to their role in reproduction, Fleming is wary that she will be viewed as "a cliche, one of those achievement-oriented, liberation-intoxicated, narcissistic baby boomers who forgot to have babies until it was too late."[59] She identifies neither with "fervent feminists" who judge "high-tech baby making to be invasive, inorganic, patriarchal, [and] anti-female," nor with those she considers imbued with a "reflexive pro-family frat-pack phallic fear." It is her belief that abortion and the women's movement as a whole had given both women and men fuller lives and had produced women who "were alive to their own pleasures . . . happier, sexier, nicer, more vital, more supportive," and more challenging than "those who had been circumscribed by the old roles."[60]

Her view of our mothers and grandmothers is as inaccurate as it is uncharitable. The women of those generations I've known are not humorless, sexless creatures. They were no more circumscribed by old roles than we are circumscribed by new roles. Unlike perhaps the most self-indulgent generation in recent history, our mothers practiced self-restraint as a part of civility. Their lives, as I have witnessed them, are as vital, interesting, useful and beautiful as any of those of my contemporaries.

In her "celebration of maternity, of femaleness, of fecundity, of family," Fleming draws attention to the "non-coercive joy" of the woman who has stepped "out of the confines of our sex, the second sex, and then, down the road, after fighting to adjust marriages and get jobs and hold them, to reembrace our femaleness, not in a corny, doctrinaire, reactionary way, but hopefully, joyfully, expectantly, fleshily, protectively. . . ."[61] In this instantiation of we-are-better-or-better-off-than-our-mothers, Fleming manages to illustrate the confines of our generation while casting a condescending backward glance at the women who went before us. The constraints may differ from generation to generation, but every person faces some limitations. One of Fleming's limitations is her infertility. She finally does experience one brief pregnancy—unfortunately, a tubal one that requires surgical removal. "As the months went by and became years," Fleming explains,

> I began to understand that I would not ever completely heal, that I would carry with me always the child I had never had —in times of sorrow, in times of

exuberance, in new and foreign places when I wanted that specific someone to show things to. That daughter. Some days I let go of it. But some days I saw her everywhere, not as a baby, a newborn, not as a toddler, or a ten-year-old even. I saw her always on the cusp of adolescence. . . . I studied young girls as they cavorted through malls, giggly and bumptious, and I saw her among them, mouthy and hopeful and yet still strangely shy, as I had been. And I wondered then whether I could leave it alone, let her exist as my figment, while I mothered or at least mentored other young women who came my way, or whether I would still have to assuage this longing.[62]

In the end, her bylines are her only babies. She recognizes that her "unrequited baby-longing" in no way diminished the thrill of her full-fledged participation in advancing the cause of women on this planet.[63]

SOCIAL PARTICIPATION

Many women see full-fledged participation in life on this planet as including giving birth to children. Nearly 2.3 million U.S. couples are infertile; each year some of them spend $10,000 or more for in vitro fertilization procedures at one or more of the three hundred fertility clinics in the nation. Americans spent $2 billion in 1993 "in their quest for a child."[64] High-tech babymaking is not only expensive, it can also be emotionally draining and physically painful for couples who submit their psyches and their bodies to surgeries and hormonal manipulation.

In contrast to the gadgetry of fertility specialists, those who contracept or abort rely on relatively low technology to maintain their preferred participatory pattern in the life on this earth and in women's "liberation."[65]

Women usually believe that they can be better mothers at some time in the future, though they seem to understand that the pregnancy terminated was the only chance for that specific being forming within to be born. Anne Archer had an abortion "because I viewed having a child at that time as an end to my life. All my hopes and dreams for myself would have had to be put aside. I had planned and worked hard all my life to be an actress. . . . I know now that I certainly wasn't emotionally ready to give the full-time attention and nurturing to a young child that each and every one so rightly deserves."[66] It seems counterintuitive to suppose that aborting one child is good preparation for nurturing another at a later date. As a teenager, actress Jill Clayburgh had two abortions, noting that at the time the question of whether the fetus was a living being never occurred to her. After giving birth as an adult, however, she says that

the fetus is alive from the moment of conception. I don't think that we should say it isn't alive until such and such a week or month . . . it's always alive. Women know the first week they're pregnant. . . . You're not a little bit alive, and you're not a little bit dead.

> It's alive, but that still doesn't make it your responsibility to sacrifice both your life and this child's life. The position is not about whether or not it's alive; it's about whether or not someone wants to give birth and have the responsibility of another human being with them for the rest of their life.[67]

Clayburgh's position is that it is morally acceptable to sacrifice the life within the woman rather than accept the responsibility to care for the child during gestation. Given their relative level of sacrifice—the woman's loss may be reducible to nine months of significant discomfort versus the child's loss of a probable seventy years of pleasures and pains—it is understandable that many sympathize more with the aborted unborn than with the healthy mother who aborts.

Having a baby, as Stefinee Pinnegar notes, isn't like getting cancer.[68] "Even with an unwed teen," Pinnegar remarked, "many good things can come from the birth of that child."[69] The image of the unborn as an approaching scourge which leaches a woman of opportunity and achievement prompts many women to abort as a backup to contraception. Feminist actress Kathy Najimy attributes some of her feminist passion to seeing her mother—a brilliant, talented, creative woman—stay home and take care of four kids, "so her whole life got sidetracked." Najimy had her abortion wondering whether she'd "regret it in later years or just a week later." She finds it sad that pro-choice women suppress their grief over their abortions because they're afraid "they would be giving anti-choice people more ammunition to use in trying to take away our right [to choose abortion]."[70] It turns out that women who abort retain victim status; the unborn are the sidetrackers of careers, orphaned through their own importunity. In this view, guilt or grief is not an index to the morality of the act of abortion.

Film star Margot Kidder's illegal incomplete abortion "haunted" her and "scarred" her deeply, though she did not regret the abortion, "I cried for the loss. I went through the grief. But I always knew I would not have been a good mother then. I knew that having that baby would have been wrong for the baby, and that you don't do that to children."[71] She remembers saying, "I want my baby back"; she remembers the "horrible, horrible nightmares" after the abortion. "They were constant and went on for a long time—images of children running at me with slashed wrists, of dead babies . . . coming out of my vagina. . . . The nightmares stopped when I had my child."[72]

POETIC IMAGES OF THE UNBORN

The unborn aborted are an unforgettable theme of some modern poetry.[73] These refrains of sorrow, pain, and sometimes self-pity portray the presence and absence of the unborn child. Anne Sexton's "The Abortion," begins with the poem's refrain: "Somebody who should have been born/ is gone." The Pennsylvania landscape is described in inorganic terms, a projection of the woman's flat emotional state and the unnaturalness of the induced abortion. She is witness to the fragility of love and of "the fullness that love began." Her conclusion is stark: "such logic will lead/ to loss without death. Or say what you meant,/ you coward . . . this baby that I bleed."[74]

The women who abort in the poems may be castigated or justified, but they always suffer. Gwendolyn Brooks's "The Mother" notes that "abortions will not let you forget," the unborn she describes as "The damp small pulps with little or with no hair,/ The singers and the workers that never handled the air." The mother of the poem insists that she "knew, though faintly" all of her aborted children and loved them all. Speaking to them, she explains: "Sweets, if I sinned, if I seized / Your luck / And your lives from your unfinished reach, / If I stole your births and your names, / . . . Believe me that even in my deliberateness I was not deliberate." The mother admits to her "crime": "how is the truth to be said?/ You were born and you had body, you died / It is just that you never giggled or planned or cried."[75]

It is the ability to see the unborn as formed like us and to see them in the world with us that lends poignancy to stories of the unborn who die. Yet abortion itself is at the same time an attempt to deny our likeness in the unborn, to make abortion bearable. David Sutton, the male "voice" of a poem in which a man convinces his lover that their life within her womb was "no different . . . from a rat's or chicken's," muses, "How should the never-born be long remembered?"[76] Some are never forgotten.

Some not-yet-born are long awaited. When Rachel was childless, she envied her prolific sister and cried to Jacob, "Give me children, or else I die!"[77] One feminist interpretation of this anguished demand suggests that women in patriarchal societies learned to value themselves only as childbearers. The social emphasis on motherhood sparked rivalry among women—even between sisters—and led to isolation and self-alienation.[78] That seems a not entirely implausible reading, but it certainly is not the whole story. It strains credulity to believe that description of the lives of women, and it denies to the women who lived before us subjectivity and status as moral agents. Even if we grant that women may have been used or abused as mothers,[79] it is also true that a mother's love for her child has been characterized as the central component of human love; a mother's rejection of her child a prime example of perversity, a sign of madness, or a symptom of a society in the grasp of death.[80] While our knowledge of Rachel's time is incomplete, we know that even in cultures which valued childbearing, where a nation's destiny was tied to the coming of promised children, some parents offered their children to be burned as a sacrifice to their gods. Rachel's longing and children as sacrificial objects mark antithetical contemporary attitudes toward children and mothering.

The texts containing these stories give only a glimpse of what the people of those times did, thought, and felt. Nevertheless, we can read ourselves between the lines. It may be that the children were offered as sacrifice not because they weren't valued in their own right, but because their parents found a way to reconcile the desire to protect a child with the demands of an idol-worshiping society. Rather than a sign of ambivalent feelings toward children, it may be they felt that in dedicating their children to be burned they were giving them up for what they thought was a higher good. Those sacrificed were sometimes thought to have achieved a glorious status by serving as an offering to the gods.

Stories of parental longing for offspring are present not only in biblical accounts of Sarah, Rebekah, Hannah, and Elizabeth, but also in some versions of folk tales such as Sleeping Beauty, Tom Thumb, and Rumpelstiltskin. So, too, has the failure of parental or filial compassion been chronicled: Hansel and Gretel, Theseus and Hippolytus, Absolom and David, Medea's treatment of her brother and her children. These sometimes terrible tales of complex loyalties, mistaken identities, and the revenge of those crazed by love or power are echoed in our contemporary culture.

In spite of all the technology we count on to separate our construction of family life from that of the bronze or the middle ages, we are everlastingly like our forebears. In our vanities and in our travails, we are nothing new under the sun. Rachel's desire for children is not unlike the yearning that prompts infertile couples to use various methods of high-tech babymaking, the contemporary substitute for Leah's mandrakes, or Bilhah's surrogacy. We can hardly attribute the modern baby hunger to a society that values women only as mothers; children are now a financial liability rather than an asset: "consumption goods."[81] But Rachel's longing for children may be the simple human impulse to love and be loved, to leave the world a child of her own flesh, lest she die and leave no living trace.

Rachel's death in giving life to her child is a literal parallel to some current accounts of motherhood in which mothers' lives are said to be sacrificed in caring for their children. A woman's struggle to accept the child growing within her seems a modern variation of Rebekah's puzzlement over the twins she carried: "If this is how it is with me, what does it mean?"[82] Rebekah carried two nations within her; her unproductive womb became fruitful through Isaac's faithful entreaties. Today nations confer in solemn assemblies: people are becoming as numerous as grains of sand upon the seashore; is there no way to shut up the wombs? Reproductive research, Janus-faced, works toward making the poor and fecund sterile, the rich and barren fertile. The contemporary practice of aborting children rather than giving birth in economic or emotional duress may be the modern equivalent of an offering to Molech: giving up the life of the child in order to achieve some other "good" end. Sacrificing children to idols is barbaric foolishness in our sight. Yet unborn children are sacrificed daily in women's efforts to maintain employment, to smooth social relations and to prevent maternal distress.

Some women today see themselves in the stories of the past as they grapple with images of themselves, their mothers, and their own children. Jungian analyst Naomi Ruth Lowinsky works toward an image of mothers that acknowledges the negative as well as the positive aspects of maternal experience, incorporating the "personal, the cultural, and the archetypal" in ways that will not leave mothers blamed. She believes that "mothers get saddled with cultural baggage or with archetypal expectations. Because the gods are dead, mothers are expected to stand in for them, taking the blame for much that more truly belongs to fate."[83]

More precisely, since psychology has for this generation largely replaced religion, guilt is removed through therapy rather than through repentance. Embarking on what Lowinsky terms a "heresy" against both "Judeo-Christian religious tradition" and "twentieth-century psychological thought," she sets out to "conceive the human story from within the mammalian experience of mothers."[84] She seeks to validate "what has been forbidden and repressed . . . the bloody side of women's nature, the fierceness."[85] She appeals to the goddesses and to women we know only dimly—Demeter,[86] Lilith, Asherah, the Black Madonna, the Shekina, Kali, and the Celtic goddess Sheela-na-gig.[87] She invites women to recognize the "red, fiery, passionate, bloody aspects of our nature, and the black, death-dealing, underworld aspects of women [which] have been demonized," by patriarchal religions.[88]

According to Lowinsky, "Every woman has a Kali side; every mother has a secret devourer, a baby killer in her soul."[89] Tracing ourselves through our mothers and our daughters, Lowinsky notes that knowledge of the goddesses allows women to bear knowledge of life, "to know that though we have our human responsibility, we are not in charge of destiny."[90] Kali, she says, "tells us that we are flesh and blood; that we give life and take life, nurture and destroy, suckle and poison; that these are in the very nature of existence, not the terrible fault of women."[91] Lowinsky concludes that

> At a psychological level the abortion issue is about our capacity to confront Kali consciously. Those who would deny women the right to choose abortion seek to control Kali by forcing women to bear children. Kali will then take other forms: ruined lives, neglected and abused children, women maimed or killed in illegal, back-alley abortions. However, those who support a woman's right to choose abortion also need to face the truth that [Sue] Nathanson's book [*Soul Crisis*] addresses. Abortion is not merely a medical procedure. It is the tearing from the womb of our own flesh and blood. It is a sacrifice of life, hopefully for life.[92]

In an age that condemns the will to power as a male defect leading to societal suicide, this odd but not uncommon appeal to respect the goddess-like power to give life or destroy it seems an attempt both to acknowledge responsibility for death by abortion and yet to evade condemnation. Lowinsky and Nathanson believe that severe "damage . . . is done to women in our culture by our refusal to honor the terrible aspect of the Great Mother."[93]

On the whole, we do not honor the power to kill; rather, we seek to prevent killing on the theory that unrestrained killing is uncivilized and bad for everyone in general. The plea that we esteem the destroyer is itself a whimper of inconsistencies, as may be seen in Nathanson's narrative of her own soul-searing abortion: "what a different world it would be if we could each become aware of and take responsibility for our capacity to annihilate others! In such a world we would be less likely to judge women for making the impossible choice between the life of an unborn child, her own life, and that of other family members."[94]

What? Is the powerful goddess herself vulnerable? Are we to pity her as she kills her own? The annihilator loves those whom she destroys, and exults in her unhappy deed:

> I wish now that my fourth child could have been sacrificed with my love and tears, even with my own hands, in the circle of a family or a community of women, in the circle of a compassionate and loving community of men and women who might be able to perceive my vulnerability as a mirror of their own, and not as it was, in a cold and lonely hospital room with instruments of steel.[95]

Is sacrificing our own children with our own hands gentler, more loving, than turning the deed over to a doctor, or infant sacrifice to Molech? We offer our most vulnerable in propitiation of our own weakness.

KNOWLEDGE OF THE UNBORN

Both science and experience support the view of the unborn as individuals fundamentally like us. Many women have some personal knowledge of their unborn children. Unsurprisingly, many women who abort, and some who contracept beyond their fertile years, carry the image of their unborn children with them. Most grieve for their loss, even as they defend their right to reproductive freedom. It doesn't take a prophet to anticipate that over time the grief and anger of a million desolate voices will be heard, like Rachel weeping for her children, refusing to be comforted over children who are not.[96]

Using technology to atone for human failing is a losing proposition and one we lose repeatedly. Such loss is illustrated in Peter Dickinson's *Eva*, the story of a comatose girl whose soul, "to save her life . . . has been put into the body of a chimp. Of course, Dickinson does not use that word; he talks about reprogramming her neuron memory into the body of Kelly the chimp."[97] She is an allegorical figure; like Eve, she becomes the mother of all living.

"Morality is the study of consequences," and Dickinson "is working through the ecological/environmental/social questions of man, the most endangered species," Thomas Kent Hinckley states in his review of the book. The consequences of this technology which sacrifices both chimp and "human" life to save human life has destructive effects that few anticipate. Like parents faced with pregnancy and abortion, Eva's mother is shaken; her father adjusts quickly to the technological possibilities.[98] Scientific manipulation of people is dehumanizing and demoralizing; the technology that placed her into the chimp's body ultimately separates her from her human mother.

The demoralization of the human race is represented by the attempts to "integrate" other humans with chimps but "rejection of transfer" occurs "very close to the unconscious, the boundary where the human mind has to mesh with the autonomous systems of the animal host."[99] "There had been the girl called Sasha and a chimp called Angel"; the team of scientists had let them "wake with their whole mouth working, and they had screamed all the time they were awake. They had done this for nine days, and then they had died."[100] The scientific breakthroughs that were to sustain life could not provide within the race the desire to live. While Eva teaches her chimp colony how to survive in what is left of the wild, groups of people give up on life. At one "community meeting . . . they passed a resolution to stop eating. Kept it too. Starved themselves to death. Nobody stopped them."[101]

Some humans, like Eva's mother, "adopt" children, or parents; but the natural biological ties within families are severed unnaturally. While the human race commits suicide, Eva gives life to her children. This grim tale of human failure demonstrates that human problems cannot be solved by technology.

While we can imagine scientific scenarios sufficient to give us pause, much of the technology we use daily is familiar and friendly. The temptation to try new machinery and new scientific techniques to cure old failings is always with us. Feminist faith in abortion technology as a means to social equality is not entirely unexpected, even in a society that frequently distrusts technology. We think every time that we have learned our lesson; then the watchdog committee churns out belated reports on scientific experimentation too lightly regulated. Reproductive medicine has targeted the female body for manipulation—for our own good, of course. Many women suffered from a too eager use of an either poorly understood or insufficiently tested Pill, from IUDs known by their makers to carry risks never communicated to the users, and from the too-often trivialized after-effects of abortion, including the link to breast cancer.

Despite this record, pro-choice feminists have welcomed the testing of RU-486, downplaying its potential dangers to women. Even if the formidable physical hazards are conquered, this new technique presents another problem. The women who abort chemically may expel the fetus any time over the course of several days. Such abortions may make it harder for women to avoid the image of the unborn child they will likely deliver whole, unlike suction abortions, frequently performed only after women are at least partially anesthetized, which pull the unborn into a mass of blood and less easily recognizable body parts.

Whether the unborn die chemically or surgically, their representation may persistently accompany the mother and father in whose image they were cast. One image of the child unborn yet living was captured by the Russian author Fedor Sologub (1863—1927), whose protagonist keeps the details of the abortion out of conscious memory but is periodically visited by a small child.

> She knew his face—it was her own child, even if he had not been born. She saw his face clearly—the dear and terrible combinations of her features with those of the one who had taken her love and discarded it. . . . It is as if someone cruel and dear opened up a deep wound with a tender, pink little finger—it is so painful! But it is impossible to banish him.[102]

In this somewhat surrealistic tale, the mother wonders whether this half-life that she gives the child in her memory will be enough for him, musing "My dear, poor unborn one!. . . . You live, but there is no you. . . . So alive, and dear, and bright—and there is no you."[103] She does not consider that the "small, unformed, wrinkled fetus which she had discarded, remained just that—an inanimate lump of matter, a dead substance to which the human spirit had not given animate form."[104] She worries instead that as he grows up he'll compare himself with a living child and "reproach his mother," though now he merely teases her, sometimes hiding from her embraces, then throwing his "warm tender little arms around her neck," and kissing her cheek.[105] As she hurries to comfort her sister, whose fifteen-year-old son has shot himself in despair at the terrors of the world, she reflects on the loss of her own son, and begins to cry. Then she hears the familiar, light step of her own child. He kisses her cheek and tells her "You're not guilty of anything. . . ." I don't want to live here. I thank you, dear mama. . . . It's true, believe me, dear mama, I don't want to live. . . . You aren't guilty of anything. But if you wish, I forgive you." Filled with joy, the woman reaches for her unborn son, who lays his hands on her shoulders and presses his lips to hers before he disappears.[106]

These no longer living unborn may return to thank their mothers for keeping them from life in a violent world, but it seems more likely that their mothers may live to rue their deaths. In Japan, many women who abort place in shrines small effigies of their aborted children, remembered and honored.[107] We have no similar cultural practice for capturing our regret after abortion. Some feminists and therapists are working on rituals that women can use to put the ghosts of their unborn to rest. Perhaps we then can rest; but so deeply ingrained in our culture are the beliefs that "Children are the keepers of the future" that "each generation has a sublime and transcendent duty to do everything it can to improve the potential for a better life in the next,"[108] that it may not be possible to turn our unborn dead into serene clay images through ritual absolution. Their image is too near our own, their living and their dying are in our hands. It is not impossible that the collective grief and fury of a generation of women bereft of their children will produce mothers who will not deny or be denied their children any longer. In a voice as weary as was Rachel they will speak: "Give me children," and they will turn their hearts and their lives to that task.

MOTHER LOVE

The shifting image from the passive to the heroic mother arising to save her children may already be with us in some of the books made to be read to children. Although their authors might puzzle at my interpretation of their words, it may be that we can read a better way for mothers and children in some books that have nothing explicitly to do with the image of the unborn or their mothers.

Maurice Sendak's *Where the Wild Things Are* was first published in 1963—the year Betty Friedan published her critique of motherhood, *The Feminine Mystique*, and the time the pressure for abortion law revision gathered prestige. Sendak's story, on one level, is the feminist theme of the invisible mother, whose demands apparently conflict with her needs. But also there is a reworking of the way the child enters the parents' world from the time of conception until the child more firmly asserts independence. Also illustrated are the tensions between maternal love, maternal weariness, and childish love learning from parental love.

The mischievous Max has been called by his mother "WILD THING!" and has responded with the frowning, wolf-suited threat (known to feminists and mothers alike): "I'LL EAT YOU UP!"[109] His reasonable and never pictured mother in control of his eating and his existence sends him "to bed without eating anything." But Max will not remain where his mother puts him: "That very night in Max's room a forest grew . . . and the walls became the world all around . . . and an ocean tumbled by with a private boat for Max and he sailed off through night and day and in and out of weeks and almost over a year to where the wild things are." Max's "ocean" and "private boat" are arresting parallels to the unborn surrounded by amniotic fluid in utero, where the developing child experiences at least something of day, night, and the wild, probably uninterpretable sounds of the mother's body and the world outside of her.

Max sails for more than nine months (a year) to "the place where the wild things are." The wild things, their "terrible roars" and the gnashing of "their terrible teeth," the rolling of their "terrible eyes" and the showing of their "terrible claws" contradict the Sendak drawings; if these be "terrible" creatures, then they are like humans at the "terrible twos." Their eyes and heads are large, their legs and arms small, in proportion to their bodies. They greet him with arms upraised like the toddler greets a parent, in their eyes a mixture of timidity and anticipation. With his own magic, his own wildness, Max tames them. Like his mother, he tells them "BE STILL!" As their king he orders the start of the "wild rumpus"; he leads it, and he orders it to stop. Like his mother, he sends the "wild things off to bed without their supper." Then in his kingly loneliness, wanting "to be where someone loved him best of all," he returns to his mother as she returns to him, signaling she loves him best of all by leaving his supper in his room. He doesn't see her, but when he smells "good things to eat," he begins his journey home.

The ominous entreaties of the wild things ring out as had Max's words to his mother, "Oh please don't go—we'll eat you up—we love you so!" Any mother who has ever felt her energy and her time eaten up by a child who loves her so can finish the rhyme of pleasure and dismay. And Max said, "No!" That his separation from his mother has been brief is seen in the simple consistency of the mother feeding the child; in this case, when Max returns to his supper in his very own room, he finds that the food is still hot. His unseen mother nurtures him even in his unruly demandingness.

In some ways, Sendak's book is a combination of discontents: the mother is unseen, Max is not quite lovable, and the wild things are a fierce and childish combination of the loving and dreadful. Our everyday familial duties and reluctances summon us, as did the wild things Max, to stare "into all their yellow eyes without blinking once." And we are none of us content until we do.

Audrey and Don Wood's picture-book expansion of the sixteenth century story "Heckedy Peg" is more a tale of our time.[110] This single mother braves the workplace, then battles with evil social forces for her children. Although she didn't know it when she left for the marketplace, she was trading her children for food, just as women who abort to improve their financial situation or in order to keep a job, may, in effect, be trading their children for money or food.

"Down the dusty roads and far away, a poor mother once lived with her seven children named Monday, Tuesday, Wednesday, Thursday, Friday, Saturday, and Sunday." Poor though this mother may be, she is strong, beautiful and wise. There is no father in this story, only children who "helped with all the chores" every day "before the mother went to market." Their cottage is full of light, and life shines in the children's faces when their mother is at home with them. Because they are "such good children" the mother tells them they "may ask for anything you want and I will bring it home from the market." Indeed, this is a woman of our day; she fulfills her children's needs, bringing home the bacon singlehandedly. The children, glorious in their simplicity, state their wants: a tub of butter; a pocket knife: a china pitcher; a pot of honey; a tin of salt; crackers; a bowl of egg pudding.

The mother—never named in this tale (surely her name is Deborah)— "kissed her children good-bye and said, 'now be careful, and remember—don't let a stranger in and don't touch fire.'" When the mother leaves, much of the light goes with her, and the children are left to their own smaller lights. Like all good latchkey children, they locked themselves in and "began to play."

Before long a "witch hobbled up the road pulling a heavy cart. She rapped at the window and called out:

I'm Heckedy Peg.
I've lost my leg.
Let me in.

Refreshing in its reflection of the folktale genre is the way in this story that the qualities of heart are seen in the image of the person: the good are beautiful and the evil are ugly. Heckedy Peg is ugly, misshapen; the sunlight that surrounds the home is weighed down by her darkness of heart. Huddling their light together, the children peer out the window at Heckedy Peg's murky visage.

They remember their mother's words: "Mother told us not to let a stranger in." "Come now, sweet chickens," Heckedy Peg replies, "All I need is a light for my pipe. Bring me a burning straw." The children do not forget. "We can't. Mother told us not to touch fire." The witch is wise to the ways of the children of mothers in the marketplace. She bargains; she offers gold if they'll let her in and light her pipe. "Gold!" they cried. "For a sack of gold we'll let you in and light your pipe." And they do. They are children of the marketplace. Each child hurries to do what the mother cautioned them against. Each grasps a fistful of burning straws, twirling and dancing toward the witch. Once her pipe is lighted, once the bond with their mother is broken, the children are no more their mother's; they belong to the witch—Kali making a house call. Like the offerings of food for the vengeful gods, the children become shadows sinking into a witch's feast, of bread, pie, milk, porridge, fish, cheese, and roast rib to be loaded into Heckedy Peg's cart and dragged from their mother's house and protection to the witch's domain deep in the woods.

When the mother returns, her basket brimming with good things for her children, she finds only "the witch's broken pipe, and burnt pieces of straw on the floor. Tears flow from her eyes. 'Who has taken my children?' she cries." Grabbing her basket, she follows a blackbird who has seen everything and leads her into the woods to the hut where the witch is about to take her first bite.

The mother pounds on the door of the hut, "Let me in!" she called, "I want my children back!" In dark celebration the witch refuses the mother until she believes the mother to be more crippled than the child devourer. This is a pro-choice baby killer, giving the mother an ultimatum: Pointing to the table laden with children shaped like food the witch gloats: "Here are your children. . . . If you can't guess them right the first time, I'll eat them for my supper."

Initially the mother is perplexed, then she acts with confidence: "I know my children by what they want," she says, matching the things in her basket with the food-children before her. Her knowledge of her children breaks the witch's spell, and "Quick as a wink, the children turned back into themselves." The mother takes her vengeance, "I've got my children back, Heckedy Peg. Now you'll be sorry you ever took them!" With that, the mother chases the witch out of the woods to a bridge; Heckedy Peg jumps from the bridge into the river "and was never seen again." The mother and her children, arms around one another, walk in sunlight to their home. This heroic mother felled the enemy of her children, the witch who saw them merely as meat. Even when they were not in their own comely forms, she saw them as they could and ought to be. Even in their non-sentient state, they were the children of her body, and she made them in her own/their own image again.

This mother sings a victory song. Her actions are not those of the ancient lament, in which the women seem to eat the fruit of the womb, and their children of a span long.[111] Women who find no wholeness in their lone subjectivity will yet be free of those shrewish impulses that would consume their "sweet chickens" kindly, taking their children's lives for their own sustenance. They may find to their own astonishment compassion for the child they carry whose single need they know in their own flesh, if in no other way. These mothers will not bring the unborn into the world because they have no sense of self, nor because they fear. They will rejoice in the birth of their children.

No one woman is a world in herself, although she may feel the world is made for the child that becomes hers. "On the eve of your birth," Debra Frasier tells each child, "word of your coming passed from animal to animal." From the Arctic to the Pacific, then to Europe "the marvelous news migrated worldwide."[112] "While you waited in darkness, tiny knees curled to chin," the earth, all creatures, the sun and moon were "each ready to greet you." When the child slips "out of the dark quiet/ where suddenly you could hear," she is welcomed by "a circle of people singing/ with voices familiar and clear." After they wash and wrap the small one they've waited for, they hold her close and whisper, "We are so glad you've come!"

Our children are wonderfully made in our own image, in the image of our betters. If our love for each other grows cold, if we have little natural affection for our own unborn, if we take pleasure in our power to destroy "the fullness that love began," we betray the sacrifices our parents made for us; we give to death those who might have brought us life more abundant than our lights can limn.

The images of mothers and children, still disputed, still taking shape, will take our configuration. We see, as it were, through a glass darkly. We do not have the power to see any being as he or she really is. We cannot see the unborn exactly as they are any more than we can see ourselves precisely as we are. We see glimpses of the unborn mixed with what we know of infants, toddlers, teenagers, young marrieds, the middle-aged, women and men full of years. We see them through our frailties, through our fears—just as we see the philosopher and her disquisition on desert and death. We feel the pull of obligation, an invitation to suffer with this being in the making—this child, this sister, this parent, friend. Which of us has the prescience to say "I will see you through your making?" We give what poor we can: one more day in this world so dependent on more than human grace.

NOTES

1. As quoted in *The New York Times*, 10 May 1988, cited by Francis J. Beckwith, *Politically Correct Death: Answering the Arguments for Abortion Rights* (Grand Rapids: Baker Book House, 1993), p. 176.

2. Brad Stetson, interview with William B. Allen, 5 October 1992.

3. Shannon Brownlee et al. "The Baby Chase," *U. S. News and World Report*, 5 December 1994, p. 86. Figure for 1988.

4. "Around 8.4 percent of all women between the ages of fifteen and forty-four (that's one out of twelve couples) are affected by infertility, but the numbers go up with age so that 20 percent of women and 36 percent of childless couples between thirty-five and forty-four have fertility problems. (That's one out of every six couples, up from one out of seven just since 1982.) And interviews with successful women of [the baby boomer] generation show that many postponed marriage and/or childbearing for their success until it was too late, until they...hit the brick wall of infertility." Anne Taylor Fleming, *Motherhood Deferred: A Woman's Journey* (New York: G. P. Putnam's Sons, 1994), p. 35.

5. Faye Ginsburg, *Contested Lives: The Abortion Debate in an American Community* (Berkeley: University of California Press, 1989). Ginsberg interviewed women in the pro-life and pro-choice movements, and analyzed their respective approaches.

6. This is the obligatory note acknowledging that there are many feminisms advocating a variety of goals and methods. Despite the claim that the movement is multifaceted, there is remarkable agreement among feminists liberal, radical, lesbian, eco-, and even post-, that legalized abortion is either necessary to women's equality or a positive good. Of all nonreligious national women's organizations, Feminists for Life of America is perhaps the sole feminist organization with a pro-life agenda— and that organization has been criticized as a front for patriarchy by other feminist organizations. See Rita J. Simon and Gloria Danziger, *Women's Movements in America: Their Successes, Disappointments, and Aspirations* (New York: Praeger Publishers, 1991), pp. 113–114. Diversity in feminism has its limits after all.

For an excellent refutation of the notion that abortion is central to equality for women, see Paige Comstock Cunningham and Clarke D. Forsythe, "Is Abortion the 'First Right' for Women?: Some Consequences of Legal Abortion," in J. Douglas Butler and David F. Walbert, eds., *Abortion, Medicine, and the Law*, 4th ed. revised (New York: Facts on File, 1992), pp. 100–158.

7. In interesting contrast to the self-congratulatory attitude we take to putting women in the workforce, E. F. Schumacher contends in Chapter 4 ("Buddhist Economics") of his book *In Small Is Beautiful: Economics as If People Mattered*, that to the Buddhist sensibility "the large-scale employment of women in offices or factories would be considered a sign of serious economic failure. In particular, to let mothers of young children work in factories while the children run wild would be as uneconomic

in the eyes of a Buddhist economist as the employment of a skilled worker as a soldier in the eyes of a modern economist." E. F. Schumacher, in *Small Is Beautiful: Economics as If People Mattered* (New York: Harper and Row, 1973, [the year Roe's economic view of motherhood was decided]), p. 57.

The social costs of releasing parents from the burden of rearing their own children are still being counted. Thomas Kent Hinckley, a volunteer counselor to emotionally and mentally ill patients states that "all of the children and youth that I see at the State Hospital come from *smashed* homes. Their problems are the result of family failure. The costs of this failure are about $70,000" per patient per year.

8. Diana Tietjens Meyers, *Kindred Matters: Rethinking the Philosophy of the Family* (Ithaca, N.Y.: Cornell University Press, 1993), p. 94. Of course feminists of the last century made that same point in their push for "voluntary motherhood," even though contraceptive technology was limited.

9. Ibid.

10. "You cannot devalue motherhood without devaluing everything else women do. You cannot declare the primary work of most women throughout most of history to be beneath serious consideration without sending women the covert message that it is really women who are beneath serious consideration. You cannot train a whole generation of women in contempt for their mothers without training them in contempt for themselves." Orania Papazoglou, "Despising Our Mothers, Despising Ourselves," *First Things*, no. 19 (January 1992): 19.

11. Deborah L. Rhode, "Reproductive Freedom," in Patricia Smith, ed., *Feminist Jurisprudence* (New York: Oxford University Press, 1993), p. 309.

12. Bonnie Steinbock, *Life Before Birth: The Moral and Legal Status of Embryos and Fetuses* (New York: Oxford University Press, 1992). She cites in Chapters 1 and 2 the philosophies and arguments of Jeremy Bentham, Peter Singer, Immanuel Kant, Thomas Nagel, Mary Anne Warren, H. Tristram Engelhardt, Jr., Joel Feinberg, Judith Jarvis Thomson, Michael Tooley, and others; see pp. 9–88.

13. See Joan C. Callahan and James W. Knight, "On Treating Prenatal Harm as Child Abuse," in Meyers et al., eds., *Kindred Matters*, pp. 143–170.

14. See the summary of the prejudice argument advanced by Germain Grisez, in Stephen D. Schwarz, *The Moral Question of Abortion* (Chicago: Loyola University Press, 1990), pp. 229–230.

15. Ibid., p. 70.

16. Ibid.

17. Steinbock, *Life Before Birth*, p. 71.

18. Ibid., p. 190, which contains part of the discussion of the morality of experimentation on living fetuses.

19. Ibid., p. 194. Steinbock continues: "It is thus not surprising that many people should be deeply distressed to learn of experiments involving the decapitation or immersion in salt solution of living second-trimester fetuses. In addition, performing such experiments is likely to take a toll on researchers, who may have to suppress their own protective responses to carry out the research. Given the social and evolutionary value of these responses, suppressing them seems a dangerous path. Such

considerations argue for a ban on research using living fetuses *ex utero*. However, symbolic concerns or a speculative risk of brutalization should not be allowed to ban research using nonviable and nonsentient fetuses, if such research is likely to have important scientific and medical benefits. While societal feeling of protectiveness toward fetuses should not be ignored, neither should they be emphasized at the expense of the interests of actual interested persons."

20. Donald H. Regan, "Rewriting Roe v. Wade," *Michigan Law Review* 77 (August 1979): 1569.

21. Judith Jarvis Thomson, "A Defense of Abortion," *Philosophy and Public Affairs* 1 (1971): 47–66.

22. Warren M. Hern, *Abortion Practice* (Philadelphia: J. B. Lippincott Co., 1990), p. 10.

23. Kimberly Sharron Dunn, "The Prize and the Price of Individual Agency: Another Perspective on Abortion and Liberal Government," *Duke Law Journal* (1990):81–117. Dunn discusses descriptions of the unborn on pp. 102–108.

24. Marielouise Janssen-Jurreit, *Sexism—The Male Monopoly of History and Thought* (New York: Farrar, Straus and Giroux, 1976), as quoted by Susanne V. Paczensky, "In a Semantic Fog: How to Confront the Accusation That Abortion Equals Killing," *Women's Studies International Forum*, 13 no. 3 (1990): 183.

This approach may accurately reflect the feelings of some women, but is not logically consistent for two reasons. Depending on which authorities one believes, effective contraception has been available for anywhere from thirty to four thousand years. This means that human beings have always had some (albeit limited) control over conception. Furthermore, an unwanted pregnancy does not necessarily result in ego damage to the mother.

For a refutation of pregnancy as self-alienation, see Camille S. Williams, "Thoughts of a Pro-Life Feminist," *World & I* 6 (October 1991): 569–585.

25. Rhode, "Reproductive Freedom," pp. 311–312.

26. Ibid., p. 312.

27. *Planned Parenthood v. Casey*, 112 S.Ct. 2791, 2807 (1992).

28. Ibid., p. 2809.

29. Susan Edmiston, "Here Come the Pregnancy Police," *Glamour*,[who else?] August 1990, p. 203.

30. Paczensky, "In a Semantic Fog," pp. 180–181. E. Ann Kaplan identifies "four groups of fetal images," all of which, she claims, present "the fetus as already human, white, and a subject...The images depict the fetus as a small human with all the outward signs that mark it as such: eyes, nose, hands, fingers, legs, feet, toes. Often, the fetus has a little smile on its lips, and a peaceful, babylike look. In addition...the `baby'[is imaged] as white and sexless, but somehow implicitly `male.'" Representations of zygotes or embryos in pictures larger than life "become moral determiners, misleading readers/viewers about the *actual* status of the zygote, and negating race/gender specificities." See E. Ann Kaplan, "Look Who's Talking, Indeed: Fetal Images in Recent North American Visual Culture," in Evelyn Nakano Glenn, Grace

Chang, and Linda Rennie Forcey, eds., *Mothering: Ideology, Experience, and Agency* (New York: Routledge, 1994), p. 125.

31. Kaplan, "Look Who's Talking, Indeed," pp. 126–127; see also discussion on pp. 124–135.

32. William P. Smotherman and Scott R. Robinson, "Dimensions of Fetal Investigation," in idem, eds., *Behavior of the Fetus* (Caldwell, N.J.: Telford Press, 1988), p. 19. These technological views of the unborn child have led some to believe that adult "fears and psychological disorders can be treated by recognizing or recreating the prenatal traumas that produced them," a pseudoscientific variation of old wives tales in which whatever traumatic events the pregnant woman witnessed would mark her child.

33. Robert H. Blank, *Fetal Protection in the Workplace: Women's Rights, Business Interests, and the Unborn* (New York: Columbia University Press, 1993), pp. 1–2.

34. Steinbock, *Life Before Birth*, p. 70, uses this term of embryos and preconscious fetuses.

35. Blank, *Fetal Protection in the Workplace*, pp. 8–9.

36. "Panel Backs Federal Funding of Human Embryo Research," *Deseret News*, 2 December 1994, pp. A1, A4. Both public opinion polls and abortion narratives illustrate the widespread belief that the unborn are alive and deserving of protection.

37. Kaplan, "Look Who's Talking, Indeed," p. 123.

38. Ibid., p. 134.

39. Ibid.

40. Ibid. Needless to say, this state of affairs is attributable to male fears and fantasies in a capitalist economy, and could have been related to the need to dispose of the property of the dead in an orderly and nonviolent manner.

41. *Planned Parenthood v. Casey*, 112 S.Ct. 2791, 2807 (1992).

42. Ibid., p. 2807.

43. Kaplan, "Look Who's Talking, Indeed," p. 129. Her remark is made in reference to dolls which either allow a child to pretend to be pregnant, or "Mommy-to-Be" dolls "whose pregnant body can be dismantled to produce the `baby' from inside." Taking our cue from the animal-rights movement, I suppose illustrators of the unborn might venture a small disclaimer, similar to that assuring us that no harm was suffered by animals used in films. It goes something like this: Any fetus depicted was conceived only after informed consent of the mother, and in no way resembles any fetus, living or dead, who was unwanted by his or her mother.

44. If we grant the premise that women have been the most oppressed class, how do we avoid charging them with participating in their own oppression? Why didn't women rise up against men or against offspring? As Stefinee Pinnegar expresses it: "*My* grandmothers weren't stupid." Even with few resources, truly oppressed women could have killed themselves rather than submit (and some did); killed their oppressors (some did; even the passive might have used poison); or they could have destroyed their children at birth (some did). That so many women have done so much good mothering—in the process keeping themselves, their men and their children alive—suggests either that they may not have viewed themselves as oppressed, may

not have actually been oppressed (or no more oppressed than others they saw), or that despite their unhappy circumstances they behaved better than they might have done, returning good for evil.

45. Marcel Proust, in Gabriel Marcel, *Homo Viator* (New York: Harper and Row, 1963), p. 8, as quoted in Sarah Hinze, *Life Before Birth* (Springville, Utah: Cedar Fort Inc., 1993), p. 130.

46. As quoted by Hinze, *Life Before Birth*, p. 78.

47. William Wordsworth, "Ode on Intimations of Immortality," as quoted by Hinze, *Life Before Birth*, p. 9; Osage Traditions, at 108.

48. Sherri Devashrayee Wittwer, *Gone Too Soon: The Life and Loss of Infants and Unborn Children* (American Fork, Utah: Covenant Communications, Inc., 1994), p. 22.

49. Jeanie Russell Kasindorf, "A Call to Murder," *Redbook*, August 1993, p. 114.

50. Serrin M. Foster, "F[eminists] F[or] L[ife]-Ohio Sponsors Controversial Art Show," *The American Feminist* 1 no. 2 (Fall 1994): 4.

51. Jana B., as interviewed by Hinze, *Life Before Birth*, pp. 5–11.

52. Name withheld by request, Hinze, *Life Before Birth*, pp. 138–140. See also the story of the unborn child who saved the life of an older sibling in the Skidmore family, pp. 13–23.

53. Janet M., Hinze, *Life Before Birth*, pp. 83–89.

54. Ibid., pp. 86–89. See also "A Cry in the Night," Debbie C., as told to Hinze, *Life Before Birth*, pp. 27–28.

55. JoAnn B., Hinze, *Life Before Birth*, pp. 93–97; Cheryl C., pp. 101–104; Jerry and Dorothy, pp. 107–108.

56. Fleming, *Motherhood Deferred: A Woman's Journey*, p. 15.

57. Ibid., pp. 24–25.

58. Ibid., pp. 18–19.

59. Ibid., p. 31.

60. Ibid., p. 245.

61. Ibid., p. 249.

62. Ibid., p. 255.

63. Ibid., p. 256.

64. Brownlee et al., "The Baby Chase," p. 84.

65. Fleming actually used that term, ironically, perhaps.

66. Anne Archer, as interviewed in Angela Bonavoglia, ed., *The Choices We Made: 25 Women and Men Speak Out About Abortion* (New York: Random House, 1992), p. 105.

67. Jill Clayburgh, as interviewed in Bonavoglia, ed., *The Choices We Made*, p. 56.

68. Conversation with Camille S. Williams, 16 December 1994.

69. Ibid.

70. Kathy Najimy, as interviewed in Bonavoglia, ed., *The Choices We Made*, p. 189.

71. Margot Kidder, as interviewed in Bonavoglia, ed., *The Choices We Made*, p. 99.

72. Ibid., pp. 98–99.

73. Like most modern poetry, much abortion poetry is written in the first person. Needless to say, the "I" of the verse is not necessarily the author of the poem.

74. Diane Wood Middlebrook and Diana Hume George, eds., *Selected Poems of Anne Sexton* (Boston: Houghton Mifflin Co., 1988), p. 56.

75. Gwendolyn Brooks, "The Mother," in Mary Kenny, *Abortion: The Whole Story* (London: Quartet Books Ltd., 1986), p. 258.

76. In Kenny, *Abortion*, p. 253.

77. Genesis 30:1, KJV.

78. See, for example, Simone de Beauvoir, *The Second Sex*, translated by H. M. Parshley (New York: Vantage Books, 1974). See Jeffner Allen's "Motherhood: The Annihilation of Women," in Joyce Trebilcot, ed., *Mothering: Essays in Feminist Theory* (Totowa, N.J.: Rowman and Allanheld, 1984), pp. 315–330, for a discussion of some feminist philosophers' attitudes toward mothering as socially constructed.

79. Reva Siegel, "Reasoning from the Body: A Historical Perspective on Abortion Regulation and Questions of Equal Protection," *Stanford Law Review* 44 (1992):261. For an alternative view see Camille S. Williams, "Abortion and Equality under the Law," in Gary C. Bryner and A. D. Sorenson, eds., *The Bill of Rights: A Bicentennial Assessment* (Provo, Utah: Brigham Young University Press, 1994), pp. 125–162.

80. Isaiah 49:15.

81. Rolf George, "On the External Benefits of Children," in Meyers et al., eds., *Kindred Matters*, p. 209.

82. Genesis 25:22, *New English Bible* (New York: Oxford University Press, 1970).

83. Naomi Ruth Lowinsky, *Stories from the Motherline: Reclaiming the Mother-Daughter Bond, Finding Our Feminine Souls* (Los Angeles: Jeremy P. Tarcher, 1992), p. xiv.

84. Ibid., p. 18.

85. Ibid., p. 186.

86. Ibid., pp. 6–13.

87. Ibid., pp. 179–207, *passim*.

88. Ibid., p. 188.

89. Ibid., p. 195.

90. Ibid., p. 206.

91. Ibid., p. 207.

92. Ibid., p. 197.

93. Ibid., p. 196.

94. Sue Nathanson, *Soul Crisis* (New York: New American Library, 1989), pp. 217–218, as quoted by Lowinsky, *Stories from the Motherline*, p. 196.

95. Ibid.

96. Jeremiah 31:15; Matthew 2:18. This theme is developed in James T. Burtchaell, *Rachel Weeping: The Case Against Abortion* (New York: Harper and Row, 1982).

97. Thomas K. Hinckley, *Brigham Young University Children's Book Review*, X:

1 (September/October 1989), p. 9.

98. Shades of Mrs. and Dr. B. F. Skinner?

99. Peter Dickinson, *Eva* (New York: Delacorte Press, 1989), p. 134.

100. Ibid., p. 136.

101. Ibid., p. 214.

102. Fedor Sologub, *The Kiss of the Unborn and Other Stories* translated and with an introduction by Murl G. Barker (Knoxville: University of Tennessee Press, 1977), p. 195.

103. Ibid., p. 196.

104. Ibid.

105. Ibid.

106. Ibid., pp. 200–201.

107. William R. La Fleur, *Liquid Life: Abortion and Buddhism in Japan* (Princeton, N. J.: Princeton University Press, 1992).

108. Peter W. Nathanielsz, *Life Before Birth and a Time to Be Born* (Ithaca, N. Y.: Promethean Press, 1992), p. 214.

109. Maurice Sendak, *Where the Wild Things Are* (New York: Harper and Row, First Harper Trophy Edition, 1984), unpaginated (at what would be p. 5).

110. Audrey Wood, *Heckedy Peg*, illustrated by Don Wood (San Diego: Harcourt Brace Jovanovich, 1987), unpaginated.

111. Lamentations 2:20.

112. Debra Frasier, *On the Day You Were Born* (San Diego: Harcourt Brace Jovanovich, 1991), unpaginated.

Chapter 6

Sex and Consequences:
An Anthropological View

Olivia Vlahos

Abortion, infanticide, and neglect, unless confined within safe limits, threaten the entire community.

—George Peter Murdock[1]

Culture emphasizes rather than overrides natural tendencies. It remakes the family into the same pattern we find in nature. Culture does not run riot.

—Bronislaw Malinowsky[2]

In 1984, rising abortion rates were beginning to prompt discussions in the popular media. A January 28 editorial in *The New York Times* attributed unintended pregnancies to contraceptive failure, ignorance, or innocence. Margaret Amer, a teenager from Cleveland Heights, Ohio, wrote to disagree. Her letter to the editor said,

> I am 16, and I know several girls my age who have had abortions or had planned to have abortions when the possibility of pregnancy arose. They knew what was happening to them, and what the results might be. They have had sex education classes in school but rarely bother with contraceptives. It seems that what they do not understand is the seriousness of sex and the creation of new life.[3]

She didn't know, she added, what would be the proper solution. Outlawing abortion would only complicate matters. The real problem, she thought, was society's attitude toward sex: altogether too casual in view of the serious consequences.

"Out of the mouths of babes," I said as I clipped her letter. "Trust a child to see the real reasons for a dilemma." If other *Times* readers had similar reactions, none of them wrote to say so. Doubtless Margaret's letter was dismissed as the odd maunderings of a repressed teenaged puritan bent on taking all the joy out of life.

Sex as joy. Sex as health, mental or otherwise. Ten years ago these were images dear to educated elites and were purveyed by the media, in popular entertainment, even in scholarly treatises. The freedom to express one's sexuality had by then become a *de facto* addition to the Bill of Rights. The only problems then admitted were quirks and hangups, curable with counseling—privately or on television—and various diseases, preventable with the magic condom. The wonders of modern medicine had already dealt with the procreative side effects—with unwanted pregnancies which could now be reliably forestalled or aborted as one chose. What consequences of sex remained to be taken seriously? Enjoy!

Sophisticated readers of *The New York Times* might then have been surprised to discover that Margaret's views of sex as serious business with serious consequences were shared, not merely by religious fundamentalists, but by practitioners of the biological sciences who look at life on earth from an evolutionary perspective. Procreation, they warrant, is Nature's First and greatest Law. Species unable to fulfill the law, species which ignore the law or flout it, will soon find themselves on the road to extinction. Nor is the human species above the Law. Whatever the unique human capacity to create culture, patterns of culture themselves depend on procreation. Without sufficient numbers to sustain tradition, a people inevitably lose vitality and their way of life. They do not survive.

The phrase "survival of the fittest" used to be associated with evolutionary theory, conjuring up vivid images of mortal combat in which superior strength and cunning gave some beings an edge over their rivals. Evolutionists have learned long since that the fittest beings are not necessarily the best fighters but rather the best breeders. And, more than that, they are breeders best equipped to produce offspring with a high likelihood of being good breeders themselves.

SERIOUS SEX: STRATEGIES OF REPRODUCTION

To understand why sex is truly serious business it is necessary to consider briefly the lengths to which adaptation can take a life form—all in the interests of perpetuation. Over the long haul, natural selection has sometimes favored species geared to mass production, and sometimes those specialized for limited births of slowly maturing young, dependent on intensive parental care for a head start in life.

The presence of predators on the scene is a challenge requiring of vulnerable beings an appropriate reproductive response. Animals preyed on as adults are apt to produce lots of babies as quickly as possible before being eaten. Animals whose progeny are attractive to carnivores tend to produce later babies, fewer babies, and bigger ones, the better to thwart predators on the lookout for small fry. Researchers in Central America discovered that when fish such as guppies were moved to stream environments with predators quite different from those in the original home, they were capable of switching reproductive strategies in as little (to us) as eleven years, or, for them, some fifty generations.

Environmental or even social pressures can trigger a procreative response. The ability to calibrate the sex of offspring to a given setting is one such ploy. Consider the female red deer whose breeding success is related in large part to her size and dominance in the herd. The breeding success of a stag is proportional to his superior fighting ability, the better to seize, defend and inseminate a large harem. Thus are his genes transmitted. But his size and strength depend, in turn, on inheritance from a large, healthy, and dominant dam, and, as it turns out, high-ranking hinds produce more sons than daughters. Subordinate hinds have more daughters who will survive more readily than their less-well-provided brothers and do a better job at transmitting Mum's lower order genes.

Savannah baboon mothers employ the opposite strategy. High-ranking females produce more daughters than sons and tend to be neglectful mothers, knowing well that subordinates will take up the slack. The latter bear more sons than daughters and, since they can't give offspring anything but love, they provide lots of that, the better to sustain the youngster who must one day leave both Mum and his natal group to establish himself in a foreign band.

SERIOUS SEX: THE HUMAN STRATEGY

So implacable is the need to procreate successfully that it accounts in large part for the profusion of forms and behaviors on view in Nature. Each represents the reproductive advantage its peculiar characteristics have conferred. The human form itself—upright, bipedal, long-legged, short armed, and eventually big-brained—may owe as much to the initial reproductive advantage conferred on individuals able to carry things for great distances as to the greater success in making tools or escaping predators upright posture made possible.

Carrying what? one must ask. Carrying where? And for whom? Why, food, of course. Back to home base with meat from a kill or a scavenging raid. Back to feed a waiting female and her offspring. So provisioned and sustained, a near-human female could reproduce at shorter intervals than could her counterpart among the apes, who, having to fend alone for self and baby, could afford to give birth only at five-year intervals.

And the near-human female? What would she need to carry? Why, her infants, born increasingly more helpless (thanks to obstetrical difficulties attendant on increasingly erect posture) and helpless for longer than the offspring of apes. Even if one supposes the little creatures had, like their primate cousins, the muscular equipment permitting them to cling to Mum's hair or ride astride her bent back, one must then ask, *what* hair? *what* bent back? Near-human Mum was straightening up, walking on her two hind feet and acquiring the evaporative cooling system that goes along with bipedal locomotion. Since sweat glands do not work well under wraps, we may assume a loss of body hair. Mum *carried* junior perforce, in her arms or in a sling made by her now freed and increasingly clever hands. Burdened by a child in hand, another by her side, and still another in utero, Mrs. Hominid could gather plant foods close to home, but her brood ate better when Mr. H. brought home the bacon, carried in his freed hands. And her babies thrived with the care and tutelage of a male protector always on the scene.

He had potent inducements to remain. Along with upright posture, both Mr.and Mrs. H. acquired unusual distributions of body hair, the prominent display of secondary sexual characteristics which rendered each continuously attractive to the other. What is more, since Mrs. H. had lost those perineal swellings which periodically announce ovulation in the female ape and consequent readiness for action, she was continuously receptive to Mr. H.'s sexual attentions. (Generosity in this department was necessary to ensure successful transmission of his genes). And the result: the bonded pair, a duo anticipated among the higher primates only by gibbons and siamangs.

The bonded pair represents the human strategy for successful reproduction. We read it not only in surviving bones but also in comparison with apes closely related to ourselves in biochemistry and mental capacity. We read it as well in the reproductive behaviors of people everywhere. ("Culture," said Bronislaw Malinowsky, "emphasizes rather than overrides natural tendencies.") The bonded pair: for the most part sexually exclusive and mutually supportive; dividing labor, sharing food, caring jointly for offspring. It was a pattern that placed a premium on learning and social skills, acquisitions that gave humankind eventual primacy over primates and all other beings on earth.

The role of pair-bonding in human evolution has been championed by anthropologist C. Owen Lovejoy. He notes that, apart from freed hands, erect posture and bipedal gait offer no great benefits, and certainly not in locomotion. Getting around on four feet, he says, is far more efficient, not to mention safer, than on two. And yet, balanced on two legs, humankind has flourished. Why? Because, says Lovejoy, "when a trait proves to have so powerful a selective advantage, it almost always has some direct bearing on the rate of reproduction."[4]

SERIOUS SEX: THE POWER OF TWO

Locating the bonded pair at the beginning of human evolution helps to explain some attitudes and beliefs common across cultures. Whether innocent of modern biology or conversant with it, people nearly everywhere think of the developing embryo as equally representative of mother and father. Her blood, his blood: together they form the child. Her blood, his spirit. Or her blood, his semen, which must be liberally supplied up to some stipulated point in the pregnancy so as to complete the child's growth and to ensure an ample supply of mother's milk. The Sambia of New Guinea are very clear on this point.

The expectant American father whose sympathetic labor pains or morning sickness are mocked by his friends might take comfort in the universality of such complaints. Indeed, in some quarters they are institutionalized. Anthropologist Ian Hogbin, who has studied the Wogeo[5] (inhabitants of the Schouten Islands off New Guinea), says several of his expectant friends, all healthy and sturdy sorts, regularly vomited after meals. What is more, they complained of being tired and "heavy," of losing their hunting skills. Just as well, perhaps, since they were supposed to avoid strenuous activities for fear of harming their babies. During his wife's labor, the Wogeo husband was responsible for performing rituals to secure a safe birth, and he permitted no knots to be tied in the house lest these block baby's entrance into the world.

Food taboos during pregnancy are very common, often for Dad as well as Mum. The expectant Wogeo Dad, for example, must not eat shark meat; baby's mouth might then be over-large. Among the Semai of Malaysia, the woman lax about food taboos will be chided by her husband, "You don't love the baby!"[6] (American fathers make the same comment to pregnant wives who sneak a beer or a cigarette against doctor's orders.) Rather than scold his negligent wife, a father among the Borneo Dusun simply assumes the avoidance chores on her behalf, turning his head away when offered choice bits of this and that and murmuring, "I cannot for the baby."[7] He will even produce the odd food cravings and food aversions expected of pregnant women if his own wife experiences none of these.

Nowhere is the procreative partnership of man and wife revealed more clearly than during the birth process itself. And nowhere is the ritual participation of fathers more complex and profound than among people who follow a hunting and gathering way of life. Our stereotype pictures birth among the primitives as being a minor matter. The parturient female simply drops out of the line of march, has her baby, and hastens to catch up. Consider instead the rituals associated with birth among the Washo, a foraging people who once lived in America's Great Basin region, rather near what is today Lake Tahoe. In the old days (we are told by anthropologist James F. Downs),[8] after a woman gave birth, she was laid in a bed of warmed sand, there to remain until her body had healed. Her husband, meanwhile, rushed to bathe in the nearest stream, leaving on its banks a deer skin or some other gift to be taken by anyone who came along. While Mum rested, he was required to be hyperactive, hunting every day, hauling wood for the fire. By so doing, he could ensure that his child would be industrious in life. He must not gamble or smoke. He must avoid meat, salt and fat. He must stay awake at night. All this to give his child an added measure of virtue, fortitude, and endurance. When baby's umbilical cord fell off, Dad hunted frenziedly so there would be plenty of meat to distribute among relatives and friends. He further stimulated the flowering of generosity in his child by inviting everyone to take whatever of his possessions they wished, up to and including everything he had.

Fathers in other cultures have attempted to protect their newborns by doing absolutely nothing. There is a name for such behavior. It is called *couvade*, and countless anthropology students have dined out on stories of drudging women, newly risen from childbed, replaced there by their lazy mates, groaning with simulated labor pains. They did so, at least, until such stories elicited more gasps of feminist outrage than amused chuckles. What is not so easy to explain or understand in this profoundly alien behavior is the underlying motivation: to take part equally in a burdensome and painfully experience which would seem to feature Mum alone.

So ingrained in the human psyche is the image of partnership in procreation and the nurturing of children that it appears even in the beliefs of people wholly ignorant of biological paternity. Among Australian aborigines of the Outback, there is no concept of fatherhood. There is only the husband of the pregnant woman. She is thought to be independently fertilized by the baby spirit, a lovely being who enters loins, her mouth, her fingernails, and is hers alone, just as the developing child is hers alone, her flesh, her blood. Even so, aboriginal belief holds that every child must have a male protector. Every female, therefore, is married or promised from cradle to grave lest the spirits suffer from myopia and choose an improbable vessel such as a child or a crone. It is to this protector that the baby spirit usually gives prior notification, appearing to him in a dream, often asking directions to the proper mother-to-be. Husband is thus enabled to be the first to announce the impending blessed event.

In the Trobriands Islands off New Guinea, babies were believed to be gifts of maternal ancestors selected from among spirits floating on tidal driftwood and debris, awaiting rebirth. It was the Trobriands husband's duty to help his pregnant wife "turn her mind away from men,"[9] for sexual thoughts would later be displayed when baby's skin turned out to be less shining and clear than it might otherwise be. It was the Trobriands husband's role to "receive the baby in his arms,"[10] to love it passionately, to feed and cuddle it, to clean up its messes, to boast of its beauty and achievements. If an acquaintance were so ill-mannered as to point out the resemblance between him and his sister's children who were, technically, of the same flesh as his own, he was enraged and insulted. For between himself and his nieces and nephews hostility prevailed. When the resemblance between himself and his wife's children was noted, however, he swelled with pride, believing that his care and devotion had created the similarities. Thus did the Trobrianders underscore the power of two in the maintenance of life, if not in its creation. Thus did they praise the essential nature of partnership.

THWARTING NATURE'S FIRST LAW: ABORTION

So powerful, so culturally pervasive is the image of partnership in procreation, so strongly felt the need for two in the nurturing of a child that the lack of a mate is, among most of the world's women, the prime motivation for abortion. It is as true here and now as it has ever been then and there. Here lies a major distinction which sets humankind apart from other beings. While a pregnant animal under severe stress may miscarry, she cannot consciously choose to terminate a pregnancy. But then, animals cannot feel shame at breaking a social taboo. The human mother, unwed and deserted, does. She feels shame because she bears the consequences of sex not taken seriously enough; shame because the social code dictated a socially recognized and responsible father for each child. Nowhere is the mother-child unit considered socially complete. Everywhere the child of such a union bears a social stigma and suffers social disabilities. In some societies, the remedy is immediately to marry the pregnant girl to her lover ("shotgun wedding" was the old American term for this) or to a substantial older man happy to add another branch to the family tree. Otherwise, the child born out of wedlock not only upsets the proper ordering of relationships and the obligations associated therewith, but usually represents as well an undue burden on the maternal family and community. Certainly this last figures prominently in the calculation of more complex societies. Peter Laslett and others have demonstrated in the book, *Bastardy*,[11] how public attitudes toward illegitimacy have always hardened with the perceived drain on the public purse. No wonder women who have loved not wisely but too well have preferred abortion to shame.

How common is the knowledge of abortion techniques across cultures? How widespread the practice? George Devereaux, who wrote in 1955 the definitive study, thought the knowledge was probably universal but conceded that there was no way of being certain, much less of quantifying the data. Ethnographic material for forty percent of the two hundred societies then fully described in the Human Relations Area Files at Yale University carried no information about abortion. For those remaining the data were often, in Devereaux's words, "skimpy and unreliable."[12] Anthropologists may not always have asked the pertinent questions. And if they did, women may not have chosen to tell secrets kept from their own menfolk. This probably owes to the fact that all cultures consider abortion discreditable to one degree or another, a violation of the natural order of things. The incidence of abortion seems to be pegged to social attitudes and social consequences. Attitudes range from mild disapproval to deep horror; punishments for the aborting woman from gossip to stigma to execution. Among American Indian tribes such as the Hopi and Arapaho, ghosts of aborted children were thought to haunt the aborting mother forever. For the Cherokee, Aztec, and Cheyenne, abortion constituted a capital crime. The Cheyenne held that the unborn had a legal personality and legal membership within the tribe, which must offer protection, or at least vengeance. In the religions of more complex people—Jews, Christians, and Muslims—abortion was also labeled a crime, as it was in ancient India.

In other societies, ambivalence prevailed. Some kinds of abortions were tolerated, others not. It was winked at if the unborn had been fathered by a demon, if it were a bastard or the consequence of incest. In some circumstances abortion might even be required. The hierarchical system of ancient Tahiti—or more properly, the Society Islands —placed entertainers in a separate caste. Though beloved by all elements of society, feted and honored as if royalty, entertainers were nevertheless required to marry among themselves and, unless promoted to the highest ranks of their profession, to terminate all pregnancies.

ABORTION ON DEMAND

The institutionalization of abortion often seems to accompany the institutionalization of gender hostility. Nowhere is the battle of the sexes pursued with more vigor than on the large island of New Guinea. Men and women, it is believed, have very different natures, forever at odds with one another. Women are thought to be by nature polluting to men. Yet, secretly, men envy women's power of fertility, and they strive to imitate and acquire it in many rituals forbidden to female eyes. Among the Gahuku-Gama of the central highlands, women are supposed to dislike bearing children, and so to do everything in their power to terminate pregnancy. Thus they deprive men of much wanted progeny. The men claim special magic to force conception and the birth of their children whether women desire it or not. They must be doing something right else the Gahuku-Gama would long since have become extinct.

Abortion is institutionalized today in the People's Republic of China, not because women hate men, but because the state fears the continued growth of a population already the greatest among the world's nations. Not content to let the forces of modernity and participation in a global economy prompt families voluntarily to limit offspring (a long-time trend in the West), the Chinese government has striven to lower the birthrate in advance of modernity. State reproductive policy has therefore decreed later marriages, few births and later births. The legal age for marriage was early on set at 26 for men and 25 for women. All pregnancies out of wedlock—whether or not the couple intended to marry —were automatically terminated. A waiting period of four years after marriage and the permission of a couple's commune or work group were necessary before a pregnancy could be planned. In other words, there were to be no babies unlicensed by the state. Although one child per couple was the ideal in urban settings, a second child was theoretically possible in the countryside. It was possible, at least, in 1980 when anthropologist Steven W. Mosher lived with the 8,000-member Sandhead Production Brigade in Guangdong Province. Of course, it all depended on the quota of births allocated by the central government to each commune and work unit. If quotas were in danger of being exceeded, cadres quickly stepped up the abortions for women bearing second offspring or for those without a license to bear. Women seven and eight months pregnant were aborted first. After all, the others might well miscarry all by themselves, leaving cadres without evidence of their zeal in implementing state directives. The process was described to Mosher as follows: "We begin by injecting Rivalor, an abortifacient, into the uterus to destroy the fetus and cause birth contractions to begin. The fetus usually expires within 24 hours, and is expelled on the second day. In the cases where expulsion does not follow within 40 hours, we have no choice but to perform a caesarean."[13]

Viewing the mute suffering of women mourning the deaths of their unborn babies or the equally mute fear of those awaiting the knife, Mosher thought of the very public American confrontations between pro-choice/pro-life advocates. None of that here. Severe punishment was the price of dissent, as it remains today.

What if a live child were removed from the womb? He was told that never happened. He did learn, however, of cases in which Rivalor was injected only after labor pains had begun. And, of course, couples who somehow managed to conceive a third child were told the child must be delivered in the commune clinic where, it should be understood, accidents might happen. In a 1983 article published in *The Wall Street Journal*,[14] Mosher wrote about officially sanctioned infanticide. After he left Guangdong Province he learned of one young mother who, in her first pregnancy, gave birth to twins. Told to choose which would be allowed to live, she could not. The choice was made for her.

Government policies of birth limitation (as yet unchanged according to Mosher's most recent publications) have given rise to private infanticide. Among rural Chinese, having a son means guaranteed security in one's old age; the birth of a daughter means hard work until death. A girl goes elsewhere in marriage, is part of her husband's family, and is responsible for his parents. It is sad, but not surprising, that in rural homes a bucket of water is placed beside the bed of a woman in labor. If the newborn turns out to be a girl, she is drowned like a kitten.

THWARTING NATURE'S FIRST LAW: INFANTICIDE AND NEGLECT

Infanticide is an act officially condemned by members of the Chinese central government and in the Chinese press, but condoned by local officials who play by the numbers and therefore find the line between abortion and infanticide a hard one to draw. It is so elsewhere. In many other cultures, the elimination of progeny is deemed murder only after the child has been suckled by its mother, or after it is named and acknowledged, or after it walks, or after some other turning point. Only then is it fully human. Americans who are horrified by infanticide can often accept and even champion the abortion of tissue that is, after all, only potentially a living being. When *is* the unborn a person? When *does* it have a soul? These are questions that fuel the pro-choice/pro-life debates. Uncertainties of cultural interpretation regarding personhood and its beginning incline many specialists to label as infanticide the killing of progeny, born or unborn.

The problem of labels does not arise when one is dealing with nonhuman reproduction. Animals do not abort, and, unless in situations of great stress, seldom do animal parents kill their offspring. Infants may be in danger from other relatives, however. The strongest baby bird often manages to deprive a weaker sibling of food and even push it from the nest. Infants may be endangered by males of their own species. The conquering male lion routinely kills all infants in a pride thereby bringing their mothers immediately into heat, ready to propagate *his* genes. The infant is, of course, always in danger from predators not of its own species.

Among human beings, it is most often the parents who kill. And why? For some but not all the reasons that would impel a woman to abort. A baby in hand may present problems that the baby still unborn may not. What problems? The baby born deformed or defective. The baby born in a time of famine. The baby born untimely before its predecessor can be weaned. Because the child is the wrong sex—as in modern China or in India where dowries must be provided for girl children; too many would beggar a family. Increasingly amniocentesis allows some mothers to abort defective fetuses or those of the wrong sex.

Infanticide is in some societies the fate of the baby perceived to be a supernatural threat. The Bariba in the People's Republic of Benin (a country formerly known as Dahomey) attribute illness and every sort of misfortune to witches who are, often unwittingly, sources of evil. The witch is not made but born with the marks of that evil condition plain to see. The premature baby, the baby born with teeth or whose teeth appear first in the upper gums, the baby whose emergence into the world is "not normal" should be given to a person authorized to dispose of it. Squeamish parents might prefer to hand the little witch over to the nomadic Fulani or to expose it in some lonely place. In recent years the Muslim Bariba have taken to depositing witch babies with local Christian missionaries. Allowed to remain alive at home, such a child will inevitably wreak havoc in its family. But, says anthropologist Carolyn Sargeant,[15] who lived among the Bariba on and off from 1976 to 1983, some witch babies, if born without a midwife's help, can be hidden by a mother and allowed to live. It is much harder to hide the eruption of baby teeth from Dad and other close relatives who are likely to insist that the child be exposed.

   Exposure was the method by which people of the Classical World rid themselves of excess children, deformed children, girl children, and children born to a family too poor to keep them. There were specific locations in Hellenic cities and in Rome where babies were left "to the kindness of strangers,"[16] childless strangers who would provide a home. Always, says John Boswell in his book on the subject, the hopeful expectation was that someone would rear the abandoned child to adulthood and that, indeed, the child would prosper. Many were the legends based on such a beginning—the story of Oedipus, for instance, or of Jason or of Romulus and Remus, foundlings and yet founders of Rome, suckled by a she-wolf. The same method of disposal continued into Christian times when infants were left on the doorsteps of monasteries or convents or dedicated to a life of service to the Church. Modern analogues of exposure range from the orphanage (now out of style) to adoption to foster care. Outcomes for the child are sometimes benign, sometimes a good deal less so.

Broadening the definition of infanticide to include abortion requires the further addition of neglect, passive or aggressive—the withholding of food or medical care (with or without design), periodic abandonment, or the administration of brutal beatings that bring about the death of a child. Susan Scrimshaw,[17] who has documented infanticide across cultures, notes that neglect as a means of eliminating children has superseded murder in many societies. Nevertheless, even in this society, outright child killings do occur. Statistics recently released by the Justice Department indicate that of all family murders (which constitute 16 percent of the homicide total), more than one-fifth involved parents killing their children. What may surprise readers caught up in feminist theology is the fact that infanticide by weapons or by neglect is more often committed by mothers than fathers. These findings are consonant with data from Canadian sources which reveal some similarities among infanticidal mothers. They are most often young and unmarried; they tend to kill offspring when they are infants, not later. Older children are more at risk when living in step-parental households—which category includes, one must suppose, the live-in boyfriend.

EXCEEDING THE LIMITS, SMALL TIME

Many years ago, George Peter Murdock, the great anthropologist who founded the Human Relations Area Files, wrote at length on the subject of social structure. The nuclear family, he held, is the basic, universal unit on which the whole interlocking web of society depends. And procreation is the essential family function. So essential that he asserted confidently,

> Even if the burdens of reproduction and child care outweigh the selfish gains to the parents, the society as a whole has so heavy a stake in the maintenance of its numbers, as a source of strength and security, that it will insist the parents fulfill these obligations. Abortion, infanticide, and neglect, unless confined within safe limits, threaten the entire community and arouse its members to apply severe social sanctions to the recalcitrant parents.[18]

One has to wonder, however, whether a people always realize when safe limits have been reached. Can they perceive how much rule breaking is too much rule breaking? And then there is the matter of the rules themselves. What if, with all the best will in the world, the rules do not serve to affirm and enhance life but rather to debase and reduce it? Unlike all other animals, human beings are capable of choosing rules that threaten their own survival. This is because, unlike all other animals, human beings are actuated by the meanings they create, and it is from these meanings that rules derive. A people's own views of ultimate reality may thus run quite counter to the First Law of Nature. Wedded to meaning, such a people may actually be unable to connect cause and effect, may be quite oblivious of what they do.

Case in point: the Tapirape, South American Indians with whom anthropologist Charles Wagley lived in the 1940s.[19] Hunter and manioc farmers, they lived in a secluded forest region in central Brazil. In 1909, when first reported by European observers, the tribe had included five villages, each with upwards of 200 people. By the time of Wagley's stay, the Tapirape had been reduced to one village of some 147 people. Of course, they had suffered from European intrusion and the epidemics newcomers had introduced. That was not in Wagley's view, however, the sole cause for depopulation. Some people, after all, are able to withstand the shock of new disease, new technology, and maintain not only their numbers but their culture intact.

Just such survivors were the Tenetehara, a people of northeast Brazil, similar in every way to the Tapirape and linguistically related to them. The Tenetehara had suffered as much from European-introduced disease and more from Europeans themselves. Where the two groups differed was in the matter of reproductive patterns. The Tenetehara practiced infanticide only when twins were born or when a woman was suspected of having consorted with demons. And although they knew of several abortifacients, they rarely used them because they so valued lots of children and large families. The Tapirape believed a woman should bear no more than three living children, and that these should not be of the same sex. So a third daughter born to a family with two already would have to be sacrificed. Ditto a third son. Fourth pregnancies were routinely terminated. In spite of diminishing numbers, the Tapirape refused to leave off their mode of family planning. In 1945 when Wagley's study was conducted, Tenetehara numbers were around two thousand, the same as when originally noted; the Tapirape were even then in severe decline.

They were not the only South American tribe already, in the 1940s, fading from view. When Claude Levi-Strauss, the famous French anthropologist, visited the Gran Chaco region, he found only remnants of tribes once dominant in the region, tribes whose ways lived on only in the tales of their descendants or in European ethnographies. Many of these tribes, like the Tapirape, had favored small families. Gone were the Mbaya, an aristocracy of warriors mounted on horses stolen from the Spanish conquerors. Of them Levi-Strauss wrote,

> The idea of procreation filled them with disgust. Abortion and infanticide were so common as to be almost normal—to the extent, in fact, that it was by adoption rather than by procreation, that the group ensured its continuance.

One of the main objects of the warriors' expeditions was to bring back children. At the beginning of the 19th century, it was estimated that not more than one in ten of the Mbaya-Guacuru group were Mbaya-Guacuru by birth.[20]

A similar depopulation was reported for the Micronesian island of Yap where, in the late 1940s, anthropologist David M. Schneider[21] lived and worked. There were at that time 2,500 people on an island which had once supported a population of 50,000. Men mourned that so few candidates for public and religious office were available, wondered sadly why more babies were not being born, but could offer no reason for the decline in numbers. Schneider, however, soon found an answer in the very patterns of the Yapese dating game.

Every pubescent girl was allowed to entertain as many lovers as she chose and in a house constructed by Dad for the purpose. There she could play the sexual butterfly—without commitment, without household chores (Mum took care of those), without a thought for tomorrow. Until a child was conceived. Then came marriage and drudgery. The Yapese knew several forms of contraception and disliked them all. But a woman could extend playtime almost indefinitely by way of self-induced abortion, and although this was severely sanctioned in Yap society, every girl knew the local abortifacients and could use them without fear of discovery during her monthly seclusion in the menstrual hut. Yapese women routinely delayed maturity and the reproductive urge until after the age of 30 when men began to find their charms resistible. For many that was too late. Cervical injuries, infections, age itself had rendered conception difficult. The barren woman, desperate for children, tried to adopt. There were no surplus babies to be had.

EXCEEDING THE LIMITS, BIG TIME

The decline and fall of complex societies, especially when literate, when populous and diverse, cannot so easily be attributed to a single cause. There is no doubt, however, that patterns of reproductive behavior have their own part to play, even in the shifting fortunes of great nations. And in such nations, not everyone will remain ignorant of the threat or the nature of its source. There will be prophets of decline.

By the second century B.C., writers and philosophers in the Roman world had begun to issue warnings about the sorry state of both mortality and births. Some worried more about the latter, for how could the legions be properly manned and led when the ranks of Roman citizens were on the wane? In the old days, Romans had considered procreation a prime duty, not only to the state but to the clan, the tribe, and above all to the family. Indeed, it has often been noted that Family constituted the real Roman religion. Never mind the great gods in their marble temples; it was the household deities that mattered most.

By the second century B. C. the old patterns were beginning to lose their authority. Roman conquests were pouring wealth into the capitol. Wealth and the leisure wealth made possible, together with the new ideas learned from conquered peoples, were changing Roman ways. And it was not only ideas that traveled, but people themselves. The population of the Italian peninsula did indeed grow from the beginning of the second century to the Augustan Age, but it was largely thanks to the influx of slaves and immigrants. These brought with them their gods and their languages, making Rome increasingly polyglot and factionalized (much like today's multicultural United States). What is more, the immigrants multiplied enthusiastically. Slaves did not. Neither did their Roman masters. Giddy with luxury, many Romans of the elite classes neglected their duties—martial, civic, or procreative—in pursuit of pleasure. Their womenfolk, having long since achieved *de facto* freedom from onerous legal and marital restrictions, joined in the fun. Nobody much wanted to be burdened with children and had few of them in consequence. Contraceptives were much in use. Any failures in this department were remedied by abortion, which became so common a procedure that women who did not resort to its use were congratulated.

Long before Julius Caesar came to power, Cicero had recommended to him the following policy: "Less lust, larger families!"[22] In 26 B. C. the Titus Livius we know as Livy began his *History of Early Rome* to celebrate the old family virtues and values that had made Rome strong and to mourn their passing. He said,

> I would then have [the reader] trace the process of our moral decline, to watch, first, the sinking of the foundations of morality as the old teaching was allowed to lapse, then the final collapse of the whole edifice, and the dark dawning of our modern day when we can neither endure our vices nor face the remedies needed to cure them. . . . Of late years wealth has made us greedy, and self-indulgence has brought us through every form of sensual excess, to be, if I may so put it, in love with death, both individual and collective.[23]

Caesar's nephew and heir, the Emperor Augustus, moved quickly to implement the pro-family measures his uncle had planned. Happy hedonists who resisted marriage or flouted its obligations were burdened with many civil penalties. The parents of multiple children were praised and rewarded. Augustus even strove to revive the old religious forms. Alas, nothing availed to effect a wholesale restoration of family values or to stem the population slide.

A century or so later, during the time of the Flavians, the historian Cornelius Tacitus found it necessary to echo Livy's sentiments. He contrasted Roman moral fiber with that of German tribes then resisting Roman legions at the frontiers of the empire. "No one in Germany laughs at vice, nor do they call it the fashion to corrupt and to be corrupted. To limit the number of their children or to destroy any of their subsequent offspring is accounted infamous, and good habits are here more effectual than good laws elsewhere."[24]

SOCIAL STIGMA AS SOCIAL CONTROL

Clearly the Romans did not take sex seriously. Not, at least, in its procreative aspects. Of course this was not true of *all* Romans, perhaps not even most Romans. That there were life-long marriages is demonstrated by tombstones bearing messages of devotion from a surviving spouse. These same inscriptions, nevertheless, include comments noting how few marriages *did* last without divorce. There were certainly conscientious parents who brought up their children in the good old ways. But we do not hear much about them. The tone of any period in history is set by the fashionable elite. It was the dissolute behavior of Rome's elite that so outraged Early Christian sensibilities and eventually trickled down to more workaday folk or to folk without work at all.

In time the ideals of family limitation reached the countryside with an accompanying decline in rural population. Births simply did not keep up with deaths, especially since many of those were of infants vulnerable to the diseases of childhood. Soon there were food shortages in a land which retained its fertility and suffered no change in climate. Shortages made the bearing of fewer children economically as well as fashionably correct. At the end of the second century A.D. the Emperor Septimius Severus outlawed abortion, but to no effect. By the third century A.D. decline had reached Roman Gaul and had proceeded apace, says historian Arthur Boak, until there were not sufficient personnel to fill critical occupations and maintain the economic and political structure of the Western Roman Empire. Unable to defend itself against disintegration from within and invasion from without, it staggered slowly to its inevitable end, which is pegged to A.D. 426.

"Once the birth rate of a people starts to decline," says Boak, "it continues to do so in a geometric and not an arithmetic ratio."[25] So profound was the population loss that accompanied Rome's demise that it would take a thousand years to restore the number of people in the West to what they had been during the Roman heyday, especially since the infertility of dissolute Rome was followed by the virtuous infertility of Early Christians among whom celibacy was all the rage.

For all its inevitability, the decline of Rome took as many years to accomplish as the entire life span of many nations. Even so, one cannot but wonder about causes and turning points. If all the literature of Rome had survived intact, would we be able to locate in it the truly crucial moment, with its array of contributing circumstances, at which the long slide began? Probably not. Changes in conditions and attitudes at that time spread so slowly from class to class, region to region, always leaving behind shoals of families still struggling to live by the old virtues, always recovering and reforming in fits and starts and falling back again.

We might have more luck with our own society, which has undergone profound changes of a similar nature. And these have taken place, not over hundreds of years but in only thirty. There is no telling whether the patterns now set in motion will prove to be temporary or lasting. In 1955 David Schneider offered the following observation in his case study describing abortion and depopulation on the island of Yap:

> Let us suppose that young Americans in their twenties emulated Yap and consistently preferred to engage in love affairs than to assume adult responsibilities. Quite apart from morality, such a shift would set in motion a series of other changes disrupting what we regard as our way of life.[26]

The advent of the Sexual Revolution in the 1960s would soon render his views prophetic.

EXCEEDING THE LIMITS, AMERICAN STYLE

Driven in large part by the vast numbers of the baby boom generation just then entering sexual maturity, patterns of reproductive behavior changed drastically, taking on an eerie similarity to the anything-goes amatory style of Roman gilded youth and the procreative ideals of the Communist Chinese: late marriage, late children, few children. And all accomplished not by compulsion but by the dictates of fashion. First came the prolongation of youth; sociologists began to peg the arrival of maturity to age 30 instead of 21. Serial cohabitation displaced marriage, and when marriage did occur, it was likely to be of short duration. Indeed, marriage became something of a passage rite for many women eager to try their feminist wings. "Alternative life-styles" gained considerable cachet, including those that featured sexual adventuring of all sorts, the heterosexual variety being underwritten by the newly invented "pill." To accommodate those unable or unwilling to contracept, abortion was not only legalized but de-stigmatized. The numbers of these procedures quickly rose from 586,800 in 1972 to 1, 680,000 in 1990.

Media images changed first to reflect and then to amplify the new realities. Language, behavior, costume once considered beyond the bounds of good taste became standard fare. Portrayals of the model married couple—committed to each other and to their generally well-behaved offspring, portrayals which had once both reflected and amplified family values of the 1950s—gave way to more up-to-date sexual combinations. Not everyone approved of change. Not everyone followed the dictates of fashion. There were enough converts, however, to alter quite quickly the nation's demographic profile and to produce some disturbing statistics.

First of all there were the plummeting birthrates. After the procreative high of the years from 1946 to 1964, children were suddenly nowhere in view. Schools were closed. Shops selling maternity wear went out of business. So did the manufacturers of baby food. The Total Fertility Rate went from 3.7 children per woman of childbearing years to 1.8, a rate at which a society declines in population. Ben Wattenberg has dubbed this period of low reproduction the "birth dearth."[27] That was not the only index of change. The rates of marriage fell; those of divorce rose. The rates of illegitimate births rose; those of legitimate births fell. The ages at which young people married rose; the age of sexual initiation fell. Doubtless many adults benefited from the repeal of convention. But behavior that may be good for some individuals may be, at the same time, bad for society as a whole and certainly bad for the society's children.

When sex is no longer taken seriously, it is always the children who are the first to suffer the consequences. Many of the unborn do not get born. Many of those who are born grow up in broken homes or in homes headed by unwed mothers able to offer children so little in the way of adequate nurture as to risk their chances in life up to and including life itself. The growing number of low-birthweight babies, babies born alcohol-or drug-addicted suggest nothing less than infanticide through negligence.

The long-term results of neglect and inadequate socialization show up in the numbers of children who rape and murder other children and in rising rates of juvenile crime in general. Already in 1965 Daniel Patrick Moynihan had predicted the consequences of illegitimacy and neglect.

> A community that allows a large number of young men to grow up in broken families dominated by women, never acquiring any stable relationship to male authority, never acquiring any set of rational expectations about the future— that community asks for and gets chaos. Crime, violence, unrest . . . that is not only to be expected; it is very near to inevitable.[28]

Neglect has never been a monopoly of the underclass. High rates of drug and alcohol abuse, early sexual initiation, early incidence of sexually transmitted disease, high incidence of abortion, high rates of suicide and accident among children of the educated elite say something about absentee parenting, the frequency of divorce, and the stress of life when both parents are running on the fast track.

Have we now exceeded the limits, the point at which abortion, infanticide and neglect are perceived to threaten the entire community? Will we now, as George Peter Murdock confidently predicted, impose sanctions? Have we reached the point when people will insist that the consequences of sex require that it be taken seriously again? Or will the fear of AIDS turn out to be a more profoundly motivating factor than the need to secure for offspring a more orderly future?

RESTORING LIMITS—TOO LITTLE, TOO LATE?

There are some hopeful signs on the horizon. Since 1987 the Total Fertility Rate has risen to 2.1 children per woman of childbearing age, thanks in large part to the crop of late babies produced by boomers in their thirties and forties. Thanks also to new immigrants with fertility rates higher than those of the locals. It is true, of course, that additional dips may lie ahead as the "busters"—the twenty-somethings whose generation is smaller in size than that of their predecessors—begin to reproduce.

In the last year or so, the general public has begun to express concern. Or rather, the media mavens have begun to take note of it. The "family values" issue has ceased to be the sole province of conservative political philosophy and has been adopted by politicians of other persuasions. We begin now to hear of efforts to reform welfare, long thought to provide perverse incentives for illegitimacy. We hear of grass-roots movements among religious adults and teenagers seeking to legitimize abstinence. These, it must be said, have garnered only lukewarm support from government agencies. We hear of organized efforts to curb the media's glorification of violence and free-wheeling sex. We hear of tentative meetings at which Pro-Life and Pro-Choice groups have sought to define common concerns.

One has to wonder whether these efforts may be too little, too late. Have we now reached and passed that crucial point after which no return is possible? It is, after all, a matter of numbers. How many people still abide by the old rules and taboos which were, however restrictive, successful in protecting the family context in which the future could safely dwell? Are the numbers of children born to intact families (now about two-thirds of the total) enough to ensure social stability? What if we approach a fifty-fifty split, as many specialists foresee? Is the divorce rate (now one in two) too high to guarantee that enough of those initially intact families will remain so while children are growing up? Is a 50 percent rate of virginity among girls under fifteen enough to contain the incidence of sexually transmitted diseases among adolescents, whose age group now holds the greatest potential for disease escalation? And this includes not only AIDS but also the pelvic inflammatory infections that will render many a girl barren before she ever marries. Already the hopes of stemming the AIDS epidemic through the discovery of cures and vaccines are fading. A high incidence of the disease is now predicted, especially among those whose behavior is "safer but still risky, such as individuals who have five or six partners over the course of a lifetime."[29]

The Alan Guttmacher Institute reports that the annual rate of abortion has fallen from 1.6 million to 1.53. Does that represent a change in the attitudes of women in the age group of 15 to 24 year olds who account for two-thirds of the abortions? Actually not, writes James A. Miller in a letter to *The Wall Street Journal*.[30] (He is director of research for the Population Research Institute.) It represents, rather, a diminished number of young women due to the "birth dearth" years from 1968 to 1977—in 1992 three million fewer than in 1980. There are fewer abortions today, he wrote, because there are fewer potential aborters aged 15 to 24. So many fewer that the decline in abortion rates should be steeper. It seems likely—as Margaret Amer suggested in 1984—some women and girls are still using abortion as the preferred method of birth control.

The likelihood is underscored by the disappointingly slow sales of contraceptives. Late in 1992, *The Wall Street Journal* was reporting that unit growth of condom packages had increased only 5 percent compared to the 40 percent to 50 percent annual gains manufacturers saw during the late 1980s. These figures bore out the findings of a telephone survey of ten thousand heterosexual Americans. "Although as many as one-third of respondents reported they had incurred some risk of exposure to AIDS," the *Journal* reporter noted, "few use condoms regularly."[31] Only 17 percent of respondents with multiple sexual partners used condoms, and some of these had high-risk partners.

Sales were still flat by July 1994, when the *Journal* published a similar story about female contraceptives.[32] Their sales were in decline. Manufacturers of the new female condom, which has difficulties in application and a 26 percent failure rate, were planning enthusiastic marketing efforts but were not themselves enthusiastic about results.

For all the weakly hopeful signs that old-fashioned middle-of-the-road Americans are attempting to restore family values, there is little evidence that society at large is ready to do what is necessary to set limits, ready (as Livy said of the Romans) to face the remedies needed to effect cure. For setting limits requires the application of stigma to behaviors that neither affirm life nor enhance it.

And that's the problem. In today's society, stigma is itself taboo. In today's society, tolerance, even affirmative permissiveness, is the dominant tenet of morality, and "choice" is its watchword. Only in matters of public health are we willing to apply stigma, and even then application is highly selective. We are very willing to stigmatize smoking and to limit a smoker's freedom of choice. Why? Because smoking can be deadly. (Never mind that those afflicted are mainly past the years of bearing and begetting children.) Because smoking burdens the health care system. Because smoking endangers nonsmoking innocents. Should *their* health be placed in jeopardy? The answer has been a resounding no. Smoking has been stigmatized. Successfully. The number of smokers has declined.

But what about other behavioral choices equally hazardous to health? What about promiscuous life-styles or those of drug addiction that make some populations repositories for disease? Should innocent sexual partners be put at risk? No comment. Should stigma be applied? Unthinkable.

We will, in fact, condemn no exercise of free choice in sexual behavior even when such choices result in the endangerment of children. Even when they drive up the costs of health care. Even when their side effects debase the quality of life. Clearly we are not ready to take seriously the consequences of irresponsible sex.

Except for members of the pro-life movement, we do not as a society condemn abortion although polls indicate considerable public discomfort about the
subject, particularly in view of the annual numbers. No wonder that, during his
campaign for the presidency, Bill Clinton was often moved to make this pro-
nouncement: "Abortion should be safe, legal and rare." He has never suggested
how rarity should be achieved or even how the rates could be marginally reduced.
He has never suggested limits of any sort and would certainly never countenance
the application of stigma.

But what does a rate of 1.53 million abortions annually say about a society,
particularly when that society possesses the most sophisticated contraceptive
technology and pharmacopeia on earth? Does such a rate bespeak carelessness on
a grand scale or callousness on a grand scale or both? What can be said of a society in which too many parents bring about their children's deaths simply by way
of their own feckless choices in life? What can be said of a society in which too
many children are neglected and no one held accountable? What can be said of a
society so riven by the competing claims and ideologies of feminism, multicul-
turalism, homosexualism, and environmentalism that common cultural ground
cannot even be acknowledged, much less common morality? What can be said of
a society with norms so uncertain and eroded that its vital center will not hold?
What can be said of a society in which nobody is quite sure what family is, let
alone what it is supposed to do? "Culture emphasizes rather than overrides natural tendencies," said Bronislaw Malinowsky. "Culture refuses to run riot."[33] Was
he too optimistic?

Well, we can't say we haven't been warned. From social scientists like Daniel Patrick Moynihan to sixteen year olds like Margaret Amer and by preachers,
pundits, and professors in between, we have been warned. In one way or another,
they have all spoken to a society which, in its willingness to let anything go,
has let everything go. They have spoken to a society which has ignored, forgotten, or flouted Nature's First Law. Some day or other, late or soon, the reckon-
ing must fall due.

Are we prepared to face the consequences of that?

NOTES

1. George Peter Murdock, *Social Structure* (New York: Free Press, 1965), p. 9.

2. Bronislaw Malinowsky, *Sex and Repression in Savage Society* (London: Routledge and Kegan Paul, Ltd., 1927), p. 217.

3. Margaret Amer, Letters to the Editor, *The New York Times*, 14 Feb. 1984.

4. C. Owen Lovejoy, "The Natural Detective," *Natural History Magazine*, (October
1984), p. 26.

5. Ian Hogbin, " New Guinea Childhood from Conception to the Eighth Year," in

L. L. Langness and John C. Weschler, eds., *Melanesia* (Scranton, Pa.: Chandler Publishing Co., 1971).

6. Robert Knox Dentan, *The Semai: A Nonviolent People of Malaya* (New York: Holt, Rinehart and Winston, 1979), p. 97.

7. Thomas Rhys Williams, *The Dusun: A North Borneo Society* (New York: Holt, Rinehart and Winston, 1965), p. 84.

8. James F. Downs, *The Two Worlds of the Washo* (New York: Holt, Rinehart and Winston, 1966).

9. Bronislaw Malinowsky, *The Sexual Life of Savages* (New York: Harcourt Brace and World, 1929), p. 201.

10. Ibid., p. 201.

11. Peter Laslett, Karla Oosterveen and Richard M. Smith, *Bastardy and Its Comparative History* (Cambridge, Mass.: Harvard University Press, 1980).

12. George Devereaux, *A Study of Abortion in Primitive Societies* (New York: Julian Press, 1955), p. 25.

13. Steven Mosher, *Broken Earth: the Rural Chinese* (New York: Free Press, 1983), pp. 254–255.

14. Steven Mosher, "Why Are Baby Girls Killed in China?" *The Wall Street Journal*, 25 July 1983.

15. Carolyn Sargeant, "Born to Die: Witchcraft and Infanticide in Bariba Culture," *Ethnology*, January 1988.

16. John Boswell, *The Kindness of Strangers* (New York: Pantheon Books, 1988).

17. Susan C.M. Scrimshaw, "Infanticide in Human Populations," in Glenn Hausfater and Sarah Blaffer Hardy, eds., *Infanticide: Comparative and Evolutionary Perspectives* (New York: Aldine, 1984).

18. Murdock, *Social Structure*, p. 9.

19. Charles Wagley, "Cultural Influences on Populations: A Comparison of Two Tupi Tribes" in Patricia Lyons, ed., *Native South Americans* (Boston: Little, Brown, 1974).

20. Claude Levi-Strauss, *Tristes Tropiques* translated from the French by John Russell (New York: Atheneum, 1964), p. 162.

21. David M. Schneider, "Abortion and Depopulation on a Pacific Island," in H. Russell Bernard, ed. *The Human Way* (New York: Macmillan, 1975).

22. Cicero, *Pro Marcello*, 23 quoted in J. P. V. D. Balsdon, *Roman Women* (New York: John Day Co., 1962), p. 76.

23. Livy, *The History of Early Rome* translated by Aubrey de Selencourt (New York: Heritage Press, 1960), pp. 4–5.

24. Tacitus, *Complete Works*, translated from the Latin by Alfred John Church and William Jackson Brodribb (New York: Modern Library, 1942), p. 718.

25. Arthur E.R. Boak, *Manpower Shortage and the Fall of the Roman Empire in the West* (Ann Arbor: The University of Michigan Press, 1955), p. 113.

26. Schneider, "Abortion and Depopulation," in H. Russell Bernard, ed. *The Human Way*, p. 365.

27. Ben Wattenberg, *The Birth Dearth* (New York: Pharos Books, 1987).

28. Daniel Patrick Moynihan, "Defining Deviancy Down," *The American Scholar*, (Winter, 1993): 26.

29. David P. Hamilton, "AIDS Conference in Japan: A Symbol of Epidemic More Than Breakthrough," *The Wall Street Journal*, 8 August 1994.

30. James A. Miller, Letters to the Editor, *The Wall Street Journal*, 25 July 1994.

31. Kathleen Deveny, "Despite AIDS and Safe-Sex Exhortations, Sales of Condomsin U. S. Are Lackluster," *The Wall Street Journal*, 25 November 1992, pp. B-1, B-5.

32. Kevin Goldman, "Marketing Female Condom Is a Challenge," *The Wall Street Journal*, 27 July 1994, p. B-4.

33. Malinowsky, *Sex and Repression*, p. 217.

Part III

Personal Perspectives

Chapter 7

Motherhood in the 90's: To Have or Have Not

Maria McFadden

[*Roe v. Wade*] is alleged to have empowered women; in fact, *Roe* legally disempowered women from holding men accountable for their sexual behavior where that behavior had unplanned results.

Roe's cultural message has been even more potent than its legal impact, for it effectively eliminated any real world consequences for men who use women as mere instruments of male sexual gratification. . . . *Roe* not only changed our law; it changed the moral culture of America. And it did so to the great disadvantage of women.

—George Weigel[1]

On September 15, I became a mother. Or, more exactly, my son was born on that day, lifted out of my womb via Caesarean. I became his mother long before that moment when I heard his first cry. Sometime in early December James Anthony's life began, weeks before I knew he was there.

This is actually the second time of motherhood for me: last year I lost a child in an early miscarriage. The embryo was hardly recognizable as one and perhaps the heart never did beat, but from the moment I knew I was pregnant, I was different—a mother. I was aware of sheltering a developing life within my body. When I lost that early life, the grief was unmistakably for the loss of a person. Not a person I really knew of course, but a person I hoped to meet, a person I imagined, and a person I already loved.

Were these beginnings of my children real, or mere romantic fantasies, because my pregnancies were wanted? And even if they *were* actual beginnings, do the rights of such beginnings take precedence over the rights of women who, unlike me, don't want to be pregnant? These questions are part of the great and emotional debate in our society over what it means to be a mother, of a fetus and of a child. Unfortunately, there is no consensus on the answers. While I firmly believe that the unborn deserve protection, and that motherhood is a central and positive event in a woman's life, there are many who view the fetus as disposable and question the positive nature of motherhood.

THE MARGINALIZATION OF THE UNBORN

The abortion debate in this country is, or should be, about whether or not these beginnings of children *are* real: do the rapidly-developing cells deserve protection as persons, or are they, however regrettably, disposable, because they are *potential* people. Because abortion undeniably stops these beginnings, it should, as I say, matter mostly whether or not what is being destroyed is human. But the original question of whether the results of conception are human or a "clump of cells" has been overshadowed by "rights talk." Even if an embryo is human, do its rights outweigh those of the woman? Should women have the right to end pregnancies?

The prevalent answer in our culture and law, and in contemporary feminism, is yes, women should be able to control their pregnancies. Debate over whether or not the fetus is human has taken a back-seat to discussion of women's rights. The sexual revolution and women's liberation have made it both easier to become pregnant accidentally and harder to make room in one's life for the accidental baby. So abortion is the only answer, the one that allows women to have sex without desire for conception and to keep jobs and careers without interruption, as men do. The ability *not* to be pregnant has become so crucial to some women's life-styles that feminists will go to any length to defend abortion, in the face of ever-increasing evidence from science and technology that the fetus is indeed human and even feels pain.

Denial of the humanity of the fetus allows women and men to act as if pregnancies are only the responsibility of a woman to herself. But what happens when a woman gets pregnant is that she becomes, willingly or unwillingly, responsible for *another* life. This doesn't mean it will be an easy situation or a desirable one—it does mean, however, that she can no more do away with that life than she could murder a baby left on her doorstep (and, except for a case of rape, the woman did have some responsibility in creating the baby).

In many ways, the responsibility for a separate life is more apparent than ever. In our super health-conscious days, pregnancy, if it is wanted, is a time full of restrictions. We no longer smoke, drink, or even take aspirin, for fear we will harm the developing fetus. A mother is expected to sacrifice her habits to give her child a good start. The focus of responsibility can even be seen and monitored, through ultrasound, for example, and the Doppler device for monitoring the fetal heartbeat.

For some who are fixated on the necessity of abortions for women, even this ability to monitor the fetus is a cause for anger. Katha Pollitt, a poet and feminist critic, wrote in an article for *Glamour*[2] that we as a society are *un*healthily obsessed with the fetus, with our sonograms, advertisements using ultrasound photos, and theories on how parents can teach their children *in utero*. She sees, rightly, that these might be contradictory attitudes for a society of easily accessible abortion. Rather than reexamine the abortion question, she claims that all the attention given the fetus is detrimental to women: for example, the sonogram demeans the woman, by rendering *her* invisible. This idea is echoed by other feminists: Barbara Duden, a professor of social sciences in Frankfurt, Germany, wrote a book titled *Disembodying Woman*. The entire book is dedicated to the idea that "ideological gynecology" has created, through ultrasound images which "skin" women, a "public fetus" whose rights supercede the woman's.[3] Duden concludes that in the face of these scientific developments, which she claims are nonetheless more about images and imagination than facts, a woman needs to be able to "ruefully smile at this phantom. Then one can speak an unconditional **NO** to life, recovering one's own autonomous aliveness."[4] In a new American book, *The Myths of Motherhood: How Culture Reinvents the Good Mother*, author Shari L. Thurer writes: "Mothers are now being usurped in the public consciousness by their fetuses. . . . To doctors, the fetus is now an 'unborn patient,' and a mother a mere 'fetal container,' the empty place in the sonogram."[5]

Focusing on the fetus, to these feminists, is anti-woman. But how can focusing on a woman's unique ability to carry a child demean her ? Isn't motherhood a large part of the essence of being "feminine"? And what is a sonogram? A picture, produced by sound waves. It is a factual thing, a part of reality, difficult to manipulate. Which doesn't mean that it doesn't involve emotion. When I saw James's first sonogram, at 4 1/2 months, I fell hopelessly in love. I could hardly feel him moving inside me yet, and I had been worried, after my miscarriage, that there would be something wrong. But on the screen my husband and I saw a perfectly round head, a beautiful spinal cord, little legs kicking, and hands grasping. As we watched, the baby (we didn't know the sex) opened its hand and proceeded to suck its thumb. Incidentally, we also saw James kicking against *my* bladder—I was hardly rendered invisible. What makes sonograms so dangerous and emotionally troubling for abortion advocates is the obviousness of a *separate* life inside a woman's body, not an appendage. The fetus seems so happy in its own little world, so safe and unconcerned in a close, warm womb where all its needs are automatically met.

The view of the womb we get from a sonogram illuminates what ought to be the safest time in a human's life. Instead, the sanctuary of the womb is invaded routinely, with the support and even encouragement of society. The Planned Parenthood clinic across the street from our apartment offers abortions up to sixteen weeks—just about the age of James's first photo, which I have lovingly placed in his first photo album. In the sonogram, he held his hand with his thumb out and his fingers tucked in; he still holds his hand that way. In my womb he was active at night and had hiccups several times a day; he still does. His sonogram was simply an introduction to the person we are getting to know. How can doctors deliberately tear out little beings who are able to move around and suck their thumbs? And how can their mothers allow it?

MOTHERHOOD

There *is* an obsession with the fetus in our culture today: to have or not to have. The event of birth seems to be a matter of control and relativity. Ever since birth "control" became a right, we have sought to perfectly control whether and when to have children. We have an abortion about every 20 seconds in this country, and at the same time we have couples spending tens of thousands of dollars on medical procedures to conceive one biological child. The more frustrated we get at the lack of control, the more we try. Take, for example, a woman who has successfully *not* gotten pregnant for years, but cannot conceive when she wants too. This isn't what she expected. So she spends years and thousands of dollars and tons of emotional energy trying to conceive. The value of a fetus, or sperm or an egg for that matter, is relative, not judged by an objective standard of life or not-life, but by whether or not the people who conceived it want it. If a woman wants an abortion, she is ridding her body of tissue; if she desperately wants a child, the products of conception are precious, and she hopes for a birth.

But birth itself is only one point in the process of development from conception. When James was born, at that moment did all his organs and bones suddenly snap into place? Did he in a matter of minutes develop his father's chin or his uncle's forehead? Were his characteristics—facial expressions, for example—instantly infused? Of course not: all these things had been developing from the beginning. The development of the person from conception is an awesome series of events, and those who respect the process do not dare say a life isn't present. People try to manipulate this life in opposite ways: abortion and some other types of birth control prevent a conception from becoming a birth; in vitro fertilization and other procedures attempt to conceive and bring about a birth from a conception. (The anti-birth procedures are much more effective than the pro-birth, as more and more women sadly know.)

Many think that we are not meant to have such control over life, which holds such mystery and wonder. Birth itself is often referred to as a miracle. When I looked at my baby son in his first weeks of life, I was amazed that his tiny body could have all its parts inside—it seemed impossible. The fact that he is here does seem miraculous, it has to be more than a result of a biological equation. It's as if he came to us from heaven, and he proves to us that there *is* a heaven, that there has to be more to this life than the physical. The proof is in the wonder of a whole new person, and how he can make his parents feel, that they alone couldn't have produced such perfection.

There isn't much time to reflect on the miracle of life when we are so busy pitting the rights of fetuses against the rights of their mothers. Questioning the worth of a fetus also has serious repercussions on how one views motherhood. It has become so important for women to have the right *not* to be mothers that even if they do decide to have a child it is not expected to completely change their lives. Women who are lawyers, ad executives, or bankers are described as such first, mothers second, and it is not the norm for motherhood to be a career, or for a career to be put on hold. Rather, one tries to squeeze childbearing in almost as an extracurricular activity. Making motherhood only one choice among many, however, leads one to believe that it isn't the all-encompassing thing it used to be. But it is! Pregnancy involves major changes, labor is painful and may involve complications, and motherhood is the most challenging, exhausting and rewarding job there is, especially if a first baby is followed by siblings. But most of all, it is important: we don't often speak about this, but our children are the world's future. Women who try to do everything as they did before they had a child end up exhausted and feeling cheated, or the children are cheated by spending more time in daycare than at home. In the name of women's fulfillment, we are skimping on the care of our most precious commodity.

We are also, ironically, skimping on the experience of motherhood itself, which can transform us. Now that I have James, I see myself quite differently. I have someone who thinks the world of me! I have someone who, as long as he lives, will be able to say "my mother. . . ." and mean me! I have someone who must be put *first*, and that's a relief. And I have someone who, God willing, will live beyond me, which makes the world seem a more comfortable place. And right now I have an adorable baby whose smiles melt my heart and whose perfect little face brings tears of joy. I wouldn't have missed this experience for anything.

Many women who have missed the experience of mothering so far are finding, despite all the avenues they have traveled for fulfillment, that they don't feel fulfilled *without* a child, that not being able to have a child when they *want* to severely threatens their happiness and their life goals. They find that the career that was so important isn't enough to make their lives feel worthwhile, and that having a child is more than a career choice; they also find that, for reasons of infertility or lack of a supportive partner, it's not always that easy to have a baby when you want one.

The 1994 movie *Babyfever* gives an interesting look at these issues.[6] The scene is a baby shower, and the documentary-style movie interviews the women attendees' attitudes about babies. Although the setting is fictional, the comments are real. The protagonist, Jenna, is agonizing over whether or not to have a baby, with a man she's not really in love with, because her biological clock is ticking (her friend's shower makes her agonize all the more). Some of the women present say they *don't* want children, and a woman who has two children frets about not having a chance to get her singing career off the ground before she had kids. But the majority of women interviewed, all seemingly in their late 30s or early 40s, are having problems having a baby: most have achieved a liberated, career-woman status, but find something missing. They now want a child, but either they haven't met the right guy, or they have, but he doesn't want children (perhaps he has some from a previous marriage and doesn't want more), or they have a medical problem with conceiving. Some without men discuss being impregnated with a friend's, or an anonymous donor's sperm, as does a lesbian couple. One well-dressed career woman talks about her demanding job and her loneliness. She says of the women's movement: "We have gotten so good at taking care of ourselves, but now we have no one else to take care of. We are highly evolved, sensitive . . . men."

That struck me as a profound comment: relentless "feminism" renders women anything but feminine, because it downplays women's need and capacity for relationships, and relegates mothering to a minor role in their lives, something to be planned only at certain times, to be put off, something not to be expected as a norm. As one woman in the film poignantly related, she expected to have a family someday, and, as her hopes for that fade, she sees other women leading the life that should have been hers. One day she looked around and it was too late. Maybe her story would have been different if the feminism she bought into had been more affirmingly feminine.

Some female reviewers of *Babyfever* took issue with precisely the notion that it is natural for women to be essentially concerned with children. Like the feminists who complained of an "obsession" with the fetus, they saw the film as representing an unhealthy obsession with babies. Charla Krupp wrote in *Glamour* that "Babies are reducing sensible women to blithering idiots"; she says that the idea that you're not truly a woman if you don't have a baby is "50-s think."[7] And Julie Salamon in *The Wall Street Journal* reported that her friend found the movie tiresome: "explaining that she had no interest in having children, she said she found nothing in *Babyfever* that appealed to her. 'Watching this movie,' she said, 'was like watching a bunch of men talk about carburetors. Fascinating for them I'm sure.' "[8]

I suppose if we reduce babies to the status of carburetors it is easier to wonder what the fuss is about (and look the other way when they are destroyed). The message of Krupp and Salamon is that childbearing should be reserved for those women who are really interested, and even the subject should not be forced on women who are not. There are certainly women who don't feel called to be mothers, and women who aren't mothers who are truly fulfilled women. But this used to be the exception, not the rule. I suspect the distaste for *Babyfever* is another angry and fearful reaction to an uncomfortable picture. Like a sonogram showing a fetus as human, this film, in its own way, shows that making babies is a central part of the experience of what it is to be a woman.

I am sympathetic to the pressures, demands and desires of modern women in American culture; after all, it's my culture too. I was lucky enough to get pregnant when I wanted to, and I have a husband and a job with flexibility. And even with a very-much-wanted pregnancy, I wasn't prepared for how difficult pregnancy can be, and what a completely life-altering process it all is. Toward the end especially, when I was weary, anxious, and uncomfortable, I realized how hard it must be for women who didn't want to get pregnant to carry the pregnancy to term, or how hard it must be for single mothers to have a baby alone. Pregnancy and childbirth are not meant to be easy or involve easy choices. Unplanned or planned, pregnancy is a major life event. Which ought to lead one to the inescapable conclusion that sex was not meant to be casual.

Sex without responsibility or without commitment does not help women; neither does abortion, nor a negative view of children. Women, and men, need to be encouraged in positive relationships, and supported in childbirth. Frederica Mathewes-Green, in her new book *Real Choices*, found that the one thing that would have made a crucial difference to women who had abortions (and later regretted them) wasn't money, or shelter, or baby clothes, but rather the existence of at least one person to really support them, someone to say: "Yes, you can have that baby, and I will stand by you and help."[9] This is all too often missing, as so many parents, boyfriends, husbands and friends buy into the abortion mentality: they "chose" a quick solution without thinking of the life-long consequences. Pope John Paul II, in his new best-selling book, *Crossing the Threshold of Hope*, writes that the only "honest stance" in dealing with an unwanted pregnancy is "that of *radical solidarity with the woman*. It is not right to leave her alone." Although some situations can be extremely difficult, if a woman has support, "she is even capable of heroism."[10]

Women *are* capable of heroism, especially where their children are involved. As any new mother understands, there is nothing you wouldn't do for your child. You look down into a perfect little face and you think : "I would do anything for you, I would give my life for yours, I would protect you at all costs." This is the essence and the beauty of motherhood, this is the way it should be. It is unfair to tell women, before they get to hear a first cry or see a tiny flailing foot, that motherhood is about protecting yourself against your own new beginnings.

NOTES

1. George Weigel, "Women Reap the Rewards of Roe in Abuse," *Los Angeles Times*, 29 November 1992, p. M5.

2. Katha Pollitt, "Why Do We Romanticize the Fetus?," *Glamour*, October 1992.

3. Barbara Duden, *Disembodying Women: Perspectives on Pregnancy and the Unborn* (Cambridge, Mass.: Harvard University Press, 1993). These terms are used throughout the book.

4. Ibid., p. 110.

5. Shari L. Thurer, *The Myths of Motherhood: How Culture Reinvents the Good Mother* (Boston, New York: Houghton Mifflin, 1994), p. 294.

6. *Babyfever*, directed by Henry Jaglom, written by Henry Jaglom and Victoria

Foyt.

7. Charla Krupp, "Baby Mania," *Glamour*, June 1994.

8. Julie Salamon, "Bringing Up Baby, Again and Again," *The Wall Street Journal*, 5 May 1994.

9. Frederica Mathewes-Green, *Real Choices: Offering Practical, Life-Affirming Alternatives to Abortion* (Sisters, Oreg: Questar Publications, 1994).

10. His Holiness John Paul II, *Crossing the Threshold of Hope* (New York: Alfred A. Knopf, 1994), p. 207.

Chapter 8

Pregnancy Care Centers: Sisterhood is Powerful

Frederica Mathewes-Green

Men tend to take abortion lightly; they regard it as one of the numerous hazards imposed on women by malignant nature, but fail to realize fully the values involved. The woman who has recourse to abortion is disowning feminine values, her values. . . . Her whole moral universe is being disrupted.

—Simone de Beauvoir[1]

The [pro-life] message should be: We care about women in crisis; alternatives are available. Getting that message out helps people in need; it also helps rebuild a hospitable American community capable of sustaining legal protections for the unborn.

—George Weigel and William Kristol[2]

The toughest thing about Marilyn Szewczyk isn't her name.[3] You can forget everything you learned in grammar school and rattle off "Seff-check." Keeping up with Marilyn's determination, energy, and vision is not so easy.

Marilyn arrives late for our lunch appointment, her ample silhouette filling the door. Outside it is a blistering white summer noon; inside, darkness and plush chairs. She makes her way to the table leaning lightly on her cane, a souvenir of the stroke two years ago. The waitresses know her ("Hiya, Marilyn, hon, howya doin'?"). Marilyn asks for a table for three; she has scheduled a *second* luncheon meeting with someone else later. Marilyn doesn't have a lot of spare time.

Once seated, she begins laying out on the table her luncheon necessities: a smoky-transparent pill case, with yellow, orange, and gray pills; an insulin injection kit; a pack of cigarettes. A cigarette comes first; as the blue smoke curls overhead, Marilyn's latest meeting has begun.

Few would begrudge Marilyn the title of the Mother of the Pro-Life Movement in Maryland. As this state has dealt with the abortion issue over the decades, she's always been near the front lines. But most of her energy goes not into fighting to make abortion illegal, but into working to bring women hope and help. Abortion is a grim, unhappy choice. Marilyn believes that, by offering shelter and clothing and a kind word, she can help women make a happier choice, one they (and their babies) can live with. Over and over, she's been proved right.

"'I was pro-abortion when *Roe v. Wade* was decided," she says. "I thought it was a matter of religion: you know, 'Mine says it's not OK, yours says it is.'" Then a friend showed her photos of children in the womb, 4 weeks, 5 weeks, before the earliest abortions are done: tiny limbs blooming out like rosebuds, a heart tripping fast as hummingbird wings. "There's no way anybody could say 'We don't know when life begins,'" she insists. Her gravelly voice is touched with simple sweetness. "That was life. There's no question when life begins."

PREGNANCY CARE CENTERS

By the mid 1970s Marilyn was volunteering with several of Maryland's pregnancy care centers. These centers offer pregnancy tests, material aid and emotional support to women who decide to continue their pregnancies. Largely staffed by volunteers, the centers give away free whatever services they can offer and material help they can gather to help women choose life.

Pregnancy care centers are an admirable embodiment of the early 1970s slogan, "Sisterhood is powerful." The fight to defend or defeat legal abortion is no doubt overpopulated with male lawyers in suits; when women think about the issue, they are more likely to picture a friend in tears. While the political players thunder that abortion is a callous convenience or right,these women think it's something else: a tragedy. Very few women want to have an abortion. Who would want to undergo an expensive, awkward, and humiliating medical procedure, and gain from it only the death of her child? If pregnant women find themselves faced with that last choice too quickly, it is because other women have not reached out with love and support, filling in more first choices at the top of the list. The more these other women think about pregnant women's sorrow, the more they think about the little torn bodies going into clinic dumpsters each day, the less they feel they can do nothing.

Pregnancy care centers operate on the venerable American tradition of barn-raising: neighbors help neighbors in need, and the job gets done. Since there is no income from clients, everything must be begged and borrowed. A typical center will have a lending closet of second-hand maternity and baby clothes, perhaps some baby furniture, a list of a few doctors willing to take on another charity patient, a list of families willing to take in a pregnant guest. One local grocery donates diapers and another gives some formula; a church pays the phone bill and a benevolent association covers the electricity. And, every month, the rent must be scraped together with donations from friends who've been asked too many times before.

Contrast this with the business-like approach at the abortion clinic down the street. Here there is a commodity which can be sold, and over 1.5 million are sold each year. At $300 per abortion the proceeds near half a billion dollars; add in the much higher fees for late abortions, about ten thousand of them per year, and the figure rises dramatically. No wonder the promoters of abortion can afford salaries, office space, even full-page ads in major newspapers and magazines. The pregnancy center director can just afford to run off "We can help!" flyers at the local quick-copy, then thumb-tack them to the bulletin board at the laundromat.

But can they help? How much good can a pregnancy center do? When a pregnancy is difficult, there is usually a tangle of reasons, some easy to solve, some impossible. Abortion has the appeal of smashing all the problems at once, wiping the slate clean. It is brutal in its efficiency, however; the solutions are roughly yanked out through the woman's aching heart. Her right to abort is noisily and publicly celebrated; her long years of pondering the cost are more privately endured. Abortion is forever.

The pregnancy care center offers a patchwork quilt of help that is thin in many places—not enough housing, not enough car seats, not enough medical care. Too often the deepest problem is one beyond the mending of any stranger's kindness: the woman's need for the baby's father to love and cherish her, to give her the protection and provision that the center, a poor substitute, scrambles to supply. But what the center can give is encouragement, the strength of sisterhood, the strength of other women who know what it's like and who won't let you down. When hope mends the quilt, sometimes it is enough.

Marilyn puffs, and squints through the smoke to line up her pills. She's got twenty years of not letting you down. When a heart attack landed her in the hospital last year, her co-laborers would get furtive, whispered phone calls at moments seized when the doctor and her husband were out of earshot. Now she's back running the Auburn Center, a toll-free hotline that crosses Maryland and unites its forty-one storefront pregnancy care centers. Women phoning in are given information about help available at their nearest center, plus plenty of kind words and reassurance on the spot. Each call is logged, and tagged as belonging to one of twenty request-categories, with 2,300 to 2,800 calls received each month.

The Auburn Center's phones are staffed "in the garage—I mean the annex" behind Catonsville's Pregnancy Center West. A staffer answers calls from 9:00 A.M. until 11:30 PM with short breaks; at other times a service answers that pages Marilyn or her daughter Barbie and can patch them in with a frightened girl unwilling to leave her number. And Barbie isn't the only other Szewczyk in the field. Marilyn rattles off a list of other kids and their spouses—Lynnie, Ann, Andy, Cathy, Richard—as well as her own mother, Kathryn, who answer phones, fold baby clothes, and keep the computer humming. When Marilyn began the hotline in 1982, she originally staffed it by asking friends and relatives,

"How much money do you need me to pay you for you to quit your job and do this?" The answer was in the range of $400 a month ("and it's still about the same" she chuckles).

Marilyn's co-worker Anne arrives as I ask about difficult calls. Anne says she just returned a call to the man who had phoned to confess that he was having sex with his daughter. He had asked for help; Anne called back with lists of resources and phone numbers. "He kept going 'Uh-huh', but I could tell he wasn't writing it down," she says, dejected. Hotline work is frustrating: no eye contact, no way to know what the caller decides to do. Marilyn describes the call from a thirteen-year-old black girl who was afraid she was pregnant. "I said, 'Listen, honey, even if you're not pregnant, you have got to stop doing this.' The girl said, 'I do?' like she was completely surprised. I said, 'Yes, you don't have to do this.' 'I don't?' She didn't seem to know it was OK not to have sex."

Do people abuse the toll-free number? Does she get rude or obscene calls? Marilyn and Anne, who have seen it all, laugh. "We had one young boy from Frederick who called every day. We were able to find out who he was. So the next time he called, I said, 'Now listen, Allen. . . .' He hung up and never called again!"

Marilyn's office is a cheerful little square building that bears no resemblance to a garage. Inside it is crammed with desks, books, videotapes, audiotapes, posters, fax, phones, and a monster copier. She sits at her desk rolling off anecdotes, pausing every few minutes to answer the phone. When the phone rings, she turns her back on me and covers the phone like a mother hen; her voice drops and becomes confidential and gentle.

Right now she is annoyed with one of the centers in her phone network. A woman had called after her husband suddenly walked out; she had children 3, 2, and 1, as well as 14-week-old twins. She had no money and no diapers or formula; for the last few days she had been feeding the twins sugar water. Dependent on public transportation, she had been making rounds at public assistance offices, with the three year old carrying one of the twins.

Marilyn referred the woman to her nearest center—but they told her that she would have to produce a birth certificate and other documentation before they would help her. "Can you imagine it?" Marilyn asks, angry and amused at the same time. "They're afraid someone will take advantage of them. Who cares? I'd be afraid that someone who really needs my help would get by. I don't care if some people take advantage. I'm not going to miss *your* baby." Her finger jabs for emphasis.

When the woman called back, Marilyn took it on herself to help. She bought a carload of groceries and took some baby furniture, clothes, toys, and set out to find the section of Baltimore called Westport. "It's near Cherry Hill—you know, that's always on the news for another shooting?" When she stopped to ask directions at a gas station, the black attendant pleaded with her, "Lady, you don't want to go there! *We* don't even go there!" But Marilyn and Barbie found the place: past overflowing dumpsters and abandoned cars, "But inside it was neat and clean as a pin, with nice furniture, not expensive but nice. How she keeps it that clean with five little kids I don't know. I have three grandchildren living with me, and I know my house doesn't look that good!"

PRACTICAL HELP

North and west from Baltimore the hills begin to roll, lapping up at the base of the Appalachian Mountains, with farmland, woods, and vacant businesses dotting the route. Just before the Pennsylvania border lies Taneytown, founded in 1754, a cluster of worn brick buildings with white wooden porches, glowing rose today under a drizzly pearl sky.

Taneytown was the home of Supreme Court Chief Justice Roger Taney, whose infamous *Dred Scott* decision (1857) decreed that blacks were not citizens; many have suggested a parallel to *Roe v. Wade's* denial of personhood to the unborn.

Marilyn's daughter-in-law Gloria has set up the Carroll County Pregnancy Center right at the town's crossroads. Her building is one-room-wide, going back deep into the block. The front section is the "Bear-ly Used Boutique," the town's thrift shop, with an extra-large rack of maternity clothes. Prices are posted, but are negotiable down to free. The next room back is a waiting room/lounge shared by clients and volunteers; then come the computer room, pregnancy testing room, a large closet where layettes are stored, and an inviting counseling room in apricot and blue with a well-cushioned couch and a pillowed rocker. Tucked around the L by the back door is Gloria's "office"—a cluttered desk.

Gloria is a willowy blond with large, limpid eyes. She explains that the thrift shop is a unique feature for a pregnancy center; it was begun as a source of funds and has become a mission in its own right. "It gives some dignity back to the young girls who come here—they can pick out the clothes they like."

Dignity is important to the families, mostly white, mostly farming, that live around here. The area is economically depressed, and many businesses have closed. But, as Marilyn had said, "They're too proud to admit that they're hungry." She had described how Gloria has had to buy up a load of groceries and go to a client's house with a white lie: "Somebody gave me all this food, and I have to give it away or it will just go bad! Can you take some?"

Gloria says that her average client is an eighteen-year-old girl in a steady relationship with a boy she plans eventually to marry. What they didn't plan was for pregnancy to complicate the picture. "They're naive, following the trend for teen sex, and have an unrealistic idea that they can have sex and everything will be fine."

Gloria describes a case where the girl came in with the boy, together with both mothers. She giggles a bit at the memory; the mothers were furious with each other, fighting over the kids' heads and volleying the blame back and forth. Gloria took the girl aside for a long talk about abstinence, while the mother listened in. "But I've been saying those same things for years!" she exclaimed. Gloria sits back. "Sometimes they'll hear it from me, where the parents were never able to get through."

The center's funding is cobbled together from many sources. In 1992 the Boutique brought in $4,363 as clear profit. It is staffed by volunteers and sells donated goods, so it has no expenses. (Rent and utilities are covered by the pregnancy center.) Another $11,800 was raised in various ways: a ham raffled at Easter raised $500, and the annual Walkathon brought in nearly $3,000. The Walkathon is a fixture of pregnancy center fundraising across the country, probably the most popular money-making tool. In Taneytown, about one hundred walkers signed up supporters to donate so much per mile to the center. On a sunny Saturday, pushing strollers and wearing T-shirts with the center's name, the walkers followed the designated route in a festive throng, and later collected the pledged donations. In past years, volunteers have delivered business lunches to raise funds, canvassing area offices and taking orders for home-made sub sandwiches. Gloria says she also has two churches which give regularly, and a number of individuals give $5 to $25 a month. In 1992 she served 392 clients.

During the last ten minutes an incessant "Mrow? Mrow? Mrow?" has struck up outside the back door. Gloria opens the door, and in walks a very tall, very thin cat: on an oversized frame designed to carry 20 pounds of burly catflesh is stretched about 8 pounds of hungry orange kitty. Gloria gives him a skeptical look as he begins pounding his head against her ankles, purring like a furnace. "Mr. Bones. He belongs to the people upstairs, but I don't think they feed him," she confides. "We've sort of adopted him, but I keep his food out on the back porch." Gloria, like all those in her line of work, is constantly making decisions about what kind of help helps and what kind of help ultimately hurts. I ask how she keeps clients from becoming overdependent. She considers this question with an air of regret.

"We took a hard look at our files awhile back and realized that we were enabling some people to use us. If they ran out of money at the end of the month, they'd call us—we've paid electric, fuel, given diapers," she said. "We decided that, once we'd helped people three times, we would require them to get involved with the services the county offers, teaching budget planning, job training, and so forth. Obviously those sort of skills are not there. If somebody has $20, but they decide to spend it on cigarettes, well, we're not going to support that decision."

Gloria is looking to move to bigger quarters. At the edge of town stands a big house on a hill, and she imagines using every corner: the clothes closet will fill the basement; a Christian book and gift store on the main floor; pregnancy care services on the second floor, and on the third floor two bedrooms for emergency housing ("Sometimes we need up to 30 days to get a client into services"). The owner, she thinks, would rather sell to a ministry like hers than have the house torn down for a commercial building. The mortgage is not prohibitive, but she has to raise $25,000 for the down payment. She's writing letters to friends.

I ask how she got into this line of work, and she laughs and shakes her head. "Marilyn is just relentless! Every gathering always turns back to a discussion of the issues." She smiles as she recalls. "When we lived closer to Baltimore, I volunteered at the center there, but when we moved way out here I thought, 'Thank goodness, I've gotten away from all that!' There's no abortion in Carroll County. But soon after I got here a neighbor's child called up; she said a friend was pregnant and wanted her to drive her to Hagerstown for an abortion. I hated to admit it, but I realized that we needed a pregnancy center. I told Marilyn, and do you know what she did?" Gloria's really laughing now. "She gave me a grocery bag—just a plain, plastic grocery bag—with about 30 pieces of literature in it, and a check for $50. And she said, 'Go open a pregnancy center.'" She shakes her head at the memory. "How did I get into this line of work? From just being stupid and not knowing that I should not listen to Marilyn."

"Nobody warned me that I should not listen to Marilyn," she laughs.

Heading south out of Baltimore, almost to Washington, D.C., you will arrive at the oldest pregnancy care center in Maryland, the Pregnancy Aid Center in College Park. The Center occupies a rambling, two-story turn-of-the-century house, whose antique charms are now encased in sheet paneling, drop acoustical tile ceilings, and mustard-yellow aluminum siding. The center was founded nineteen years ago, director Mary Jelacic tells me, "by a group of students at the University of Maryland who were incensed about *Roe v. Wade*; they asked, 'Why isn't anyone addressing the needs of women in crisis pregnancy?' They set up a counseling center that's been operating ever since."

Unexpected pregnancies became even more of a crisis in 1988, when local hospitals cut back the number of charity patients they would accept. But the Pregnancy Aid Center was ready, having developed facilities for on-site prenatal care. In addition to the usual pregnancy center offerings of practical and emotional support, clients could come to the Center's clinic for a medical exam and be assured that they and their babies were progressing toward a healthy birth. Patients are asked to give $5 per visit, but the fee is waived whenever necessary.

Mary Jelacic believes that the center's ability to offer medical care is what makes the difference between choosing abortion and choosing birth for many of these women. The clientele is 85 percent Hispanic, and their choices are often limited by language, finances, and legal status. While they can make room for a new child, the up-front charge of thousands of dollars for the delivery is daunting. The Pregnancy Aid Center fills the gap, allowing immigrant Hispanic women the same choices that their wealthier, insured American sisters enjoy.

SISTERHOOD

Ideological partisanship does not stand in the way of serving women. Three of the doctors who previously staffed the clinic labeled themselves pro-choice; they believed that birth was a choice that should also be available and supported with quality care. All three have now moved from the area, and certified nurse-midwives from the faculty of Georgetown University's School of Midwifery have taken their place. Michaela Donohue and Becky Skovgaard will be seeing patients today.

The Pregnancy Aid Center's client load—two thousand per year, eight hundred using medical services—makes use of every square foot of space. An assortment of high chairs, squeezed out of interior storage, stand in a forlorn group outside the front door, as if hoping to be let back in. Just inside there is a sunny waiting room with six mostly-mismatched chairs and a sofa; in the next room, the office, there is a metal desk and another seven chairs. Boxes are stuffed under chairs and stacked in corners.

Notices and signs tacked to the walls are in Spanish and English, or sometimes only Spanish ("Consulta Legal Gratuita"), and pamphlets with titles like "Esta mi bebe tomando suficiente leche?" line the wall rack. Further down the hall are rooms for counseling and storage of clothing, and Mary's office in a large and utterly crammed space that was once no doubt a parlor. Now a large copier sits in the bay window. Upstairs there are two examining rooms, more storage, and another large waiting room with a doctor's scale and specimen cups.

Waiting in the office this lunchtime are two Hispanic women and a blond with two children; an African woman wrapped in bright batik represents another segment of the Center's clientele. The blond has completed her examination, and is telling the kids that the early contractions are nothing to worry about, that she's having them because "I'm on my feet with the band so much." The girl, about 10, runs over to the fetal models and brings back the one of six-month size. "The midwife said that the baby is about this size now." She shows it to her mother, a pink doll the size of her hand, curled in on itself and sucking a thumb. The mother gazes at it and beams a dreamy smile; sister and brother frown at the rival gravely with a bit more ambivalence.

I am invited to the upstairs waiting room where the staff is having lunch. Here the Wide World of Chairs theme is continued. Mary Jelacic is a bright-eyed brunette in a red cotton dress and a ponytail. Decades in America have not erased her Scottish accent, although the Croatian surname comes from her husband. She came to the Center as director in 1981, when she read in her church bulletin an offer of part-time employment. Her children were in school and it seemed a good time to take on something not overly demanding (or so it appeared at the time). Mary's training was in special education, and she says, "I considered unplanned pregnancy to be a somewhat handicapping condition."

Also lunching with us are Alicia, a new volunteer, a man named Terry (whom Mary jokingly refers to as "el jefito"), and midwife Michaela Donohue; soon the second midwife, Becky Skovgaard joins us. Everyone is downing sloppy sub sandwiches, and Terry jokes about raiding the layette closet for bibs.

How does the Center find funds to operate? Michaela says wryly, "Mary goes out on the streets and begs." Mary laughs and explains that the Center is listed with the Combined Federal Campaign and can be designated through United Way. There are also individual and church contributions, as well as grants from the March of Dimes, the Giant Food grocery chain, the Knights of Columbus, the Knights of Malta, the Archdiocese of Washington, and a few local foundations.

How busy does it get? Mary recounts the story of the infamous evening, a couple of years ago, when they had thirty-three patients come to the clinic. The doctor attending that evening was there for the first time, on loan from Holy Cross Hospital; his specialty was infertility. ("He didn't find much of that here," someone comments.) It was a chaotic time: "Number thirteen was an ectopic—that set him back a wee bit," and she was rushed off to the hospital. Apparently, the doctor had expected to finish at a reasonable hour and had to keep making trips to the phone to cancel dates and appointments. Finally, he got to number 32, who had been sitting quietly on the steps all evening with her hands folded on top of her belly. But once she got on the table, the doctor yelled, "Mary! The feet are in the cervix!" This baby was about to come into the world wrong-way-around, and such a case usually requires an emergency Caesarean. Mary called the Fire and Rescue Department located across the street, which made the short trip, sirens blazing, and arrived before the patient had managed to get back into her clothes. She was hastily dressed and sent off to the hospital with her chart pinned to her chest "because she didn't speak any English, you know."

Only when the Keystone Cops frenzy had died down did they realize that the last patient, number 33, had been sitting patiently in the back room with her clothes off all that time. As she took her leave, the doctor told Mary, "You took ten years off my life tonight!" He never returned. The next day Sister Jane Anne at Holy Cross Hospital scolded Mary: "What did you do to our boy!" The doctor moved out of state and into the relative calm of an infertility practice. Mary winds up the story by talking about that breech baby: his name is Mario and he's now 2 1/2. Every year the mother brings Mary a potted plant and a birthday party invitation; every year Mary goes.

We are interrupted by a Hispanic boy of about fifteen with headphones slung around his neck and a heart-melting bashful smile. He is the son of a patient, and he asks to speak to Mary; he wants to know whether he can become a volunteer at the center. When Mary returns, discussion ensues about this boy, whom they are afraid is becoming a "Parental Child"—he is missing school in order to take care of his mother and siblings. The room becomes an extended-family conference on the boy's welfare and family situation.

As I watch them, I am thinking about how much Mary does for women and their families. I picture Marilyn driving into Westport with a carload of gifts, and Gloria cocking an eye at the wildly purring Mr. Bones. I am thinking about the charge that pro-lifers only care about fetuses. I haven't heard any of them talk about a fetus yet.

Instead, Mary and Michaela and the others talk about the Center's clients, most of whom are between the ages of twelve and twenty five. Just over 50 percent turn out not to be pregnant; like Gloria, Mary encourages abstinence for young women: "They're adolescent, their bodies are still growing, they're not in stable relationships—abstinence is best." She says that many feel that sexual activity is almost a requirement; if everyone is telling you to use condoms, you can't use them without having sex. Some just need permission to stop.

Mary encourages teens, most of all, to talk to their parents. Yes, she agrees, when your parents find out you're pregnant they'll hit the roof. But if you have a secret abortion and get injured (like a sixteen-year-old girl in this county who died after having a legal abortion without her parents' knowledge), your parents will find out anyway, and then they'll have three shocks to endure: My child was sexually active, got pregnant, and had an abortion! Mary urges, "Tell them first."

To make this easier, Mary or volunteers will go with the child to tell the parents. They do this at the Center or the home, or they meet them at McDonald's. About a third of the time, the client chooses abortion. Some of these come back for medical care or postabortion counseling; the Center doesn't reject or condemn.

Like Gloria, Mary is hoping to move her Center to a new building. Her Scots blood makes her tenacious in a bargain; when the center was evicted from the present building years ago, she didn't leave ("We had no place to go, so we stayed") and instead got an interest-free loan and bought the building. She laughs, "The board thought it was time to fire me because they thought I'd lost me marbles." Now she has her eye on the new medical building down the street. The price is dropping fast, but she's patient enough to wait, and then there's the matter of a lack of funds to purchase it. But she believes the building is for her. It will put her a block from the local abortion clinic.

As I leave, Mary is speaking earnestly to a Hispanic client, working hard to assemble sentences in Scottish-accented Spanish. Here we have a Scot with a Croatian name speaking Spanish to a woman from El Salvador, while upstairs women with Scandanavian and Irish backgrounds are examining pregnant women from Mexico and Cameroon. All around the world, women make babies and have babies the same way. And all around the world, other women help and support them. This is how they do it in College Park, Maryland.

The abortion battle may be most loudly fought in the political arena, but few pregnant women are found there. Where women in need go, other women go to help, in Taneytown and College Park and two thousand other centers across the land. It is a subversive work, when women help women give birth, and it is the best proof yet of the power of sisterhood.

NOTES

1. Simone de Beauvoir, *The Second Sex* (New York: Vintage Books, 1989), p. 491, translated and edited by H. M. Parshley. Reprint of the 1953 edition published by Alfred A. Knopf, New York.

2. George Weigel and William Kristol, "Life and the Party," *National Review*, 15 August 1994, p. 56.

3. Frederica Mathewes-Green is a regular contributor to the Capital Research Center's publication *Philanthropy, Culture and Society*, from which this chapter was drawn.

Chapter 9

Women Who Abort:
Their Reflections on the Unborn

David C. Reardon

For two hours I could feel her struggling inside me. But then, as suddenly as it began, she stopped. Even today, I remember her very last kick on my left side. She had no strength left. She gave up and died. Despite my grief and guilt, I was relieved that her pain was finally over. But I was never the same again. The abortion killed not only my daughter, it killed a part of me.

> —Nancyjo Mann, founder, Women Exploited By Abortion[1]

Pregnancy and birth link together women all over the world and throughout all time; that earthy, vital process is the most elemental symbol of woman's strength. Disrupting it by thrusting tools deep into her body is as obscene as pouring dirty motor oil into a mountain lake. I oppose abortion because it violates women more deeply than rape, a more hideous violation because it brings grisly death into the very house of life.

> —Frederica Mathewes-Green[2]

Sit with me for a moment in the waiting room of an abortion clinic. Here you will find women who, in general, are neither philosophers nor fools—categories which admittedly include substantial overlap. Very few of these women have engaged in arcane debates about the meaning of "personhood." Fewer still are so foolish as to believe the claim that having an abortion is no worse than having a tooth pulled.

Look about and you will see women from a wide cross section of American culture. Bright and dull, conservative and liberal, religious and irreligious—all are represented. There is significant overrepresentation by adolescents, unmarried women, and racial minorities, but still, they are a cross section of America. And like all Americans, these women are uneasy, and deeply divided over abortion, more so today than ever before in their lives.

Many of these women, even now, while waiting to be escorted to the operating room, bury their heads in the sands of denial. "It will be over soon. I just won't think about it. I'll just go on with my life like before. It wouldn't be legal if it wasn't right. It wouldn't be legal if it wasn't safe. I just won't think about it."

Others, who at best consider their pending abortions to be an evil necessity, are saying goodbye: "Forgive me. Mommy doesn't want to do this, but I really don't have any choice. If only I could have you, I would love you so much."

For some their wait is unemotional, but they are intellectually tortured by the metaphysical question: "Am I doing the right thing?" Still others are carefully focused on their answers to this same question: "This is the right thing, the only thing, to do. I can always have a baby, later, when the time is right, when I can be a good mother. It wouldn't be fair to me, Jim, or even the baby, to have it now."

These women, joylessly seated around the waiting room, are just typical Americans. They share the same spectrum of American beliefs and angst over the abortion question. Polls show that approximately 70 percent of Americans believe that abortion should be legal. Yet another 70 percent (which obviously requires at least a 40 percent overlap) also believe it is immoral. Americans recognize a tension between what is legal and what is moral.

This same tension is also apparent in abortion clinic waiting rooms. Interviews at clinics report that 70 percent of the women having abortions view abortion as immoral, or at least deviant, behavior.[3] Rather than choosing according to their own moral beliefs, they are acting against their belief systems because they feel pressured by others, or circumstances, which "force" them to violate their consciences.

Why, after over twenty years of legal abortion, do Americans, including young women for whom abortion has always been legal, still have a negative moral view of abortion?

WHAT EVERYONE KNOWS

The answer to this question is the same as it was two decades ago. In 1971 the editors of *California Medicine* wrote in support of legalized abortion but noted that the moral view underlying this change would only slowly be adopted.

Since the old [Judeo-Christian] ethic [of the sanctity of life] has not yet been fully displaced [by the new ethic which places relative rather than absolute value on human lives] it has been necessary to separate the idea of abortion from the idea of killing, which continues to be socially abhorrent. The result has been a curious avoidance of the scientific fact, *which everyone really knows*, that human life begins at conception and is continuous whether intra- or extra-uterine until death. The very considerable semantic gymnastics which are required to rationalize abortion as anything but taking a human life would be ludicrous if they were not often put forth under socially impeccable auspices. It is suggested that this schizophrenic sort of subterfuge is necessary because while a new ethic is being accepted the old one has not yet been rejected.[4]

With an honesty often missing from the current abortion debate, the pro-choice editors of *California Medicine* affirm that everyone really knows that human life begins at conception. *Everyone* knows it. Every denial is simply "semantic gymnastics" offered by "socially impeccable auspices" to ease our way.

Sitting in an abortion clinic waiting room, this truth rides uneasily beneath the surface of silent submission. No one dares to speak it, but everyone knows it. It lies at the heart of the question all children eventually ask: "Where do babies come from?" While a child might be temporarily diverted from the answer to this question, no child's curiosity is completely satisfied until the full truth is revealed. Life begins at conception. Babies are created by an act of conception, the uniting (hopefully in an act of love) of a man and woman, sharing the substance of themselves, two becoming one in the flesh — both symbolically, in the sexual act, and most truly, in the conception of a new life.

The knowledge that the human fetus, the human embryo, or even the human zygote, is in fact a *human being* is as undeniable as the answer to the child's question: "Where do babies come from?" The women in the waiting room, some of whom have yet to pack away their cherished dolls, remember when they once asked that question. They remember the answer. They remember the truth. And it is this truth, no matter how much they try to ignore it, forget it, or bury it beneath slogans or philosophical quibbles — it is this truth that demands their attention.

A Feeling of Knowing

In interviews with forty women shortly after their abortions, sociologist Mary Zimmerman avoided any questions regarding the women's view of the nature of the human fetus in order to avoid upsetting them. Yet even when this question went unasked, it was clearly on the minds of the women, most of whom revealed at least some hint of their opinion during the interview. Nearly 25 percent of them explicitly stated that the aborted fetus was a life, a person, or a human being. In many of these cases, they admitted having a sense of having killed or murdered another being. Another 25 percent expressed confusion about the nature of the fetus. In these cases, the women generally believed the fetus was human but denied that abortion was killing. Zimmerman suggests that this contradictory stance was taken in order maintain their self-images as moral persons. Finally, only 15 percent maintained that the fetus was *not* a person or human life, but even these women expressed themselves in terms of denial rather than with arguments to support their beliefs, stating, for example, "I feel that it's something there, but I don't really feel that it's a life yet."[5]

The feeling of life being killed is a common thread throughout the testimonies of women before, during, and after an abortion. According to one woman interviewed in the waiting room: "It's killing. But it is justifiable homicide." Another, shortly after her abortion, said: "Like when you have an abortion you're just destroying a part of yourself. That's the way I feel anyhow. I just feel bad inside, that's all. I didn't really want to do it. It's a sin."[6] Still another woman described her feelings after an abortion, saying: "I hated myself. I felt abandoned and lost. There was no one's shoulder to cry on, and I wanted to cry like hell. And I felt guilty about killing something. I couldn't get it out of my head that I just killed a baby."[7]

For some the anticipation of guilt itself moves them toward acts of self-punishment. An example of this was reported in a *New York Times* interview with American women who have traveled to England for RU-486 abortions. A woman from Pennsylvania explained that for her there were "psychological advantages" to the harrowing experience of repeated clinic visits for RU-486 and prostaglandin injections and in the six hours or more of labor pains to expel a dead human fetus. "I didn't want to just zip in and be put to sleep and zip out in two hours with it all done," she explains. "In a way, that would have been too easy. This was a big painful decision for me. I would have felt irresponsible if it had been over with like that. I wanted to remember this all my life. I never want to do it again."[8] For this woman the price for an abortion must be measured in something more than negotiable currency. The act must be etched in one's memory with proper solemnity. Physical and emotional pain are the only fitting tributes which can be made to a life denied.

Even in those who deny the humanity of their unborn child, there is often an admission that this denial can be maintained only by a conscious effort. For example, one woman writes: "I didn't think of it as a baby. I just didn't want to think of it that way."[9] Another insists that denial is the only way to deal with it: "I made up my mind to do it, and like I could let it drive me crazy, any woman could, but you can't, because you've got to live with it and there's really no sense in letting it drive you right off the edge."[10]

For others, even the process of discussing their experience threatens their rationalization. For example, one woman interviewed in a clinic as she awaited her third abortion at first insists she has adjusted well to the first two abortions, but then she goes on to describe experiencing symptoms which are now identified as part of postabortion syndrome. She finds herself confessing that she has developed a compulsive fascination with other people's children, experienced outbursts of anger, and had periods of depression and substance abuse. As she hears herself describing these problems, which she herself attributes to her abortion, she begins to doubt what she should believe, finally concluding: "Maybe I should go to a psychiatrist, but I really don't have the money or the interest. Truth is hard to take, and I just don't know if I'm ready for it."[11]

What is the truth, which she already knows, but is too "hard to take?" Abortion destroys a human life. Moreover, this life is her own child. This human life is also the progeny of her male partner. And their parents. And their grandparents. In this way, abortion is even more than a profound moral issue; it is a familial issue. The abortion experience defines not only how she sees herself, it also defines how she sees her family.

AMBIVALENCE

Even the most ardent defenders of abortion rights are not immune to these issues. Linda Bird Francke, a professional journalist, feminist, and a pro-choice activist, describes how when faced with an unplanned pregnancy which would have interfered with her and her husband's rising careers, the couple decided "It was time for *us*," not another child. It was a relatively easy decision. Without any emotional handwringing, the logical and practical choice was made.

It was not until Francke and her husband were actually sitting in the waiting room that an unexpected ambivalence arose. "Suddenly the rhetoric, the abortion marches I'd walked in, the telegrams sent to Albany to counteract the Friends of the Fetus, the Zero Population Growth buttons I'd worn, peeled away, and I was all alone with my microscopic baby." Intellectually, she tried to concentrate on how small the fetus was, and therefore how impossible it was for it to be human, but she had given birth before and the feel of her own body kept telling her that there was real life growing within her. "Though I would march myself into blisters for a woman's right to exercise the option of motherhood," she writes, "I discovered there in the waiting room that I was not the modern woman I thought I was."[12]

By the time she entered the operating room, Francke was desperately hoping for some release from her predetermined course. She longed for her husband to valiantly "burst" through the door and stop it from happening. When he failed to do so, and the doctor began to dilate her for the surgery, she herself begged him to stop. But the doctor told her it was too late and completed the surgery anyway. At that point she gave in: "What good sports we women are. And how obedient. Physically the pain passed even before the hum of the machine signaled that the vacuuming of my uterus was completed, my baby sucked up like ashes after a cocktail party."[13]

Afterward, her ambivalence continued. During times of relaxation when she had time to reflect on the beauty of the world, she experienced the common reaction of "visitations" from her aborted child. Her benign "little ghost" would come to her and wave. And she would tearfully wave back to reassure her lost baby that if only it returned, now they would make room for it in their busy lives.

Five years after her abortion, Francke was drawn to reinvestigate her own mixed feelings about abortion and wrote a book entitled *The Ambivalence of Abortion,* in which she transcribed the reactions to the abortion experience of almost seventy women, couples, parents, and men. What she found, as the title suggests, is widespread ambivalence, and often frank admission of guilt and remorse. Over 70 percent of those she interviewed expressed some type of negative feelings about the abortion. Most believed that abortion involves a "baby." Those who denied the human fetus's humanity did so in curt assertions that belie the edge of uncertainty. Few were as well prepared for the abortion decision as was Francke, who at least had the advantage of having been a pro-choice activist who had confronted the issues and argued for the principles used to justify abortion. Instead, most have never participated in the abortion debate. Most have deep moral reservations about abortion, yet they are aborting because they feel they have no other choice.

Francke's interviews are consistent with the findings of other researchers. These findings suggest that for most women, abortion is at best a marginal choice. Between 30 and 60 percent of women having abortions initially had a positive desire to carry the pregnancy to term and keep their babies.[14] Many of these women still desire their babies even at the time of the abortion, but they are aborting only because they feel forced to do so by others or circumstances. Indeed, over 80 percent say they would have carried to term under better circumstances or with the support of loved ones. Over 60 percent report having felt "forced" to have the abortion by others or by circumstances, and approximately 40 percent of postabortion women were still hoping to discover some alternative to abortion when going for counseling at the abortion clinic.[15]

THE ILLUSION OF CHOICE

Such data suggest that rather than "choosing" abortion, many women, perhaps even most, are just "submitting" to abortion. The rhetoric of "choice" may actually be obscuring the problem of *unwanted abortions*—abortions on women who would prefer to keep their babies if only they could receive the love and support they need to empower them as mothers.

No one can reasonably deny the testimonies of women who describe how their lovers, parents, and others have pressured, badgered, blackmailed, and even physically forced them into accepting unwanted abortions because it would be "best for everyone." Even pro-choice ethicist Daniel Callahan, director of the Hastings Center, writes: "That men have long coerced women into unwanted abortion when it suits their purposes is well-known but rarely mentioned. Data reported by the Alan Guttmacher Institute indicate that some 30 percent of women have an abortion because someone else, not the woman, wants it."[16]

These data, combined with over a thousand case studies—in my files alone— demonstrate that the decision to abort is often a tentative one, or even accepted solely to please others. For many it is nothing more than an act of despair. For all, it is an intensely emotional issue which irreversibly changes the course of one's life, and touches the very depths of one's sexuality and self-perception. It is a life-marking event. Just as after a marriage one becomes a wife, or after the birth of a child one becomes a mother, so after abortion one becomes—well, "another"—somehow different than before.

As with all life-marking events, it is human nature to look back and wonder, "How would my life be different if I hadn't married Jim? How would it be different if I never had had the twins?" So the woman who has had an abortion is inevitably confronted with the question, "How would my life be different if I had had that baby?"

For many women, the abortion clearly becomes one of those key points in their lives around which all other events take reference. In their minds, everything can be clearly placed as having occurred either "before the abortion" or "after the abortion." They may even see themselves as being two completely different people before and after this defining event. In a retrospective study of 260 women, an average of nearly eleven years after their abortions, 51 percent reported having undergone a "dramatic personality change" following their abortions, of which 79 percent said the change was a negative one.[17]

POST-ABORTION TRAUMA

Abortion is such a profound event in one's life that one must either thoughtfully integrate it into one's life, or fearfully suppress it. Neither is easy. The former requires great fortitude and honesty. The latter is simply unhealthy. It is a fundamental principle of psychiatry that suppression of emotions is the cause of numerous psychological and physical ailments. Suppressed feelings create their own internal pressures, sap emotional energy, and cause turmoil in one's life until they burst forth in a way which can no longer be ignored.

These observations are substantiated by the testimony of Dr. Julius Fogel, a psychiatrist and obstetrician who has been a long-time advocate of abortion and has personally performed twenty thousand abortions. Although he approaches abortion from a pro-choice perspective, Dr. Fogel is deeply concerned about the "psychological effects of abortion on the mother's mind." According to Dr. Fogel:

> Abortion is an impassioned subject. . . . Every woman—whatever her age, background or sexuality—has a trauma at destroying a pregnancy. A level of humanness is touched. This is a part of her own life. She destroys a pregnancy, she is destroying herself. There is no way it can be innocuous. One is dealing with the life force. It is totally beside the point whether or not you think a life is there. You cannot deny that something is being created and that

this creation is physically happening. . . . Often the trauma may sink into the unconscious and never surface in the woman's lifetime. But it is not as harmless and casual an event as many in the pro-abortion crowd insist. A psychological price is paid. It may be alienation; it may be pushing away from human warmth, perhaps a hardening of the maternal instinct. Something happens on the deeper levels of a woman's consciousness when she destroys a pregnancy. I know that as a psychiatrist.[18]

Other investigators, on both sides of the abortion issue, share Fogel's concern. Researchers have reported over one hundred psychological sequelae connected to abortion stress. These include sexual dysfunction, depression, flashbacks, sleep disorders, anxiety attacks, eating disorders, impacted grieving, a diminished capacity for bonding with later children, increased tendency toward violent outbursts, chronic problems in maintaining intimate relationships, difficulty concentrating, and a loss of pleasure in previously enjoyed activities and people. One five-year retrospective study in two Canadian provinces found that 25 percent of women who had abortions subsequently sought psychiatric care compared to 3 percent of the control group.[19]

Perhaps most disturbing is the increase of self-destructive behavior among postabortion women. Women with a history of abortions are significantly more likely to smoke, drink, and use drugs. A study of 700 women found that drug and alcohol abuse subsequent to a first pregnancy was approximately four times higher for those who aborted compared to those who carried to term.[20] Another study of 260 women who had abortions found that 37 percent described themselves as being self-destructive, with 28 percent admitting having made one or more suicide attempts.[21]

Suppression and denial are the most common means of coping with abortion. Between 60 and 70 percent of women who eventually confronted negative feelings about their abortions admitted that there was a period of time during which they would have denied to others, and themselves, any regrets or negative feelings. On average, this period of denial was about five years, with a low of one month and a high of twenty years.[22]

In general, denial and avoidance behavior is readily apparent. Participants in our case study project who claimed that their postabortion adjustment was easy almost always gave only short, concealing responses that at the same time reveal volumes. Consider the following response, which arrived just today, and is typical of the pattern I have described here:

Why did you have an abortion? "I wasn't carrying the baby right and I had knots in my stomach."
How would you describe the abortion? "I didn't like it, but I did what was best."
How did the abortion affect you? "It made me feel sad because I took another's life."

What have you done to deal with the abortion, and did it help? "Nothing really. I got over it."
How do you think the abortion changed your life? "I take better care of myself."

Notably, this woman describes that what she aborted was a "baby," not a "fetus" or a "pregnancy." She further states, very matter of factly, that in having the abortion she "took another's life." These statements suggest that this woman is not engaging in any sophisticated rationalizations. To her it is not a "potential life," it is a baby, whose death warrants sadness. In the same simple and straightforward way, she copes with this death simply by "getting over it." One hopes that she has indeed gotten over it, but one fears that in actuality she may simply be engaging in avoidance behavior which prevents true resolution and integration of the experience into her life.

SELF-DECEPTION

But, then, denial and avoidance are integral to abortion. You don't have to take my word for it. Look at *In Necessity and Sorrow*, a book by Dr. Magda Denes, a pro-choice feminist psychologist.

Shortly after her own abortion, Denes, like Francke, felt drawn to spend months at an abortion facility to observe how others experienced abortion. Unlike Francke, Denes is a trained psychologist and knows to look beyond the words of those she interviews. She sees that words of bravery are used to disguise fears, and words of calm to hide doubts. For example, when introducing the interview of one patient, she writes: "All that she says sounds honest and straightforward. It is only when she refers to the abortion that she lies, not so much to me as to herself."[23] But seeing through these self-deceptions does not mean that Denes criticizes them. Instead, she justifies denial as a necessary defense mechanism by which all people protect themselves from their worst sides: "Oh yes," she writes, "these people lie, they kid themselves, testify falsely, confess in bad faith, shirk responsibility, only pretend to honor, bracket the past, and invent their lives. And who among us does differently? Especially in times of crisis. Especially in times of irreversible choice."[24]

Self-preservation is the name of the game, and Denes clearly sees that sanity in the abortion clinic can be achieved only by a strict adherence to the rules of the game. Both patients and staff collaborate in this conspiracy of self-deceptions. Describing her interviews with both staff and patients, she writes: "Above all, this is a document on the evasions, multifaceted, clever, and shameful, by which we all live and die."[25] In the abortion clinic, she adds, "reality is a matter of courtesy. A matter of agreement not to rock the tempest-torn boat."[26]

Although Denes is personally committed to the pro-choice philosophy, her book, like Francke's, was never embraced by the pro-choice movement. It is too dark, too questioning, too disturbing. In fact, despite the opposite leanings of their authors, both Denes's and Francke's books show that abortion is at best an ugly experience, at worst a heart-wrenching nightmare. Neither is able to find any substance in the stories they tell to support the pro-choice rhetoric which they themselves earnestly believe. This failure occurs because when one studies the effects of abortion on women in an intimate and personal way, it is never an encouraging story. What emerges is always much more sorrow than joy, much more guilt than relief.

The philosophy of "choice" is admirable only when stripped of its reality, only when worshiped as an ideal, believed in its abstract. When examined from the viewpoint of women filled with despair, dread, guilt, and denial, this pro-choice rhetoric is cold and uncomforting. When examined from the viewpoint of the aftermath of breast cancer, miscarriages, ectopic pregnancies, substance abuse, suicidal tendencies, sexual dysfunction, Mother's Day depressions, and impacted grieving, it is a mockery.

In sum, speaking as one who has been there, Denes favors abortion on de-mand purely on the grounds that women should be given a choice. Yet, she is uncomfortable with that choice, for even under the most ideal circumstances, even if abortion on demand were "provided free by the state, [and] supported with mercy by the church," she believes that such a pure freedom to abort would only accentuate the horrors, doubts, guilts, and other problems which are *inherent* to abortion. "For if we remove abortions from the realm of defiance of authority," she writes,

> ... if we permit them to be acts of freedom as they should be, their meaning, private and collective, will inescapably emerge in the consciousness of every person. ... I think it is a far, far lighter task to regard oneself as a martyr and to battle the world than to know the private sorrows of unique commitments and the heartache of self-chosen destiny. I wish, therefore, to be taken for what I am. A pro-abortionist with a bad secular conscience."[27]

Denes is not unique. Because "everyone really knows" that life begins at con-ception, everyone who has ever been involved in abortions, at some level, has a bad conscience—or at least a nagging one. This is true of everyone involved: the father, the parents, siblings, friends, counselors, doctors. But it is especially true for the mother because her body has been desecrated, her body has been used by another as the actual killing ground for the child her womb was designed to pro-tect.

Like many others, Denes is compelled to admit that abortion, though justifi-able, is "a type of murder" because its victim is "alive and human." For women who allow themselves to reflect on their abortions, no other conclusion is pos-sible.

Still, those women who possess sophisticated philosophies, strong coping resources, and semantic agility can keep this aborted life at a distance. They remind themselves that it was just a "potential" life whose time for fulfillment had not yet come. They can lessen the impact by sanitizing the terms with which they think about it. But for the majority of women, who lack the sophistication, the coping skills, and verbal dexterity, this aborted life is quite simply their "baby"—a person they would have cuddled and loved if only things had been different.

For this latter group of women, their abortions were an "evil necessity." Many of them feel an immediate sense of guilt, self-condemnation, and feelings of having betrayed both themselves and their child. Others try to block out their feelings through denial and suppression, focusing on the future but eventually struggling with the past. For these women, who know that what they aborted were their "babies," the need to grieve will inevitably overtake them, and this need must be nonjudgmentally acknowledged by society and shared by their loved ones.

The future of the sophisticated woman who holds to a more dehumanized view of the life lost during her abortion is less certain. If she had integrated these beliefs into her life *before* her abortion, then there would be a congruency between what she believed and how she acted. In such a case, it may be plausible that she has not been changed or affected by her abortion experience.

But in the absence of this congruency between a woman's preabortion beliefs and her "sophisticated" postabortion mind-set, her prospects for peace of mind are not good. In this case, her more "mature" and "experienced" views are likely to be nothing more than a veneer of rationalizations which conceal, but have not obliterated, the person who once knew that abortion means the destruction of a human life. Because the modernity of this woman is just a veneer, she lacks the confidence and security of those for whom this modernity runs deep and was an integrated part of their personalities before their abortions. This woman with only the veneer of modernity is easily identified by the angry energy with which she feverishly defends the abortion liberty. She is not calmly confident of her belief system, or even capable of respecting the contrary beliefs of others. Instead, she sees every challenge to her new ethic as a personal insult precisely because these challenges reverberate through the veneer of her new ethic to disturb the slumber of an old ethic which still lays a claim to her heart.

Such a woman will know no true peace until there is an accord between the person above and below this veneer. And this peace, I suggest, can only be found when the person below is freed to grieve and repent according to the old ethic, precisely because it was this old ethic which had a claim on her conscience at the time of the abortion. It is to this old ethic which she must still provide an answer. Until she does, her new ethic, like every ethic adopted to justify past acts, is polluted with rationalization. Her new self is unstable, built upon a discordant self—a self with an unreconciled past. Such a woman is a psychological time bomb. She has unresolved pressures contained within a veneer. If that veneer is ever dropped, the emotional explosion which occurs may cause irreparable damage both to her own life and the lives of her loved ones.

So it is that when I look around the clinic's waiting room, I see lives driven by despair, not hope. I see women inwardly crying, saying good bye. And I see women whose clenched teeth and fixed eyes are determinedly set on the future because they dare not look at the past.

As I look into their many faces, the philosophical debate over when a human becomes a "person" dissolves into nothing more than ethereal elevator music. Whether these waiting women listen to it or ignore it, it has no real effect on the living of their lives. For beneath the lyric of excuses and jargon, on the level of a little girl who once asked, "Where do babies come from?", every woman here knows that life begins at conception. It is a human life. It is a familial life. It is a part of her and part of another. It is her child. The only question which remains is how she will live with this truth, or how long she will be able to run from it?

NOTES

1. Nancyjo Mann, Foreword to David C. Reardon, *Aborted Women, Silent No More* (Chicago: Loyola University Press, 1987), p. xvi.

2. Frederica Mathewes Green, *Real Choices: Offering Practical, Life-Affirming Alternatives to Abortion* (Sisters, Oreg: Questar Publications, 1994), p. 24.

3. Mary K. Zimmerman, *Passage Through Abortion: The Personal and Social Reality of Women's Experience* (New York: Praeger Publishers, 1977), p. 69; Reardon, *Aborted Women*, p. 13. Portions of this essay were drawn from *Aborted Women, Silent No More*. David C. Reardon is the editor of *The Post-Abortion Review*. A free sample of this quarterly publication is available by sending a self-addressed stamped envelope to the *The Post-Abortion Review*, P.O. Box 9097, Springfield, Illinois 62707.

4. "A New Ethic for Medicine and Society," *California Medicine* 113, no. 3 (September 1970): 67–68, italics added. *(One is reminded of Norma McCorvey's embrace of the pro-life position, saying she had 'always been pro-life.'-Ed.)*

5. Zimmerman, *Passage Through Abortion*, pp. 194–195.

6. Magda Denes, *In Necessity and Sorrow* (New York: Basic Books, 1976), p. 94.

7. Linda Bird Francke, *The Ambivalence of Abortion* (New York: Random House, 1978), p. 61.

8. *The New York Times*, 23 March 1994, cited in "The Public Square," *First Things* (June/July 1994): 79.

9. Francke, *The Ambivalence of Abortion*, p. 201.

10. Denes, *In Necessity and Sorrow*, pp. 97–98.

11. Francke, *The Ambivalence of Abortion*, p. 63.

12. Jane Doe [pseud. Linda Bird Francke], "There Just Wasn't Room in Our Lives Now for Another Baby," *The New York Times*, 14 May 1976.

13. Ibid.

14. Zimmerman, *Passage Through Abortion*, pp. 110–111; Reardon, *Aborted Women, Silent No More*, p. 12.

15. Reardon, *Aborted Women, Silent No More*, pp. 14–15.

16. Sidney Callahan, "An Ethical Challenge to Prochoice Advocates," *Commonweal*, 23 November 1990, pp. 681–687, esp. p. 684.

17. David C. Reardon, "Psychological Reactions Reported after Abortion," *The Post-Abortion Review* 2, no. 3 (Fall 1994): 4–8.

18. From an interview with columnist Colman McCarthy, "A Psychological View of Abortion," *St. Paul Sunday Pioneer Press*, 7 March 1971. Dr. Fogel, who continued to do abortions for the next two decades, reiterated the same view in a subsequent interview with McCarthy, see "The Real Anguish of Abortions," *The Washington Post*, 5 February 1989.

19. R. F. Badgley et al., *Report of the Committee on the Abortion Law*, (Supply and Services Agency, Ottawa, Canada, 1977), pp. 314–319.

20. See "New Study Confirms Link Between Abortion and Substance Abuse," *The Post-Abortion Review* 1, no. 3 (Fall 1993): 1–2.

21. Reardon, "Psychological Reactions Reported after Abortion."

22. Ibid.

23. Denes, *In Necessity and Sorrow*, p. 101.

24. Ibid., p. 122.

25. Ibid., p. xvii.

26. Ibid., p. 6.

27. Ibid., pp. xv–vxi.

Part IV

Religious Perspectives

Chapter 10

When Good Men Do Nothing: Reflections From a Modern-Day *Bürgermeister*

Michael McKenzie

First, Moloch, horrid king, besmeared with blood
Of human sacrifice, and parents' tears;
Though, for the noise of drums and timbrels loud,
Their children's cries unheard that passed through fire
To his grim idol.

—Paradise Lost, Book I

Nobody ever called General George S. Patton squeamish. In his memoirs of World War II, as he fought his way across France and Germany, Patton describes destroyed German tanks, bombed-out buildings, and even hideously burned German corpses with a martial relish. To him, that was a normal part of war. But all this death and destruction which was a part of Patton's world paled next to his first encounter with what were called "horror camps" or "hell camps."[1]

In fact, the horrors of the Ohrdruf camp even caused the hardened Patton to become physically sick and to label it "the most appalling sight imaginable."[2] The evils were so incredible, and disproved so thoroughly the notion that reported Nazi evils were mere propaganda, that Patton conceived of the idea of having first American soldiers and newsmen, then the local German inhabitants come view the camps themselves.[3]

From the very first contacts between the German civilian populace and the horrors of the camps, it was clear that some seemed to know very little about what was going on there, most had a pretty good idea, and still others aided and abetted their Nazi masters. Patton himself believed that most of the local civilians were ignorant of the "infamies" which occurred at Ohrdruf, and instead placed much of the blame on the local *Gauleiter*, a minor Nazi functionary who was responsible for party control in that area.[4]

From early on, however, there was also a healthy dose of skepticism regarding the supposed ignorance of the civilians who lived near the death camps. After all, didn't they ever notice the arriving cattle trains packed with their horrible human cargo? Weren't they suspicious when the wind blew the wrong way and the unmistakable odor of burning flesh assailed their nostrils?[5] Were there ever no instances such as the unforgettable scene in the movie *"Schindler's List,"* when ash from a nearby crematorium blanketed a local town? How about the stories of various escapees and survivors? Were they given no credence whatsoever? Certainly such thoughts must have been in the back of the reporter's mind who asked Lieutenant General Walter Bedell Smith at a press conference in 1945, "And they [the local citizenry] say they didn't know about it [the horrors of the camps]?"[6]

Frankly, the just verdict of history has been pronounced upon the German *volk* who either claimed ignorance, fear, or impotence as a reason for not acting against the Nazi Reich. After all, some brave Germans *did* act. Many of the "Confessing German Church" paid a heavy price for their opposition; some indeed paid the ultimate price. Thus, the German civilians do indeed bear their own moral responsibility for what went on at the death camps. There is culpability in helping to bring Hitler to power; there certainly is culpability in support of the Nazi war effort; and there is culpability in the self-induced mass blindness to what was happening to the Jews. No respect for authority, no claims of ignorance, and no protestations of powerlessness do anything to remove the stigma which has settled over the German civilians of that period. Even silent opposition on their part was not enough. When barbarous evil is going on, those present have a moral duty to speak out, even to act.

As I studied the history of World War II, I must admit to feeling no little anger—and a little smugness—toward those same Germans who claimed ignorance in the face of such barbarous evil. I comforted myself with the thought that such hypocrisy and cowardice could never happen here in America. Then, as I began to study the abortion issue in depth, a number of disquieting propositions took shape in my mind. They came in no particular order; in fact I had believed most of them for a long time. However, I had never before put them all together. These propositions were: (1) fully human life begins at conception; (2) in America alone, abortion was therefore killing about 2 million *people* every year; 3) there were a lot of Christians in this country who believed that both the above propositions were absolutely true; 4) the vast majority of those Christians— including myself—didn't act like we believed it;[7] 5) thus, the American church is morally analogous to those Germans half a century ago who protested that they either: didn't know, didn't care, or couldn't act.

Hence I found myself in the position of a German *Bürgermeister*, lacking only the final forced inspection of the camps. What were my excuses for my own inaction? Did not the very same reasons which so justly condemned the German civilians also condemn me? Was I not a culpable spectator at a devilish circus far worse than any envisioned half a century ago? Granted, there are differences, even important ones, between the abortion tragedy and the Holocaust. But if one believes that life, real life with all the attendant moral cords and claims of personhood, begins at conception, then are there any *moral* differences in the killing? Thus, those of us who believe that abortion snuffs out the life of a human *person* have some unpleasant comparisons to face[8]

A number of proposed explanations of the dilemma never made much headway in my thought.[9] Some Christians explained their inaction by stating obvious governmental differences between the Nazi regime and ours; others made the point that abortion is legal here, and the Nazi horrors came at the expense of even their own laws;[10] still others pointed out that the Holocaust itself occurred during time of war, and is therefore disanalogous to today. Some writers focused on the entire issue of voluntarism: after all, elective abortion is not compulsory abortion. A few thinkers attempted to distinguish between human life and human personhood, believing the latter category to be of more moral worth than the former.[11] One last answer even concerned itself with the *destiny* of the aborted baby. That is, unlike the situation with the Jewish Holocaust, at least we could comfort ourselves with the fact that the aborted unborn are in heaven.[12]

I found all of these explanations not only philosophically and theologically unsatisfying but really beside the point. For one thing, none of them really deal with the heart of the matter: whether or not Christians are acting as idle spectators in the presence of mass murder. For another, many of the writers seemed quite ready to defend their own inaction, while admitting that an actual genocide was taking place. They seemed quite clearly to be saying, "Yes, abortion is murder, but the reason we're not acting as though it is, and the reason we *shouldn't act* as though it is, is because of 'X'." That is *not* the purpose of this chapter; I am not quite willing yet to believe that we *must* be relegated to passivity in the presence of genocide. My purpose is to examine part of the social pressures and forces —sometimes unseen and unfelt—that bear down upon us. This chapter does not excuse our nonbehavior; it only tells us where to look if we want to influence and change these social forces. Ultimately, then, this work serves not as a lens through which to view the evil of others, but as a *mirror* in which to see ourselves.[13]

At the outset, two broad pathways appeared as possible answers to this dilemma: either there was something peculiar to the German and American peoples—or to their respective situations—which made their (our) inaction explainable; or, what went on in Germany during the Holocaust and what goes on now in America are analogous to other periods of persecution and genocide throughout history. Since the effects of the Fall know no racial or ethnic boundaries, I suspected that the latter alternative was closer to the truth. Thus, the ultimate answer lies in the fallenness which grips all of us; the proximate answer may very well lie in how such evil is expressed in society. Or to put it better, I am focusing on how society frames and influences evil in general, and persecutions/genocides in particular.

Thus, this examination helps to explain why so many of us who call ourselves evangelical and pro-life do so little to protest the evil of abortion. Why, for example, aren't 30 million Christians marching *en masse* on abortion clinics, demanding that they close?[14] If my explanation is valid, then it can also help us to understand how persecuting societies develop, how they operate, and how they can best be opposed in their persecution. For, it is my thesis that the unborn in this country are suffering a persecution which follows the same basic sociological patterns as other persecutions; and the only way to mitigate the persecution is to attack the patterns at their own key presuppositions.

THE PATTERNS OF PERSECUTION

In a helpful work, R. I. Moore identifies the main stages in the development of a persecuting society.[15] As historical examples of various persecuted groups, he identifies heretics, Jews, and lepers. Since the stages of persecution of each of these quite divergent groups bear the same identifiable characteristics, Moore starts with the presupposition that the explanation of the persecution "lies not with the victims but with the persecutors."[16] Furthermore, any distinctiveness of the persecuted groups "was not the cause but the result of persecution."[17] Before examining the necessary stages in the beginning of any persecution, it is worth noting that the intensity of persecution usually passed through different stages as well. A group could be subject to "pursuit, denunciation and interrogation, exclusion from the community, deprivation of civil rights and the loss of property, liberty and on occasion life itself." All of these are forms of persecution, varying mainly on the sociological pressures of different locations.[18]

The first step necessary for a group to be targeted for persecution is the obvious but no less essential requirement that the group be capable of ready identification. Moore calls this process "classification," and whether it is due to clothing, location, appearance, language, or habits, the "enemy to society" must first be able to be identified as a group, so as not to be perceived primarily as individuals.[19] It is interesting to our study to make the point that such ready identification sometimes came from earlier good motives. For example, Moore points out that society had often set Jewish communities apart in order to "protect their religious and cultural identity." Tragically, this "identification for protection" was later turned against the Jews when the political and social climates changed.[20] When writing about the Armenian genocide at the hands of the Turks, Donald E. Miller and Lorna T. Miller comment that this step necessitates that the victim group be "perceived to fall short of being fully human. It is only when the victim group is dehumanized through such labeling that genocide can occur."[21]

The second stage concerns the development of a socially constructed myth which labels the identified group as a source of social contamination and danger. A key component of this stage is the recognition that this myth may be founded "upon whatever foundation of reality."[22] The notable feature is not whether the myth is true, but whether it can serve to collectively energize and mobilize the populace to recognize the danger posed by the group in question.[23]

Thus, such myths are often composed in apocalyptic language: "the threat which the victims present is omnipresent, and so highly contagious as to be virtually irresistible . . . [t]his is the language of fear, and of the fear of social change."[24] Moore sums it up by saying that "pollution fear, in other words, is the fear that the privileged feel of those at whose expense their privilege is enjoyed."[25] We can see this scapegoat language exemplified in how the Nazis held the Jews responsible during World War II for treason, treachery, weakness of the German allies, disease, greed, and weakness of German morale. In fact, for Joseph Goebbels, head of the Nazi propaganda machine, the entire war could be summed up as the "life-and-death struggle between the Aryan race and the Jewish bacillus."[26]

Clearly, the use of dehumanizing language serves as a dialectic transition between classification and myth-making. When Goebbels employed the term "bacillus," it was meant not only to classify the Jews, but also to portray them as less than human agents of fear in the Nazi myth of racial superiority. Thus, language can act as both cause and effect within the sociological forces which propel persecution. Its use is both an attempt to force people to see others in a new light and the result of new and different attitudes and presuppositions.

The Millers also make the point that genocides frequently occur in times of widespread political and social turmoil. "Mass violence often emerges out of unstable political conditions that threaten the social order: the economy is failing, political boundaries are changing, or previously disenfranchised minority groups are progressing economically."[27] In bad or perilous times, people naturally look for scapegoats on which to pin their misfortunes.

Lastly, genocide is often carried out "in conditions that discourage intervention by outside parties."[28] This is done as a tacit acknowledgment that if people *really knew* what was going on "behind those walls," they may not approve and hence attempt to intervene. This is also, of course, an acknowledgment by the persecutors that there is a universal moral sense and that their acts are violating that sense. Having discussed the social categories which shape (and are shaped by) persecution and genocide in general, let us now examine how abortion fits the historical patterns.

THE PERSECUTED UNBORN

The unborn constitute one of the most easily definable groups possible. They are dependent on another easily definable population (i.e., women) for their very survival, they make their presence known by unmistakable signs during pregnancy, they are never confused with other groups, and they are not readily thought of as individuals. The latter characteristic will quite rightly be questioned by those people who have developed strong feelings of affection for the individual unborn child. But such feelings are usually limited to those with ties to the mother or the family. My point here is only that a disinterested observer of a pregnant woman is likely to relate her (and her unborn child) to others of the same class and type, rather than thinking in terms of the unborn child and mother as consisting of two separate individuals. Ironically, as was the case with the Jews historically, such separation of the unborn was once made almost wholly for positive reasons. Recognizing the fact that pregnancy was almost universally admired and desired in this country, our entire society went out of its way to cater to the expectant mother and her unborn baby. Although it would be far from the truth to suggest that all such feelings have vanished, it is not claiming too much to notice that neither the universality nor the level of societal approval of pregnancy has maintained the level of the past. The reason for that downswing brings us to the second requirement for persecution.

It used to be that it was mainly Christians themselves who claimed that the world was about to end. This is no more the case. To see current apocalyptic works which dwarf those of, say, a Hal Lindsey, one travels not to the Christian bookstore, but to the environmental section of the local library. Here those with advanced degrees in the sciences have taken the mantle of secular prophets, warning their readers that their very existence—*earth's* very existence—is threatened with nearly inevitable doom. Of course the causes of this peril are typically legion: toxic waste, air pollution, water pollution, ozone depletion, and destruction of the rain forest all vie in a showcase seemingly designed to scare us half to death.[29] But the one crisis which always seems to lead the list, the "mother of all catastrophes" (pun intended), is the claim that overpopulation will soon lead to irreversible calamity. In fact, it is claimed that overpopulation is actually the *cause* of all the other disasters.

Unquestionably, the guru of this apocalyptic thought is biologist Paul Ehrlich of Stanford University. When I was a biology major in the 1970s, his work *The Population Bomb* was required reading. The mere fact that many of the predictions made in that book fell flat has not changed his mind as to the peril of overpopulation. In a speech given at an Environmental Protection Agency-sponsored seminar, Ehrlich claims that the "population problem" is our number one environmental crisis, that it is inevitably linked to all other environmental crises we face today, and that unless it is solved, it is in fact pointless to try and solve any other threats to the environment.[30] We must act now to limit births, he states; else nature will step in and do the same thing by global starvation.[31] Lest anyone doubt the connection between Ehrlich's views on population control and abortion, listen to how he views the Chinese policy of involuntary population control, which mandates abortions after one child: "The Chinese have been way out front on this and have been trying to deal with the population problem in ways that are not horrendous. . . . I think it [China's policy] is as moral a program as a country of 1.1 billion people, largely undeveloped, speaking a whole series of languages, could possibly put together."[32] Clearly, any moral problems that Ehrlich has with involuntary abortion are dwarfed by the immensity of the crisis as he sees it, and the answer lies in influencing society that the entire idea of growth—economic or population—must be utterly rejected in favor of what he calls "shrinkage."[33]

This same substance and tone are echoed by Helen Caldicott, who claims that human population growth is wreaking havoc on the ecosystem. She likewise cites China's population control policy as a "good example to the rest of the world."[34]. She is incensed at what she labels the "male-dominated religions" (primarily Islam and Christianity) for promoting childbirth and rejecting abortion, and she praises Ireland's new liberalized abortion policy as an example of "enlightened political change."[35] In fact, Caldicott goes so far as to heap lavish praise on the abortifacient RU-486, claiming that she would like to be a "salesperson" for the drug, for it "induces a painless, spontaneous abortion."[36] But Caldicott spends most of her energy attacking what she sees as the inevitable link between patriarchal religions and fertility: "No longer can we say that it is God's gift that we are pregnant."[37]

It is not just the overpopulation myth which paints pregnancy and the unborn as scapegoats. That is, when a woman becomes pregnant in this sort of social climate, she is more and more aware of the popular spin on population issues. If she decides to keep the baby, she obviously has decided to weather these forces, basically making her and her unborn child part of the same "team." If this truly represents a case of "you and me against the world," there are other sociological forces which attempt to pry between the unborn child and the mother, painting the unborn as a threat, not against the world at large, but against the mother herself.

These arguments originate mainly from radical feminism, with the woman's autonomy and freedom the main issues at stake. With the concept of "choice" so all-important now, it can be forgiven someone if he or she thinks that just the concept of choice itself is more important than the option chosen. It is in this vein that Judith Jarvis Thomson gives us her famous analogy of the unconscious violinist. She asks us to believe that pregnancy is analogous to a person being hooked up involuntarily to a violinist, their kidneys being needed to cleanse the musician's circulatory system.[38] Thomson gives us this portrait to attempt to show us that even if the unborn is admitted to be fully human (as is the violinist), that doesn't mean that the mother (the one with the healthy kidneys) must keep him or her alive. Thus, the unborn child is now perceived as a threat against the mother's right to choose, her right to be independent.

Another philosophical argument which pits the unborn against the mother is made by Mary Anne Warren. Warren suggests five traits which are necessary prerequisites to human personhood, and which are absent in the unborn. The absence of these traits means that a woman's right to procure an abortion—for reasons of her "happiness and freedom"—is absolute.[39] In fact, this motif of "fetus as threat" is so strong in Warren's argument, that it is only the absence of such a threat when the baby is born which allows her to argue against infanticide (since the baby can then be put up for adoption without posing any threat to the mother).[40] It is important to reiterate that this threat to the mother posed by the unborn has nothing to do with physical endangerment. It is instead framed as if the unborn is solely a threat to the mother's total autonomy, her desired way of life. Ironically, I see these arguments as themselves acting in powerful and pervasive ways upon modern women, actually influencing them *from without* in much the same way as many feminists accuse the "patriarchally dominated society" of doing.[41] Thus, true autonomy is a fiction; the real issue is an evaluation of the ideas which constantly compete to influence us.

Hence, the killing of the unborn clearly meets the two criteria of classification and scapegoat myth. The apocalyptic language is stronger in the formulation of the overpopulation myth, but it is not uncommon for "pro-choice" rhetoric to bring in similar language of fear. It is the fear of rights being taken away, the seemingly countless women killed by "back-alley abortions"; it is the fear of American women regressing into the primitive and patriarchal past. This common language of fear, and the realization that the same group is the scapegoat in both myths, convinces me that these two myths—the unborn as threat to *both* world and mother—are really two sides of the same coin. Hence, these two myths coalesce to form a doubly heavy weight: women are pressured to abort to save the world, *and* to preserve their "happiness and freedom." If one is convinced that his or her action is both morally praiseworthy *and* conducive to personal happiness, that is a powerful influence indeed. Bystanders feel these pressures no less keenly. Men are especially hesitant to speak out against abortion, fearing that they will be charged with oppressing women.

As mentioned earlier, the very way pro-choice advocates use language to devalue the unborn serves to bridge the gap between classification and scapegoat myth. Gary Gillespie analyzes the emotive power of abortion language on several levels.[42] Applying Stephen Littlejohn's cognitive grid to abortion language used by all sides of the issue, Gillespie describes four levels of language use, beginning with the least emotive: fact, value, theme, and metaphor. At the least emotive level of "fact," abortion advocates employ medical terms for the unborn such as "a spot of blood," "a specialized collection of cells," "birth matter," or "pregnancy tissue." At the more emotive level of "value," the terms become less medical and more likely to dehumanize the unborn: "devitalized tissue," "feto-placental unit," and "products of conception." At the level of "theme," the abortion advocacy rhetoric actually pits the unborn against the mother. Here, the unborn is labeled "worm," "parasite," "glob of cells," and "cancer-like cells."[43] Although in all categories the language is deliberately crafted so as to deny humanity and/or personhood to the unborn, it is clearly at the thematic level where the unborn are the most dehumanized—even demonized—and hence are most likely to fit into the scapegoat myth. After all, who would think twice about destroying parasites or cancer?

Viola Bernard, Perry Ottenberg, and Fritz Redl divide dehumanization into two types: "object-directed" and "self-directed."[44] Self-directed aims inward, devaluing one's own humanity; object-directed looks outward and identifies others as lacking the key characteristics of humanness. It is essential to see how the two forms are mutually reinforcing: one's perception of others as less than human lessens one's own sense of self; such deprecation of self leads inevitably to a lack in relating to others.[45] In the abortion tragedy, prospective parents often perceive themselves unworthy because they have dared to conceive a child (especially so, if it is out of wedlock); these feelings of dehumanization feed similar feelings toward their unborn child.

Other players in this tragedy illustrate object-directed dehumanization. Abortionists and spectators often demonstrate classic object-directed symptoms. Abortionists who perform numerous late-term abortions are forced into constructing elaborate defense mechanisms which act as a "self-automatizing detachment from a sense of *personal* responsibility."[46] To nourish this diminished sense of responsibility, they portray the unborn with classic dehumanizing language. Thus, when the unborn are viewed as inanimate objects, the abortionist and spectator can "write off" any misery or pain of the unborn as something that "just couldn't be helped."[47]

Abortion also fits the Miller's two criteria of unstable social and political climates, and the "cloisterization" of the genocide. The so-called end of the Cold War brought little in terms of long-term optimism to Americans; there remains a great deal of *angst* regarding the future. The very real threat of crime keeps many people in terror on a constant basis; there is a widespread lack of confidence in the ability of education to provide any answers whatsoever; and there is a rising attitude that government has not only failed to provide any answers, but may be *incapable* of providing any. Pervading all this discord is an attitude of complete helplessness—there is the inevitability of a Greek tragedy in the air. Certainly, the latter attitude has been helped along by those in academia who have long since given up the search for universal truths. It is in this social climate that abortion is on the rise; it is in this climate that we hear of the evils of overpopulation.

It is often said by pro-lifers that if there was a window into the womb, there would be fewer abortions. Probably so. Quite rightly, if we could see the miracle of life unfolding, there would no doubt be less desire to destroy it. But more to the point, if abortions were performed in a more accessible setting, or if attendance at an abortion were somehow made mandatory for all of society, there would doubtlessly be fewer abortions still. As it is, however, abortions are performed in places that are walled off from the public; and 2 million unborn are killed each year in this country in complete anonymity. Some of the insulation is obviously due to the abortion centers becoming focal points of violence. Nevertheless, it is valid to ask whether abortion would be as popular if all of us could see what the abortionist sees. Certainly, it cannot be questioned that abortion, like the historical examples of genocide, deliberately takes place as far away from the public eye as possible.

Thus, abortion as the persecution—even genocide—of the unborn fits the social pattern of other persecutions and genocides. The pressures brought to bear by abortion advocates are framed in much the same way as was the case with other dominant, persecuting groups: the victim group is identified and classified, and then typecast as villain and scapegoat in a foundational myth. To oppose this myth is to oppose the greater good (either world survival or the mother's autonomy). The unborn as scapegoat is fully realized in our troubled times of moral relativism; and abortion becomes our "dirty little secret," hidden away from public scrutiny. Hence, conditions are ripe for the paralysis of the public, the only ones who can stop this genocide of the truly helpless.

MUST WE STAND BY?

C. S. Lewis, in *The Problem of Pain*, helps us to refocus the issue properly. He ends the chapter on Hell with the advice to those would-be judges of others: "This chapter is not about your wife or son, nor about Nero or Judas Iscariot; it is about you and me."[48] I might put it this way: "This paper is not about Planned Parenthood or the abortion doctors; it is really about you and me." I have already described how societal pressures—personal, social, and philosophical—have combined to portray having children not only as "politically incorrect," but, in many instances, as an offense against the planet itself. These pressures not only undoubtedly influence prospective mothers, but also society at large. For example, 50 percent of those claiming to be "Born-Again Christians" label environmentalism a "very important issue" which influences their voting patterns.[49] Also, the birthrate has fallen steadily in the United States and is now at approximately 1.8 children per couple.[50] Clearly, at some level, we in this country have bought into the idea that there are entirely too many people in the world and we should do our part to correct that problem. Nevertheless, I want to turn the spotlight briefly—if intensely—on those of us who are involved with the abortion issue only as spectator. What are the specific social pressures bearing down upon us *as bystanders*?

In nearly every ethics course, students hear the story of Kitty Genovese, sadistically murdered in New York City, while thirty-eight of her neighbors watched but did nothing to help her. Why, it is asked, did none of her neighbors either intervene or even call the police from the safety of their own apartments? In the literature that arose during this time period, it is helpful to examine some of the social influences which prompt nonintervention by bystanders in emergency situations.

Bibb Latane and John M. Darley have examined the phenomenon of by-stander non-intervention, and in labeling intervention as a *process* and not a spontaneous decision, they have identified four critical criteria for intervention. The satisfaction of each, they say, is essential to any successful intervention.[51] The first criterion in the process is that the bystander must notice that something is wrong. Whether the event occurs in the subject's immediate presence, or whether he is informed by others, the subject must decide that something is not as it should be.[52] In applying this criterion to abortion intervention, since the act of abortion itself is carried out in designed isolation, it is not hard to see how even this baseline criterion may go unmet.

The bystander must next define the event as an emergency. Here, any ambiguities act to soften the possible emergency and hence dull the bystander's desire to intervene. If others are not acting, then perhaps what's taking place isn't an emergency after all.[53] It takes little imagination to see these influences at work in the nonintervention of abortion. Those who protest abortion are often portrayed as crackpots or fanatics, hardly examples to emulate. Subconsciously, many of us think: "If abortion were really that evil, wouldn't there be lots of 'normal people' out there protesting?" Also, there is a great deal of ambiguity about abortion within the Christian community. In a survey of those calling themselves "born again," nine issues ranked ahead of abortion in ranking of importance.[54] Moreover, a substantial number of us apparently have doubts as to whether *our own* position is even the correct one.[55] As a nation in general, and as the body of Christ in particular, we're just not all that sure that abortion is the sort of an emergency which deserves our active and personal intervention.

The third stage is reached when the bystander evaluates the emergency as his or her own personal *responsibility* to act.[56] It's not just the attitude of "let someone else do it" (although that undoubtedly plays a part). Rather, it is the modern American trend to defer to the expert: if doctors, nurses, and clergymen don't seem all that vexed about abortion, then what business is it of mine? In addition, the perceived status of the victim comes into play. If the bystander thinks the victim may somehow *deserve* what's happening, then he will be far less likely to intervene.[57] At first glance, it would seem as if the unborn are the undeserving victim *par excellence*, but recall the persuasive power of the over-population myth. It's not a hard stretch to imagine that many of us, when hearing of a specific abortion, may silently think to ourselves, "Well, it's a tragedy, but there's too many people already. Perhaps it's all for the best."

Lastly, even if the bystander has fulfilled all the above stages, he or she must still decide *how* to help.[58] Latane and Darley divide this final stage into two possibilities: acting *directly* to stop the emergency, and acting by way of *detour*, calling on those more qualified to deal with such situations.[59] Here, the idea of personal risk intrudes most harshly; that is, what are the possible negative consequences if I intervene? Clearly, the social pressures surrounding the abortion issue come into play here. New federal statutes have made the price of some forms of civil disobedience at abortion clinics extremely costly for the protester. He or she must be willing to risk not only personal pain and disgrace, but also financial ruin and long separation from family and friends. When such costs are weighed with the ambiguities which many Christians already feel about abortion, it is no wonder that many Christians are reticent about engaging in such active forms of intervention. The Christian bystander is also unlikely to intervene by way of "detour." It is the state, the experts themselves, who are guarding the abortion clinics and protecting both clients and doctors. If any intervention is to occur, the bystander knows that he or she must act directly and take the consequences.

If the bystander fails to take any of the above steps, he will fail to intervene.[60] As a result, the Christian bystander is faced with enormous social pressures not to intervene, not to resist the pressures of social conformity. Interestingly, Latane and Darley's findings indicate that bystanders often deny that social pressures influenced them not to act, even though it was conclusively proven that in fact it was those very same pressures which produced their inaction.[61] Another complicating factor has to do with the passage of time. The longer a bystander waits, the less likely he is to intervene.[62] Abortion in America has been legal for over twenty years; in all probability, as time passes, Christian intervention on a mass scale will be less and less likely.

TOWARDS THE FUTURE

In view of how these social pressures are formed, and how they act to influence all those involved in the abortion issue, we Christians must act to reverse their pervasive effects. First, we must strive to "re-humanize" the unborn. Whether by pointing to the strides made by fetology in showing us the remarkable abilities of the unborn, or by our own use of nonsterile language,[63] we must insist on utilizing every device possible which stresses the humanity of nascent life. This linkage between the born and the unborn serves to reduce the tendency to see the unborn as a special group, ready for classification and persecution.

Second, we must attack the foundational myth at its source. Despite the politically correct views of the day, scientists themselves are sharply divided on whether or not a population crisis even exists. There are excellent data which suggest that the entire idea of an apocalyptic overpopulation crisis is a gross simplification of a complex issue, and a rehashing of outdated and misguided theories.[64] Christians should make themselves aware of such data and dispute the doomsayers, effectively cutting the connection between the myth and the unborn.

Third, the idea that pregnancy is a gift from God and something to be cherished ought to be encouraged. Understanding the inevitable links between societal attitudes and laws, it is nevertheless the case that pregnant women should get special considerations, concerning everything from more convenient parking spaces to better seats on buses.[65] Relatedly, Christians should lobby against laws which discourage pregnancy (i.e., by taxation).

Fourth, keeping in mind the Miller's point that genocide often thrives in secrecy, Christians ought to continue exposing what goes on in abortion clinics. Whether or not abortion is "America's dirty little secret," many Christians (and others of good-will) would be horrified to see an actual abortion. Questions of taste must pale before issues of genocide—we have a responsibility to show the truth. Historically, public exposure has tended to discourage genocide; perhaps abortion will follow this pattern. I must admit, however, that I am not overly optimistic.

As I write this, the avenues open for Christians to actively protest abortion are being slowly, yet inexorably, choked. Legislative attempts by various states to restrict or modify *Roe v. Wade* have generally been overturned. As mentioned, draconian fines and prison terms have often been levied against those who dare even to *peacefully* protest at clinic locations. Socially, protesters are pariahs, cast as fanatics on the extreme fringes of society.

Within the Christian community itself, there are signs that apathy toward abortion is growing, tending to polarize evangelicals even further. Many Christians are simply tired of it all. "We tried our best, our efforts failed, it's all in God's hands now." This closure of what have always been viewed in America as legitimate avenues of protest will undoubtedly serve to energize those who see even civil disobedience as not going far enough. Violence at abortion clinics and violence against abortionists will be sporadic but will not go away. To quote Dickens's Ghost of Christmas Present, "if these shadows remain unaltered by the Future," the persecution, the genocide of the unborn will continue; and we Christians will pray, write many books and letters of protest, and continue life very much as before. But let us not do one thing: let us not point with accusing fingers at the busy German people of half a century ago and shrilly denounce them for idly sitting by while 6 million Jews went to their deaths. Instead, let us pray for strength and wisdom, asking the Lord what exactly He would have us do, and then let us quietly ask for mercy and forgiveness.

NOTES

1. We unfortunately have followed the Nazi practice of labeling such camps "concentration camps," such linguistic sterilization hiding their diabolic function. All early references to these camps, however, labeled them "hell camps," "horror camps," or "slave camps." As this chapter shows, language acts as a powerful cause and effect of societal morality.

2. George S. Patton, *War as I Knew It* (New York: Houghton Mifflin, 1947), p. 199. Patton understandably omits his illness in his memoirs, but it is mentioned by

General Omar Bradley in his own memoirs, *A Soldier's Story* (New York: Henry Holt and Co., 1951), p. 539.

3. This policy was fully approved and implemented by General Eisenhower. To Eisenhower, these camps produced the "worst memories of the war" and were "indisputable evidence of Nazi brutality and ruthless disregard of every shred of decency." See Dwight D. Eisenhower, *Crusade in Europe* (Garden City, N.Y.: Doubleday & Co., 1948), pp. 408, 441.

4. Patton, *War as I Knew It*, p. 204.

5. According to John Powell, the guides at Dachau explained that when the crematoria of the camps were operating, the odor of burned flesh could be detected for six miles. See John Powell's *Abortion: The Silent Holocaust* (Allen, Tex.: Argus, 1981), p. 22.

6. Cited by Eisenhower's naval aide, Harry C. Butcher, at a press conference on April 21, 1945, in Butcher's *My Three Years with Eisenhower* (New York: Simon and Schuster, 1946), p. 815.

7. Let me be clear that I am speaking about physical, non-violent intervention on behalf of the unborn by Christians (rather than non-physical methods such as letters to the editor, etc.). Such intervention might take the form of marches, protests, civil disobedience, and picketing. Some Christians obviously do take part in such forms of protest against abortion, but most do not. I am also not referring to taking up arms against abortionists. Although some may argue that the logic of my position leads to such conclusions, I do not agree. This essay focuses on the sociological pressures that influence Christians not to engage in traditional forms of American civil disobedience against abortion. Such pressures make their presence felt when active intervention of any kind is contemplated; the mere fact that the more involved the contemplated intervention, the more severe the pressures, does not invalidate the examination of the pressures themselves.

8. I'm fully aware that many non-Christian (and some Christian) thinkers differentiate between human life and personhood in regard to the unborn. I think such distinctions irrelevant and arbitrary. Hence, the ultimate (and unargued) presupposition of this chapter is that human personhood begins at conception.

9. The Holocaust is one of the favorite analogies of evangelicals writing about abortion.
Powell's work obviously makes the connection, as does James K. Hoffmeier, ed., *Abortion: A Christian Understanding and Response* (Grand Rapids: Baker Book House, 1987), p. 11. Many Christian parachurch and political organizations likewise make the analogy, but the stress is mainly on the acts of killing. This chapter, however, focuses on the role of the Christian as spectator.

10. Even if this explanation is valid, it is only so for part of the Holocaust. Many Jews were immorally slaughtered under the sanction of German laws—especially later in the war.

11. As mentioned, I do not follow such reasoning. For one thing, such a *tertium quid* between humanity and the animal kingdom creates more moral difficulties than it solves.

12. I have had several conversations with Christians who used this as a source of comfort (and a reason not to act).

13. I am also *not* addressing the theological reasons which many Christians cite for their failure to actively intervene against abortion. That ground has been well covered, and such reasons sound sadly similar to those cited by many German Lutherans during World War II.

14. According to surveys, 12 percent of Americans (approximately 30 million people) consider themselves "evangelical," consider the Bible the written Word of God, and read the Bible at least once a week outside church. See George Barna's *The Barna Report, 1992–93* (Ventura, Calif.: Regal Books, 1992), p. 81. Likewise, over 95 percent of those calling themselves "evangelicals" view abortion as "immoral behavior" and as "murder." See James Davison Hunter's *American Evangelicalism* (New Brunswick, N.J.: Rutgers University Press, 1983), pp. 85, 103. But I argue that there is a "soft core" to such claims, allowing society to significantly influence evangelical behavior regarding abortion.

15. R.I. Moore, *The Formation of a Persecuting Society* (Oxford: Blackwell Publishers, 1987).

16. Ibid., p. 67.

17. Ibid.

18. Ibid., p. 99.

19. Ibid., pp. 66, 68, 80, 88.

20. Ibid., pp. 27, 40.

21. Donald E. Miller and Lorna Touryan Miller, *Survivors: An Oral History of the Armenian Genocide* (Los Angeles: University of California Press, 1993), p. 45.

22. Moore, *The Formation of a Persecuting Society*, p. 99. Also, see Miller and Miller, *Survivors: An Oral History of the Armenian Genocide*, p. 46.

23. I am avoiding any analysis of whether or not the various foundational myths are valid. I do think, however, that the foundational myth for abortion—overpopulation as crisis—is vastly overblown and oversimplified. What I am mainly concerned with is the myth's power in modern society to motivate people, both to action—and inaction.

24. Moore, *The Formation of a Persecuting Society*, p. 100.

25. Ibid., p. 101.

26. Joseph Goebbels, *The Goebbels Diaries*, Louis P. Lochner, trans. (New York: Doubleday & Co., 1948), p. 148.

27. Miller and Miller, *Survivors: An Oral History of the Armenian Genocide*, p. 46.

28. Ibid., p. 46.

29. I was amazed at the sheer number of such works.

30. Anthony Wolbarst, ed., *Environment in Peril* (Washington, D.C.: Smithsonian Institution Press, 1991), pp. 110, 119–20.

31. Ibid., pp. 111–12.

32. Ibid., pp. 131, 132.

33. Ibid., p. 129.

34. Helen Caldicott, *If You Love This Planet: A Plan to Heal the Earth* (New York:

W.W. Norton, 1992), p. 115.

35. Ibid., p. 116.

36. Ibid., p. 118.

37. Ibid., p. 121.

38. As found in Thomson's "A Defense of Abortion," in Tom Beauchamp and LeRoy Walters, eds., *Contemporary Issues in Bioethics* (Belmont, Calif.: Wadsworth Publishing Co., 1989), p. 191.

39. Thomas Mappes and Jane Zembaty, eds., *Biomedical Ethics* (New York: McGraw-Hill, 1986), p. 469.

40. Ibid.

41. It is not my purpose to evaluate these arguments here. The fact that I find them weak and specious is not the issue; the issue concerns their prevalence and power in our society.

42. Gary Gillespie, "Abortion as Symbolic Action," in David Mall, ed., *When Life and Choice Collide: Essays on Rhetoric and Abortion* Vol. 1 in *To Set the Dawn Free*, David Mall, ed., (Libertyville, Ill.: Kairos Books, 1994).

43. See Gillespie, "Abortion as Symbolic Action," pp. 232, 233, 235.

44. Chapter 8 in Nevitt Sanford and Craig Comstock, eds., *Sanctions For Evil: Sources of Social Destructiveness* (San Francisco: Jossey-Bass, 1971).

45. Ibid., p. 104.

46. Ibid., p. 113. The application of these categories of dehumanization to abortion is mine. However, some abortionists and many of their nurses have stopped their involvement in such abortions, saying in effect, "We just couldn't do it anymore." In the face of the obvious fact of the destruction of a human baby, it is little wonder that most people either construct elaborate defense mechanisms or quit doing abortions altogether.

47. Ibid., p. 116.

48. C. S. Lewis, *The Problem of Pain* (New York: Macmillan, 1962), p. 128.

49. Barna, *The Barna Report*, 1992–93, p. 145.

50. See Wolbarst, *Environment in Peril*, p. 132.

51. Bibb Latane and John M. Darley, *The Unresponsive Bystander: Why Doesn't He Help?* (New York: Appleton-Century-Crofts, 1970). They actually cite five stages, but I have collapsed numbers four and five together into the final stage of decision making.

52. Ibid., pp. 31, 32.

53. Ibid., pp. 31, 33.

54. Barna, *The Barna Report*, 1992–93, p. 145.

55. Hoffmeier, ed., *Abortion: A Christian Understanding and Response*, p. 220.

56. Latane and Darley, *The Unresponsive Bystander: Why Doesn't He Help?*, pp. 32, 34, 90.

57. Ibid., p. 33.

58. Ibid., p. 34.

59. Ibid., pp. 34–35.

60. Ibid., p. 121.

61. Ibid., pp. 124, 125.

62. Ibid., p. 122.

63. In this chapter, I have consciously chosen to use the term unborn rather than the usual—and more sterile—fetus. Whatever such usage lacks in style, it makes up in pointing to the humanity of the unborn.

64. To cite just one example, see Dixy Lee Ray and Lou Guzzo, *Environmental Overkill* (Washington, D.C.: Regnery Gateway, 1993).

65. I am convinced that laws play their own part in shaping attitudes; we need not wait for the proper attitudes to arrive first!

Chapter 11

The Catholic Debate on the Moral Status of the Embryo

Tom Poundstone

From a moral point of view this is certain . . . it is objectively a grave sin to dare to risk murder.
—Congregation for the Doctrine of the Faith, *Declaration on Abortion*[1]

The Catholic Church's position on abortion, in *vitro* fertilization, and embryo experimentation is primarily rooted in its assessment of the nature of the fetus. What is that assessment, what are the grounds for its being held, and what are the objections of Catholic ethicists who dissent from this teaching?

Contrary to popular opinion, the Catholic Church does not teach that ensoulment or fully human life begins at conception. Such a misunderstanding is understandable. The official stance of the Church's hierarchical magisterium is that, since we cannot be certain that ensoulment does not take place at conception, we should act as though it does. To act otherwise in such a situation of doubt would be to risk murder.

It cannot be denied, and the Church does not try to deny, that its teaching on prenatal life has undergone numerous subtle changes. Although abortion has been consistently condemned from the earliest days of the Christian community, early Fathers of the Church such as Jerome (342-420) and Augustine (354-430) distinguished between unformed and formed fetuses, reserving the classification of homicide for abortions taking place after formation. Others like Basil of Cappadocia (330-379) rejected such "hair-splitting" differences between formed and unformed fetuses, classifying all deliberately committed abortion as homicide.

ENSOULMENT

Gradually, this line of discussion became assimilated to the discussion on ensoulment, a matter on which Jerome and Augustine had remained cautiously agnostic. For centuries many in the Church accepted a theory of delayed ensoulment. The greatest theologian in the Church's history, Thomas Aquinas (1224-1274), accepted Aristotle's view that the conception of the male was not completed until the fortieth day and the female not until the nineteenth. The Council of Trent (1545-1563) reflected this belief by restricting penalties for "homicide" to abortion of an animated fetus only. Thomas' theory remained the general belief of the Church until the nineteenth century.

With the rise of genetic and embryological studies, the idea of immediate ensoulment gradually gained support and then solidified its hold within the Church. No particular stage of development (e.g., implantation, initial brain waves, quickening, viability, birth) presented itself as so significant as to indicate that before that stage the fetus could not have been ensouled and after which it must be. Once all other alternatives were rejected, the fetus began to be viewed as having been ensouled as a fully human person from conception. The emphasis was now on the continuous development of potentialities which the ensouled individual with her or his unique genetic package possessed from the moment of syngamy.

Despite this convergence of embryological information, the Church has refrained from making a dogmatic declaration. In its strong condemnations of abortion in the encyclical *Casti Connubii* (1930) and at the Second Vatican Council (1965), the time of ensoulment was not mentioned. Interestingly, the final draft of the Council's *Gaudium et Spes* #51 changed an earlier reference from "life in the womb" to "from the moment of conception onwards" lest a question be raised about the moral status of the fertilized ovum before entering the uterus. A note by the drafting committee, however, explicitly stated that the time of animation is not touched upon.[2]

In the *Declaration on Abortion* (1974), the Congregation for the Doctrine of the Faith cites the evidence offered by modern genetics, but it refrains from drawing a conclusion on when ensoulment takes place. In a footnote, the Congregation leaves no doubt that it is not defining the moment of ensoulment. It writes:

> This declaration expressly leaves aside the question of the moment when the spiritual soul is infused. There is not a unanimous tradition on this point and authors are as yet in disagreement. For some it dates from the first instant, for others it could not at least precede nidation. It is not within the competence of science to decide between these views, because the existence of an immortal soul is not a question in its field.[3]

In that document the Congregation incorporates the modern human/person distinction to make its point. Regardless of the time of ensoulment, at the moment of syngamy there is a new, genetically distinct human life deserving of respect and protection. The moment of ensoulment, if it does not coincide with syngamy, marks the transformation from human life to human personhood. The

Congregation does not claim that there is unanimous agreement on when this takes place, but it lists no other proposed alternative occurring later than nidation, more commonly known as implantation.

In *Donum Vitae*(1987), the same Congregation stresses even more clearly that scientific evidence is clearly leading human reason to conclude that the presence of human life and personhood are inseparable. Since the thirteen years between the publication of the two documents has ushered in the age of *in vitro* fertilization, it is not surprising that the Congregation has chosen to stress its view that ensoulment dates from the moment of syngamy. It writes:

> Certainly no experimental datum can be in itself sufficient to bring us to the recognition of a spiritual soul; nevertheless, the conclusions of science regarding the human embryo provide a valuable indication for discerning by the use of reason a personal presence at the moment of this first appearance of human life: How could a human individual not be a person?[4]

Note the rhetorical question at the end of this passage from *Donum Vitae*: "How could a human individual not be a person?" To answer that question, those who suspect that ensoulment might be delayed cite a distinction between genetic individualization and developmental individualization. During the first two weeks after conception, there is a possibility of both twinning and recombination. In twinning, the multiplying cells of an embryo divide, forming two genetically identical embryos eventually resulting in identical twins. Much less common, but still documented, is the phenomenon in which two genetically distinct embryos combine to form one embryo, a chimera. Although these events are somewhat rare, our experience with *in vitro* fertilization has shown that the potential for twinning is inherent in all human embryos given the appropriate circumstances.[5]

Both of these possibilities pose severe problems for the idea of individuality thought necessary to accommodate ensoulment. In traditional Catholic understanding, the soul is unique, indivisible, and indestructible. In the case of twinning, a soul would have to be infused at a point later than conception; in the case of chimera formation, two souls would somehow have to be reduced to one through either a fusion or a disappearance of one. In response to these challenges, those in disagreement with the Vatican's stance of immediate ensoulment have postulated a delayed ensoulment taking place sometime after twinning and recombination can no longer occur, a time corresponding closely with implantation and the development of the primitive streak at a gestational age of roughly twelve days. It should be stressed that this window of doubt concerning the presence of personhood is confined to this very early stage of pregnancy.

In the *Declaration on Abortion*, despite its acknowledgment of a variety of opinions within the Church, the Congregation claims that its moral stance is independent of whether the soul is created and infused at conception or after the point of developmental individualization. It is the independent status of its moral argument which enables the Congregation to leave unanswered the time of ensoulment. The Congregation expresses its moral argument as follows: "From a moral point of view this is certain: even if a doubt existed concerning whether the fruit of conception is already a human person, it is objectively a grave sin to dare to risk murder."[6]

This argument is further elaborated on in the following excerpt from a footnote to the text:

> [O]ur moral affirmation remains independent [of science] for two reasons: (1) supposing a belated animation, there is still nothing less than a *human* life, preparing for and calling for a soul in which the nature received from its parents is completed; (2) on the other hand it suffices that this presence of the soul be *probable* (and one can never prove the contrary) in order that the taking of life involve accepting the *risk* of killing a person, not only waiting for, but already in possession of his or her soul.[7]

The shape of this moral argument might come as a surprise to a reader of the text. It acknowledges that we cannot be certain as to when ensoulment takes place, yet it is still able to establish a certain moral conclusion despite that uncertainty. Whereas many ethicists argue that such acknowledged uncertainty about the time of ensoulment might provide some leeway in terms of what actions are morally permissible, the Congregation categorically forbids such laxity. The key to the argument is determining the nature and extent of moral responsibility in situations of doubt that involve questions of human life and justice.

THE SAFEGUARDING OF THE PERSON

The fact that the Congregation has chosen to italicize the words "probable" and "risk" indicates the centrality which they play in the argument. In the tradition of Catholic moral theology, "probable" does not mean "more than likely to be true," but simply that it is "arguable." It means that strong arguments can be given in support of it. However, more than one possibility might be described as "probable," with some being more probable than others. At times, therefore, it would be more accurate to translate it as "possible, but not necessarily very likely." In this case, the proposition will always maintain its status of being "probable" precisely because the contrary cannot be proven, even though the contrary might be more likely. That is the meaning of the term when the Congregation writes, "[I]t suffices that this presence of the soul be *probable* (and one can never prove the contrary)."

In Catholic ethics, that a position is "probable" is not always sufficient for it to be held. What gives it additional weight in this particular situation is the other italicized word in the argument: "risk." Since the risk in this situation is murder, the obligation to overcome doubt before acting is imperative. Unless the doubt can be overcome, the risk of committing murder cannot be morally justifiable.

The classic example to illustrate this situation is that of a hunter who is not certain whether the movement in the thicket is that of deer or another human. Traditionally, it has been held that in such a situation of doubt the hunter may not shoot. The situation, however, may be more nuanced than that. John Mahoney notes that two circumstances are particularly relevant in responding to this case. First, what if the hunter has taken a great degree of care to eliminate the likelihood that a human is in the bush? Second, what difference does the motivation of the hunter make? Does his own survival, or that of others, depend upon his securing a supply of food, or is he simply hunting for pleasure? Mahoney thinks that the correlation between the degree of likelihood and the degree of necessity is the crucial factor in determining this case.

The Congregation's stance is that in such situations of doubt the safest course must be followed. Even if it is highly unlikely that no harm will occur, nothing can justify such risk taking. This position in Catholic moral theology, adopting the safest position even if it might be doubtful in content or in application, is formally known as "tutiorism." Kevin Kelly describes it as follows:

> As long as we are not 100% certain, it argues, we must play safe and avoid all risk of directly killing a fully human being. And since it accepts that 100% certainty on this issue is humanly impossible, it regards its position on abortion as definitive and unchangeable. Any discussion among theologians, it would claim, can at best be purely theoretical.[8]

That "theoretical" discussion among theologians which Kelly refers to questions the tutioristic or safest stand which the Church has taken. Some advocate what in Catholic moral theology has been called "probabiliorism," a stance which says that one can follow a position opposed to an obligation if and only if it is more probable than the proposition supporting the obligation, that is, when it is more likely to be right.[9]

Ethicists like Mahoney argue that the degree of moral risk corresponds to the degree of probability or likelihood that one is dealing with an ensouled human person. If it can be shown, as many believe the argument from twinning and recombination shows, that it is highly unlikely that the preimplantation embryo is not an ensouled human person, the risk that one is committing homicide is correspondingly slight.[10] Note that Mahoney counters the Congregation's assertion by looking more closely at the scientific record to support or discredit his theory of when ensoulment is most likely. The Congregation, though it initially supported its argument with scientific findings, ultimately roots its argument in a negative assertion: "[I]t suffices that this presence of the soul be *probable* (and one can never prove the contrary)."

This internal challenge to the Church's "safest" interpretation has come not in discussions concerning abortion, but in considerations of *in vitro* fertilization. Karl Rahner, the leading Catholic theologian of this century, recognized that the "safety first" argument must be weighed against other important values that might be being sacrificed in the name of unjustified safety. He writes,

> Catholic theology presupposes that at the moment of union of the male and female cells a human being comes into existence as an individual person with his or her own rights. If this is the case, such a person is no more an inconsequential possible object for experiments than the prisoners of Nazi concentration camps were. . . . A one-hour-old human being has as much right to the integrity of his person as a human being of nine months or sixty years.

> Nowadays, however, the above mentioned presupposition is no longer held with certainty, but is exposed to positive doubt. . . . Of course it does not follow from the fact of such an uncertainty that experiments with fertilized embryonic material are equivalent to morally indifferent experiments with mere "things." But it would be conceivable that, given a serious positive doubt about the human quality of the experimental material, the reasons in favor of experimenting might carry more weight, considered rationally, than the uncertain rights of a human being whose very existence is in doubt.[11]

Richard McCormick, the dean of American Catholic ethicists, thinks that the cumulative effect of the phenomena cited in opposition to seeing human personhood present at conception gives probable reason for believing that respect for life does not make the same demands at the preimplantation stage of development as it does after implantation. As a result of that conclusion, he felt himself able to vote in approval of the research and testing necessary for successful *in vitro* fertilization in his capacity as a member of the Ethics Advisory Board to the Department of Health, Education and Welfare (HEW) in 1978. However, he notes that it was a decision not made without "fear and trembling."[12] This trepidation is reflected in his insistence that the original report for HEW specifically say that the phrase "acceptable from an ethical standpoint" be understood as "ethically defensible but still legitimately controverted." The dispute, he says, is not finished. It leaves the matter open for further reconsideration and revision, but there is sufficient basis for action at the present without waiting for greater certitude.

Rahner, Mahoney, and McCormick would not agree that the doubt about the preimplantation status of the fetus is great enough to legitimate abortions. The window which they have granted *in vitro* fertilization is only the first fourteen days of an embryo's life (preimplantation, predevelopment of the primitive streak, a period of high wastage, and a period when twinning and recombination are possible). Furthermore, they do not grant a blank check to scientists. One's purpose in tampering with human life, albeit pre-personal life, must still survive strict moral scrutiny.

NOTES

1. Congregation for the Doctrine of the Faith, *Declaration on Abortion* (Vatican City: Vatican Polyglot Press), 18 November 1974, note 19.

2. John T. Noonan, "An Almost Absolute Value in History," in John T. Noonan, ed., *The Morality of Abortion: Legal and Historical Perspectives* (Cambridge, Mass.: Harvard University Press, 1970), p. 46 n. 158.

3. Congregation for the Doctrine of the Faith, *Declaration on Abortion*, note 19.

4. Congregation for the Doctrine of the Faith, *Donum Vitae* (*Instruction on Respect for Human Life in Its Origin and on the Dignity of Procreation*) (Vatican City: Vatican Polyglot Press), 27 February 1987: I.1.

5. To these arguments some attach the observation that a high percentage of fertilized eggs do not successfully implant themselves in the uterus. The assumption is that if the losses are so high, these preimplantation embryos cannot realistically be said to possess an immortal soul. John Mahoney observes that this argument, though effective in combination with other arguments, does not have probative force on its own. Its argument based on scale of loss could be applied to children born alive in countries with high infant mortality rates, thus implying that even at birth they did not possess an immortal soul. Cf. John Mahoney, *Bioethics and Belief* (London: Sheed and Ward, 1984), pp. 61, 66.

6. Congregation for the Doctrine of the Faith, *Declaration on Abortion*, #13.

7. Ibid., n. 19. Italics in the Latin original.

8. Kevin T. Kelly, *Life and Love: Towards a Christian Dialogue on Bioethical Questions* (London: Collins Liturgical Publications, 1987), p. 52.

9. John Mahoney, *The Making of Moral Theology: A Study of the Roman Catholic Tradition* (Oxford: Clarendon Press, 1989), pp. 137ff.

10. Mahoney, *Bioethics and Belief*, p. 82.

11. Karl Rahner, "The Problem of Genetic Manipulation," in Karl Rahner, *Theological Investigations* IX (New York: Herder and Herder, 1972), p. 236.

12. Richard A. McCormick, "Theology in the Public Forum," in Richard A. McCormick, *The Critical Calling* (Washington D. C.: Georgetown University Press, 1989), p. 206.

Part V

Legal Perspectives

Chapter 12

The Effective Enforcement of Abortion Law Before *Roe v. Wade*

Clarke D. Forsythe

[How] can [we] look our daughters in the eye and tell them that it is somehow consistent with freedom for them to trample on the human rights of their unborn offspring. We're going to have to find the courage one of these days to tell people that freedom is not an easy discipline. Freedom is not a choice for those who are lazy in their heart and in their respect for their own moral capacities. Freedom requires that at the end of the day you accept the constraint that is required . . . a respect for the laws of nature and nature's God that say unequivocally that your daughters do not have the right to do what is wrong, that [your] sons do not have the right to do what is wrong. They do not have the right to steal bread from the mouths of the innocent, they do not have the right to steal life from the womb of the unborn.

—Dr. Alan Keyes[1]

There must be a limit to a liberty so mistaken in its foundations, so far-reaching in its malignant consequences, and so deadly in its exercise.

—Judge John T. Noonan, Jr.[2]

INTRODUCTION

For the past generation in American life, there has been virtually no enforcement of the criminal abortion laws that were on the books in every state just thirty years ago.[3] This is due to the Supreme Court's 1973 decision in *Roe v. Wade*,[4] which legalized abortion in every state, for virtually any reason, at any time of pregnancy. Today's generation can barely remember a time when police and prosecutors regularly worked to shut down abortionists. Yet, certain images surrounding the enforcement of abortion law still retain their power—the dirty and fearful "back alley," the specter of thousands of women dying from illegal abortions, and the belief that millions of illegal abortions made a mockery of the laws. Numerous books and articles seek to perpetuate these images.[5] Whether these images are, in fact, an accurate portrait of the impact of abortion laws is hardly known.

Yet, a 1990 Gallup Poll indicates that, if it were not for the power of the federal courts, significant public opinion would even now support some prohibition of elective abortion at some time in pregnancy.[6] If the Supreme Court were ever to overrule *Roe v. Wade*, and the political authority returned to the states to enact and enforce laws against abortion, it would be necessary to assess whether such laws could effectively save lives. Would they be good public policy? Insofar as the Supreme Court in its 1992 decision in *Planned Parenthood v. Casey*[7] believed that the country could not "go back," it is important to reassess the presumptions about what it is that Americans would "go back to."

If Americans examined the history of abortion law—after 22 years of experience with legalized abortion on demand—they might be surprised by what they found. Abortion history is heavily laden with numerous myths. But a number of truths are apparent. Abortion laws were uniformly enforced against physicians and virtually never against women, who were considered second victims of abortion. The medical reasons that called for therapeutic abortions (to save the life of the mother) had steadily declined by 1960 due to advances in medical care. The number of women who died by illegal abortion had steadily declined before 1960 due to advances in antibiotics. By 1972, women did not die by illegal, "back alley" abortions to a significantly greater extent than women die today from legal abortion. Generally, abortion laws were regularly enforced before *Roe v. Wade,* and they effectively inhibited the performance of abortions.

This history, in turn, must be compared with our current experience of abortion-on-demand and its affect on women's and children's lives. What is the truth about abortion as it is practiced in this country today ? The number of abortions—and the repeat abortion rate—has dramatically increased since nationwide legalization. Most abortions are performed in high volume, assembly-line clinics. Counseling is usually done in groups, by nonphysicians, and never by doctors. The woman never sees the doctor until she is gowned and in stirrups, the abortion takes six to eight minutes, and she never sees the doctor again. If she has complications, the clinic is not equipped to serve her, but instead refers her to the nearest emergency room. Women are still killed and injured by abortion, and medical malpractice claims against abortionists are proliferating. Many women experience negative psychological consequences from abortion.

After twenty two years, abortion-on-demand has failed to fulfill its promises of reducing illegitimacy, ending child abuse, and improving women's lives. Long periods of popular frustration with failed public policies have sometimes sparked dramatic public reaction—witness the growing national consensus today (1995) on some reform of welfare and the culture of dependency. Such could be the future of the abortion debate in America if the public were educated on the reality of abortion history and current abortion practice.

THE HISTORICAL DEVELOPMENT OF MEDICINE AND ABORTION LAW

In Anglo-American culture, laws against abortion have been enforced since at least the thirteenth century. But the nature of that enforcement has been subject to constant change and development. Our knowledge about pregnancy—its onset, determination, progress, and the causes of its termination—has been limited by medical science.[8] The law of abortion and the law of homicide developed very differently in the history of Anglo-American law as a direct result of medical knowledge. The text and scope of abortion statutes, the mechanisms of enforcement, and the protection for women and unborn children have changed over the past five hundred years as medical science has improved. In addition, the target of abortion laws has changed—from midwives to doctors—as the nature of the medical profession has changed. It is seldom recognized that the language and enforcement of abortion laws have been necessarily tied to the contemporary state of medical science, and yet that relationship must be understood before any accurate analysis of the purpose, method, and shortcomings of the enforcement of abortion law can be undertaken.

THE STATE OF MEDICAL SCIENCE AT COMMON LAW

The 1990s is an age of ultrasonography, in utero surgery and transfusions, and fetal medicine and therapy.[9] Medicine can identify and treat the health problems of the unborn child in the womb earlier and earlier in gestation.[10] It is not often recognized just how new this technology is, or how radically it has changed and enhanced society's understanding of life in the womb.

The most important medical aspect of abortion law enforcement has always been determining the existence of a live fetus and the cause of any injury or death. It is clear that the mere detection of early pregnancy was quite difficult for medicine from the fourteenth to the twentieth century.[11] Pregnancy tests for the detection of HCG (Human Chorionic Gonadotropin) performed on urine were developed only fifty years ago and were relatively unreliable up to the 1960s.[12] Early treatises on midwifery (the forerunner of obstetrics) devoted entire chapters to determining the "signs" or indications of pregnancy. Consequently, for purposes of legal proof the common law fixed upon the phenomenon called "quickening"—the physical sense by the mother of movement of the child in utero—as the first true sign of pregnancy. Since "quickening" does not usually occur until 16-18 weeks of pregnancy, however, it was virtually impossible before the twentieth century for medicine to prove a live pregnancy before 16-18 weeks of gestation. Therefore it was impossible for the law to apply the homicide law to abortion.[13] Before quickening, all other primitive signs of pregnancy were considered ambiguous and uncertain.[14] Quickening was thus an evidentiary distinction, not a moral one. Because of these evidentiary problems, the law of abortion developed independent of the law of homicide.

One significant development of common law regarding abortion was the so-called "born alive rule." In the event of an assault on a pregnant woman that ended in fetal death, it would be necessary for the law to determine that the child was alive at the time of the assault, and that death was caused by the assault and not by natural means. As a result, the common law created the "born alive rule" as an evidentiary buffer against false charges and ambiguous medical evidence.[15] The term "born alive" means expulsion from the womb alive; it does not relate to any particular time of gestation.[16]

Consequently, no homicide law could be applied against an abortion unless the child was expelled from the womb (born) alive and died thereafter. It was virtually impossible for the law to prove a homicide (the killing of a human being) unless the child was expelled alive, observed outside the womb, and died only thereafter. Hence, a child could die in the womb or shortly after birth for myriad reasons. These reasons could not be easily identified, and the natural causes could not be readily separated from the criminal causes. Since homicide, at common law, was invariably a capital crime, judges and juries were reluctant to convict on uncertain evidence. Viability, though prominently emphasized in *Roe v. Wade*, was never a concern of the common law.[17]

THE LAW AGAINST ABORTION

It is now beyond any doubt that the common law prohibited abortion in order to protect the right to life of the unborn child to the greatest extent possible, given contemporary medical science.[18] It is often falsely assumed that because the law did not treat abortion before quickening as *homicide*, it did not treat abortion before quickening as any *crime*.[19]

There is an important distinction, however, between the recognition of legal rights and their enforcement. Declaring a principle and proving its violation are two different things. Thus, William Blackstone, one of the foremost common law historians, could declare the unborn child to be a person at the earliest moment that it could be determined to be alive, but enforcement of the law protecting the child's life, which depended on evidence, was entirely another matter.[20] The law was constantly hampered by problems of evidence.

Recent historical research has eclipsed the numerous myths about the history of abortion law that were adopted by the Supreme Court in *Roe v. Wade*.[21] There, the Court relied almost entirely on the work of one law professor, Cyril Means, who happened to be chief counsel for NARAL (National Abortion

Rights Action League).[22] Relying entirely on two English cases from the 1300s, Means argued that abortion was a common law liberty.[23] But Means mischaracterized those cases,[24] and overlooked many other common law cases of punishment for abortionists.[25] Yet, the Court's erroneous adoption of Means' claims has sustained the modern myth, repeatedly asserted, that English law did not treat abortion as a crime *before* quickening.[26] Several U.S. courts accepted the view of Blackstone that it was necessary to allege quickening in order to indict,[27] and state courts repeatedly held that abortion after quickening was a crime at common law, without regard to statutory authority.[28] However, there was a trend among American courts later in the nineteenth century toward reconsidering that notion and holding that abortion was a crime at common law without regard to quickening (or at any stage of pregnancy).[29] This position was supported by leading, authoritative commentators on the criminal law.[30] Today, there can be no question, if the historical facts are considered, that abortion was considered a crime of some degree by the common law at *every* stage of gestation and was *never* protected as a right.

A second myth of abortion history is that there were no abortion laws in America until the first abortion statute was enacted in Connecticut in 1821. Yet, the American colonies imported the English common law against abortion and enforced it, to the extent possible given primitive medical science. Common law abortion cases have been discovered in a number of American colonies.[31]

A third myth of abortion history is that the nineteenth century American abortion statutes were enacted to protect only the mother, and not the child. This notion has been exploded in recent years by extensive scholarship. It is now recognized that sixty five court decisions from forty states recognized that their nineteenth-century state statutes were intended to protect the life of the unborn child.[32]

A fourth myth surrounding the history of abortion is that abortion was a commonly accepted and frequent practice among American women before the nineteenth century. The independent research of Professors Joseph Dellapenna and Marvin Olasky has undermined that myth. Dellapenna demonstrates that there were no safe and effective techniques—intrusion or ingestion—throughout the nineteenth century.[33] In addition, as medical science developed, the law became increasingly sophisticated in dropping all limitations to prohibit abortion at any stage of gestation. Professor Olasky has shown that abortion was closely connected to prostitution, and was not widely dispersed through the populace.[34] Thus, due to both uniform social prohibition and practical unavailability, abortion could not have been widely accepted or practiced.

Despite the obstacles posed by primitive medical science, and the evidentiary problems that crippled effective enforcement at various times, the purpose of abortion law in Anglo-American law has been to protect the life of the unborn child and protect the mother from death or injury. These purposes have been consistent throughout Anglo-American history, even though the means for fulfilling those purposes were often technologically limited.

PROBLEMS OF ENFORCEMENT

Although abortion was consistently treated as a crime, enforcement of abortion laws required proof of the crime, and proof was dependent on medical evidence. As Professor Dellapenna explains, "The technological dimension . . . explains why there were so few reported prosecutions of abortion before 1840 and why those and later prosecutions so often resulted in acquittal or conviction for lesser offenses."[35] As medical understanding of pregnancy developed, changes in the law evolved to assist enforcement, and enforcement improved and became more sophisticated. Enforcement improved with technology.

Enforcement Against Abortionists, Not Women

A key aspect was the target of abortion laws. Male physicians did not perform obstetrical or gynecological procedures before the early-to-mid-nineteenth-century because of cultural attitudes that forbade them from attending women during pregnancy. Rather, female midwives attended to women in pregnancy. Thus, midwives, as abortionists, were the targets of the earliest abortion laws. For example, in order to prevent abortion, ordinances were enacted in New York and Virginia in the 1700s which prohibited abortion by midwives.[36] These ordinances were blanket prohibitions on the induction of abortion.

A fifth myth of abortion history is that aborting women were the target of abortion law before *Roe v. Wade*. Although some state laws in the nineteenth century allowed the prosecution of aborting women, there is apparently no reported appellate decision in American history upholding the conviction of a woman for self-induced abortion or for submitting to an abortion.[37] Dellapenna also provides evidence that treating women as a second victim was "based on both the rarity in practice of voluntary, elective abortion and the danger of the procedure when it did occur."[38] Although there is evidence that, at common law, women were occasionally subject to criminal prosecution for participation in abortion, the common law gave way to the pragmatic judgments of modern abortion law that the abortionist is the most significant culprit, that the woman is a second victim of abortion after the child, and that criminalizing women's participation undermined effective law enforcement. A parallel can be found, perhaps, in the disinclination to charge girls as accessories to the crime of statutory rape.[39]

Most states expressly treated women as the second victim of abortion.[40] This was so even for self-abortion.[41] "[W]omen were never charged with murder, only seldom . . . named co-conspirators, and still more rarely . . . regarded as accomplices."[42] Thirty nine of the forty state courts which considered whether aborted women were accomplices concluded that they were not.[43] As one commentator has aptly summarized the law:

> The primary issue in the complicity cases was not the guilt of the woman but of her abortionist. The defense—not the prosecution—sought to have such women named as accomplices because they often were the only eyewitnesses to their abortions. Since most states required that the testimony of an accomplice be corroborated before being admitted into evidence, the abortionist would typically allege that the woman was his accomplice in the performance of the abortion. The defense hoped thereby to make the woman's testimony inadmissible and thus, in the absence of corroborating evidence, to win acquittal.[44]

In other words, if the abortionist could convince the court to treat the woman as an accomplice, and her testimony could not be corroborated by another person, her testimony would not be admitted and the case would dissolve. As late as 1968, Ruth Barnett—the abortionist cast as the hero in a 1994 book, *The Abortionist*—used this tactic, unsuccessfully, in her appeal from her conviction.[45]

The most that the states did in the way of penalizing women for abortion was to prohibit any person—male or female—from *soliciting* abortion. At the time of *Roe v. Wade*, seventeen states still had such laws on the books.[46] But there is no known prosecution of any woman under these laws. Whether these laws effectively inhibited women from soliciting abortion is unknown; certainly their mere existence supported the aim of general deterrence by stigmatizing abortion as a criminal act. Some historians, like Leslie Reagan, charge that although women were not arrested, prosecuted or incarcerated for abortion, the intimate nature of the investigations was a form of "punishment." But even Reagan concedes that "[n]o evidence suggests that officials consciously designed their investigative procedures to harass women. . . .," and these same investigative procedures were applied evenhandedly to men.[47]

The policy considerations in favor of not treating women as accomplices extended beyond the evidentiary necessities. If a woman was considered an accomplice or criminally liable, she might be unable to recover for the negligence of an abortionist.[48] The inhibiting influence of negligence actions against abortionists might suggest that an injured woman *should* recover even if she submitted to an illegal act. This policy of treating women as the second victims of abortion controlled the modern enforcement of abortion law throughout the twentieth century.[49]

Questions of Intent and Evidence

Early state abortion statutes often created evidentiary problems by their own definition of the elements of the crime, but, with experience, these were often eliminated by amendment.[50] For example, Illinois adopted its first abortion statute in 1827 and, to its credit, was especially progressive in not containing any quickening limitation. However, between 1867 and 1874, the Illinois statute included a broad exception ("unless the same were done for *bona fide* medical or surgical purposes"), and experience found that it "was a comparatively easy matter to show, in case a prosecution was attempted, if an operation was done for *bona fide* medical or surgical purposes."[51] This language remained in place until 1874, when the Illinois legislature deleted the loophole, which was viewed as "uncertain, unbounded, and undefined," and replaced it with the phrase, "unless same were done as necessary for the preservation of the mother's life."[52] Similar problems of intent persisted in other states as late as the middle of the nineteenth century when states began to amend their statutes to eliminate requirements of quickening and proof of pregnancy.[53]

Evidentiary problems caused by the lack of medical proof continued to plague law enforcement. The problem of gathering evidence was commonly raised by physicians and lawyers. At a Chicago medical symposium in 1905, one physician noted:

Notwithstanding the prevalence of the crime there are few accusations or indictments for inducing abortion unless the death of the mother results when of course the indictment is for murder. In the few cases of indictment for producing abortion the action was brought because of the serious injury to the mother. Ordinarily it is very difficult to get satisfactory evidence against a professional abortionist. The relatives or others interested in the case are generally very anxious to prevent any publicity for obvious reasons and even in case of the death of the mother it is frequently impossible to get any member of the family to take action in the matter. Outside parties cannot be expected to interest themselves with such matters which can concern them only in a very indirect way and which would bring them only great annoyance and perhaps place them in a very embarrassing position. This difficulty of securing evidence and initiating an accusation is the reason why the abortion law is so much of a dead letter.[54]

Nevertheless, at the turn of the century, efforts were undertaken by the coroner for Cook County, Illinois, to increase the effectiveness of law enforcement efforts, and several abortionists were convicted and imprisoned.[55]

The Law of Attempt

The relation of an attempt to the completion of a crime has been a traditional problem in the enforcement of the criminal law.[56] To ease the problem, the law of attempt is often specifically set forth in state statutes. For example, in Illinois, "a person commits an attempt when, with intent to commit a specific offense, he does any act which constitutes a substantial step toward the commission of that offense."[57] Generally, "it is not necessary for an 'attempt' that the last proximate act to the completion of the offense be done."[58] Justice Holmes distinguished between mere preparation to commit a crime and an attempt in the following terms:

> But combination, intention, and overt act may all be present without amount-
> ing to a criminal attempt,—as if all that were done should be an agreement to
> murder a man 50 miles away, and the purchase of a pistol for that purpose.
> There must be dangerous proximity to success. But when that exists the overt
> act is the essence of the offense.[59]

The importance of the law of attempt to the successful enforcement of abortion law was demonstrated by the Amen investigations in New York in the
1940s. In New York, an offer did not constitute an attempt to commit an abortion for purposes of the criminal law, but an offer could be used in professional
disciplinary proceedings. New York Assistant Attorney General John Harlan
Amen then proposed a bill to make it "a misdemeanor to offer to perform an
abortion," but this bill failed to pass.

Prior to *Roe v. Wade*, some American courts exercised a leniency toward
finding that an attempt to perform an abortion had been committed. In *People v.
Cummings*,[60] for example, a California court held that the fact that a woman was
not pregnant was no defense to a conviction for attempted abortion, when the
abortionist had begun the performance of the abortion. Impossibility was found
to be a factual matter that was no defense to a charge of attempt.[61]

Elimination of Abortion Advertising

Another policy which states adopted to curb abortion was to prohibit the advertising of abortion. Contrary to some historical accounts, legal restrictions on
abortion clinic advertising did not begin with the Comstock laws of the 1870s.
Rather, they began at least as early as 1845, when California passed legislation
making it a felony to "willfully write, compose or publish any notice or advertisement of any medicine or means for producing or facilitating a miscarriage or
abortion."[62] Early in the twentieth century, the Chicago Medical Society began a
successful campaign to get Chicago newspapers to cease abortion advertising.[63]
At least fifteen states banned the advertisement of abortion services or abortifacients.[64]

Enforcement in the Nineteenth Century

Prosecutors in the last half of the nineteenth century were vigorous and successful in many cities, which is where abortion and prosecutions predominated.
Abortion advocates note the abortion trade of Madame Restell in New York City
and offer it as evidence of social tolerance of abortion, but they ignore the re-

peated prosecutions of her, which eventually led to her suicide before she could be tried yet another time.[65] Similarly, Dr. Isaac Hathaway of Philadelphia was convicted of performing abortions in 1883 and sentenced to seven years at hard labor.[66] Dr. McGonegal of New York City was convicted of first degree manslaughter and sentenced to fourteen years in prison in 1890.[67] In 1894, in New York City, police arrested five abortionists and ten midwives.[68] The *New York Times* reported the arrests and trials of several other doctors between 1894 and 1896 (Drs. Van Ziles, Lee, Thompson, Kolb).[69] While there may be evidence that police and prosecutors were lax in their enforcement in some cities, prosecutions were undertaken in major metropolitan areas in every decade throughout the last half of the nineteenth century.[70]

PROGRESS IN ENFORCEMENT IN THE 20TH CENTURY

The Early Decades

Prosecutors throughout the country enforced abortion laws in the early decades of the twentieth century. In the 1930s, prosecutions against abortionists were regularly noted in some newspapers. As usual, evidence was critical. Thomas P. Peters, an assistant Kings County, New York district attorney, in 1929 contrasted the prosecutions with convictions, stating, "prosecutions are frequent, but in my experience convictions are seldom obtained."[71] Dr. Maurice Sturm went on trial for abortion in March, 1930 in New York City. Prosecutions were also brought in New York against Dr. George Rothenberg, Dr. George Haley, Dr. Mulholland, Dr. William Gibson (a county coroner), Dr. Gilbert Ashman, and Dr. Edward Mandell.[72] A Pacific coast abortion ring was publicized and targeted in the 1930s.[73] In a 1936 Los Angeles trial, Reginald Rankin and others were prosecuted for operating the ring. In 1946, authorities in San Francisco prosecuted Dr. Charles B. Caldwell, who was accused of committing an abortion that resulted in a maternal death.[74] In the 1940s and 1950s, prosecutions for abortion were brought in many states, including New York[75] and Texas.

The Amen Investigations

Every state in America enacted and enforced laws against abortion in the twentieth century. However, there are a few points in history where sustained, coordinated efforts to improve the enforcement of criminal abortion laws were undertaken. One example is the campaign conducted by New York State Assistant Attorney General John Harlan Amen (1898-1960) in the late 1930s and early 1940s. Amen's investigations grew out of a three year probe that he conducted, upon the appointment of the governor, into municipal corruption in Kings County (Brooklyn), New York. Part of the corruption unearthed included bribery of assistant district attorneys to obstruct the prosecution of abortionists.[76]

Based on his investigations, Amen identified three primary obstacles to the effective legal control of criminal abortion.[77] First, abortion prosecution must deal with obtaining evidence against the abortionist. Amen noted that the abortionist, a nurse, and the aborted woman were usually the only persons with knowledge of the crime. The aborted woman would rarely come forward to provide evidence. Evidentiary problems were such that the most effective investigation and prosecution occurred only in those "rare exceptions" when the patient tragically died.

Second, Amen noted that it was difficult to "set the enforcement machinery in motion with the same vigor and efficiency which is displayed in the prosecution of crimes of violence."[78] This was affected by public opinion, and when "the moral or common sense of the community looks upon criminal abortion with complacency or toleration, it is most difficult for prosecuting officials and courts to extend themselves to the utmost in an effort to secure convictions."[79]

> We all know that public opinion plays a large part, not only in placing laws on the statute books, but also in their enforcement. When the moral and common sense of the community are in accord that some particular kind of behavior is wrong, the problem of enforcement becomes relatively simple. Violations are infrequent since there are few who wish to commit them. When committed, the violators are dealt with promptly, vigorously and efficiently.
>
> On the other hand, when public opinion is lukewarm or divided, the problem of law enforcement is tremendously increased. . . . [A] more complete solution of the problem lies in a still further aroused public opinion. Therefore, I think it is safe to say that the greatest obstacle so far encountered to the legal control of abortions is public indifference. So long as there is a widespread public feeling that under certain circumstances an induced abortion should be permissible or justified, certain results inevitably follow. There will be a large market for the services of the criminal abortionist. This practice will remain a profitable field of medical activity. These facts will aid certain doctors in convincing themselves that they are performing a useful public service. The enormous number of abortions performed and the secrecy naturally surrounding them, will impose an insurmountable burden upon the State's investigative and enforcement agencies.[80]

Third, Amen identified the difficulty of "securing punishment sufficiently severe to act as an effective deterrent."[81] He noted that, in New York, abortionists faced not only the criminal abortion statute, but also professional disciplinary provisions involving revocation of their medical license under the Education Law.[82] As a practical matter, Amen noted that an offer to perform an abortion could subject an abortionist to disciplinary action under the Education Law, but not under the criminal abortion law, where an offer did not constitute an attempt, which was narrowly defined as "an act performed in an effort to accomplish the actual abortion."[83] Thus, under the criminal law, there could "be no criminal prosecution except on proof of an abortion actually performed or attempted."[84]

To make an offer prosecutable as an attempt, Amen recommended to the New York State Legislature that the Penal Law be amended to make it a misdemeanor to offer to perform an abortion. This bill had two purposes. First, it would promote a simpler and speedier form of prosecution by allowing abortion prosecutions to be brought in the New York Court of Special Sessions, where, at that time, misdemeanor cases were tried by three judges. Second, the prosecutions in the Court of Special Sessions could use the same evidence used in the professional disciplinary hearings under the Education Law. The bill was introduced in the New York Legislature, but it failed to pass.

The problem of obtaining evidence was exacerbated in New York by the fact that women who submitted to abortion were technically subject to penalties under the law, even though this was apparently never enforced.[85] With the constitutional privilege against self-incrimination, an aborted woman could not be compelled to give testimony against an abortionist that could be used simultaneously against her, and thus defense counsel usually urged silence. This privilege could be removed, however, by a grant of immunity from prosecution for the testimony. Such immunity statutes are of two types—"use immunity" and "transaction immunity"—and the statutes compel the testimony and immunize the witness from any prosecution arising from the testimony. Consequently, Amen initiated the introduction of a bill in the New York Legislature that would have made it clear that such immunity applied to abortion prosecutions. The bill was passed and signed by then-Governor Herbert Lehman.[86]

The use of "testers" enhanced the enforcement of abortion law by counteracting the problem of witnesses. Testers are individuals who pose as prospective applicants to "test" the response of the parties who might violate the law. For example, in housing rights cases, testers pose as prospective buyers or renters before real estate agents or landowners. As long ago as the 1930s, testers (or "paid investigators" as they were called in some cases) were used in professional disciplinary investigations in New York State.[87] As Amen described it, "[i]n abortion cases, a pair of female investigators were often sent to the office of the suspected doctor with the purpose of discovering whether the doctor would offer to perform an abortion. If sufficient evidence of an offer to perform an abortion were secured, charges were prepared on the basis of the investigators' reports and the proceeding was started on the basis of such charges."[88] Sometimes a man and woman, posing as a husband and wife, would solicit an abortionist. Amen indicates that the use of testers was intimately connected with the law of attempt.

This practice of using female testers seems to have encountered some skepticism in the New York courts in the 1940s. Some courts rejected disciplinary action against abortionists based solely on the testimony of testers without some independent corroboration.[89] Finally, in 1946, New York's highest court affirmed the use of testers, holding that the testimony of two women investigators was sufficient, and did not require independent corroboration.[90] Female testers seem to have been used in Baltimore too.[91]

A fourth essential element relating to the effective enforcement of abortion law was perhaps too obvious for Amen to mention—conscientious and ethical enforcement of the law by public officials. One sociologist suggested that the abortion trade was inevitably connected with (and greatly dependent on) corruption of police and other public officials.[92] Abortion rights proponents often portray what in fact was official corruption as "official support."[93] The corruption that the Kings County New York Grand Jury documented in a 1941 report may explain the low number of successful administrative complaints reported by the New York Board of Medical Examiners between 1928 and 1934.[94] Corruption designed to obstruct abortion law enforcement also seems to have been a factor in Portland, Oregon and Los Angeles.[95] To the extent that there are any facts supporting the abortion proponents' claim that abortion law was "rarely enforced" in the 1930s but "often enforced" in the 1950s, corruption in New York and Los Angeles may have contributed.[96] By whatever name, official corruption sometimes impeded law enforcement.

Professional Disciplinary Proceedings

Another method of abortion enforcement, independent of the constraints of the criminal law and the court system, was professional disciplinary proceedings against physician-abortionists. This method was civil, not criminal, and, as a result, one advantage of this method was that a lower standard of proof—one appropriate for civil proceedings—was applied.[97] With abortion—an area of law where the nature of the offense made evidentiary proceedings particularly difficult—this lower standard of proof was significant.

Although it might be assumed that "self-policing" by physicians might be prone to abuse, New York State in particular seems to have used the professional disciplinary proceeding effectively against abortionists. For nearly thirty five years, between 1936 and 1970, New York successfully suspended or revoked the licenses of abortionists in a series of cases.[98]

As a result of his investigations, John Harlan Amen sought to increase the vigor of the professional disciplinary proceedings. Formerly, the Education Law allowed revocation of license for "a physician [who] did undertake in any manner or by any ways or means whatsoever to do or perform any criminal abortion. "The 1941 Kings County grand jury concluded that this lacked vigor because the law did not make clear that it applied to "the corner druggist, the solicitor" or a physician who did not perform abortions but referred women to abortionists. The grand jury concluded that "effective control of the problem required the imposition of some such punishment" to deter such action because the "vast numbers of criminal operations [abortions] resulted from recommendations of this kind."[99]

Amen initiated two bills in the New York Legislature to meet this problem. The first bill amended the Education Law to make a referring physician subject to disciplinary proceedings. This was passed and signed on May 8, 1942. A second bill would have amended the Penal Law to make it a misdemeanor for any person to give referral information "as to where or by whom an abortion could be performed." This bill died in the legislature. Unknown to Amen at the time, this action would have serious implications twenty five years later when abortion activists initiated an abortion referral service in New York which undermined the enforcement of the abortion law and led to its eventual repeal in 1970.[100]

Finally, Amen sought to streamline the procedures for professional disciplinary proceedings. The Kings County grand jury had found the procedures to be so cumbersome as to be inadequate to deal with the number of disciplinary cases for abortion. Delay was a most significant obstacle, and delay was in the interest of abortionists since they were not suspended during the pendency of the hearings but could continue to practice.[101] Amen initiated another bill which would have provided for four significant changes in the disciplinary proceedings: (1) establishment of a full-time medical grievance committee, compensated by the state, (2) elimination of the requirement that representatives of different schools of medicine be on the committee, (3) hearings by the full committee of each case, with the presentation of evidence and legal counsel by an assistant attorney general, and (4) the unanimity requirement for recommendation of punishment reduced to majority vote. Amen believed that such a bill would have gone a long way to "removing some of the serious obstacles to effective legal control of criminal abortion."[102] Although the bill was backed by certain medical societies, it was apparently never introduced. An alternative, compromise measure—not containing the reforms supported by Amen—was apparently introduced with support by members of the Grievance Committee. It passed but was vetoed by Governor Lehman, based on Amen's recommendation.

The result of Amen's singular attempt to invigorate the enforcement of abortion laws in New York is uncertain. Amen went off to Germany at the end of World War II as a Nuremburg war crimes prosecutor. Olasky concluded that the anti-abortion drive in New York in the 1930s lost momentum in the 1940s for three reasons: abortionists used their financial resources to fight the media and legal attack; procedural difficulties hindered the introduction of evidence; and World War II commenced. Yet, even in the early 1950s, a decade after Amen's historic investigations, the Kings County district attorney initiated a vigorous prosecution of abortionists in Kings County.[103]

"THERAPEUTIC ABORTION" COMMITTEES

One new method for monitoring physicians' decision making about induced abortion—the so-called therapeutic abortion committee—developed in the 1950s. This institution was created not by state legislatures or law enforcement authorities but by doctors and hospitals, to protect themselves from violations of the law.[104] The practice was for a physician contemplating the performance of a "therapeutic" abortion (to save the mother's life) to obtain an opinion concurring in the judgment from a committee of physicians.[105] According to Dr. Alan Guttmacher—a prominent advocate of the legalization of abortion—in a 1954 article,

> The mechanics for authorization of therapeutic abortion vary from hospital to hospital. Each institution has its own rules. These fall into four general patterns: 1. Consultation with one or two other physicians; 2. Review and decision by the chief of the obstetrical and gynecological service; 3. Review and decision by the chief of staff or the medical director of the institution, and 4. Review and decision by a therapeutic abortion committee.[106]

Guttmacher predicted that the therapeutic abortion committee would become "standard procedure in another decade."[107] It was used in other cities, including Baltimore and Chicago.[108]

The committee system seems to have inhibited physicians' individual, arbitrary approval of elective abortions. Guttmacher found that when a therapeutic abortion committee system was used, "a material reduction in the number of requests for therapeutic interruption occurs since cases of questionable merit have little likelihood of being accredited for operation."[109] He found that this was due to the fact that "the board system has the advantage of consultation among several senior physicians and does not depend on the views of one or two who frequently may have personal interests in affirmative decisions." He even "praise[d]" it for that reason.[110] He declared that "[t]he physicians with no hospital administrative responsibility for the certification and selection of cases for therapeutic abortion advocate the operation far more freely than those who do."[111] This sentiment was seconded by Herbert Packer in 1959.[112]

Perhaps for the very reason that the committee system inhibited individual, arbitrary decisions approving elective abortions, it served to protect physicians from prosecution. One physician concluded that "no adverse decisions were discovered where there was adequate consultation beforehand and approval by hospital staff committees."[113]

Enforcement Up to *Roe v. Wade*

Abortion rights proponents, relying on anecdotes by fellow opponents of abortion laws, contend that the enforcement of abortion laws before *Roe* was lax.[114] However, there is substantial evidence that law enforcement authorities regularly enforced the abortion laws until the Supreme Court's decision in *Roe v. Wade* in January, 1973. This is seen in reported appellate cases involving abortion in the states in the 1950s and 1960s.[115] There were celebrated trials of abortionists in many states. These included Dr. G. Lotrell Timanus of Baltimore, Dr. Roy Odell Knapp of Akron, Ohio, Dr. Robert Spencer in Ashland, Pennsylvania, Geraldine Rhoades in Sacramento in the 1950s, Sophie Miller in St. Louis in 1951, Mary Pagan in Cincinnati in 1953, Grace Schaumer in Wichita in 1954, and San Diego abortionist Laura Miner.[116] In 1966, in a state as "liberal" as Oregon, officials prosecuted and shut down an elderly abortionist, Ruth Barnett.[117] As late as May, 1972, seven abortionists were arrested in Chicago.[118] Massachusetts successfully prosecuted Dr. Benedict Kudish on the eve of *Roe v. Wade*.[119] This record suggests that, generally speaking, state officials were not among those advocating legalization of abortion in the 1960s.

Likewise, between 1966 and 1973, many states modified their abortion law, but none to the extent that abortion was liberalized in *Roe v. Wade*—on demand, throughout pregnancy, even in the third trimester. In 1973, thirty one states still retained their pre-*Roe* laws prohibiting abortion except to save the life of the mother. New York modified its law in 1970, but the legislature repealed the change the following year, and that repeal was vetoed by Governor Nelson Rockefeller. Two states—Michigan, by 62 to 28 percent, and North Dakota, by 79 to 21 percent,—rejected modifications of their law by state referenda in late 1972, on the eve of the *Roe* decision. In *state* constitutional challenges to state abortion laws before *Roe v. Wade*, 75 percent of the state courts upheld their abortion laws.[120] The Supreme Court shut down state prosecutions in January 1973; they were not voluntarily suspended.

The regularity of enforcement is also seen in passing references in histories of abortion. For example, in a 1993 book intended to support legalized abortion, the author notes that of the "former abortionists" she interviewed, "almost all of them had at least one brush with the law."[121] The same author cites a Baltimore doctor in the 1940s and 1950s who refused to perform abortions "because the personal risk to me was too great. There was no way in the world I was going to jeopardize my entire family and risk going to jail."[122] Although she was extolled as having operated an abortion trade between 1918 and 1968 in Portland, Ruth Barnett indicated that by 1965 "the number of women she was able to help had fallen to a 'relative trickle'."[123] Marian Faux, in her history of *Roe v. Wade*, notes that Jane Roe never got an abortion (but placed her child for adoption) because she could not find an abortionist in Texas, despite her original claim (later admitted to be false) that she was pregnant by a gang rape.[124] Reagan records that persistent police investigations even without prosecutions served as an effective deterrent.[125]

THE EFFECTS OF ENFORCEMENT

An essential function of law is social control. In evaluating law as a method of social control, lawyers and policy analysts reflect on what conduct should be considered criminal, what goals are served by making the conduct criminal, and whether making the conduct criminal is a means well adapted to serving the end of the law.[126] The criminal law can have both an individual prevention effect and a general prevention effect. Individual prevention involves "the effect of punishment on the punished."[127] General prevention involves "the ability of criminal law and its enforcement to make citizens law-abiding."[128] Punishment is understood to have three distinct effects of general prevention: "it may have a *deterrent* effect, it may strengthen *moral inhibitions* (a *moralizing* effect), and it may stimulate habitual *law-abiding conduct*."[129] The effectiveness or ineffectiveness of a law is not usually relevant to its constitutionality.[130] As a matter of policy, however, if these questions are *neutrally* applied to the enforcement of abortion law, in the *same* manner they are applied to other areas of law enforcement, they demonstrate the effectiveness of abortion law enforcement up to the time of the Supreme Court's decision in *Roe v. Wade*.

In the assault on abortion law in the 1960s, however, these enforcement questions were *not* neutrally applied to abortion law. The movement to abolish abortion law in the 1960s focused its attack on the effects of enforcement. Opponents contended that the effects outweighed the utility of enforcement. Two themes drove the attack: the number of illegal abortions and the number of women killed or injured by illegal abortion (maternal mortality and morbidity). Usually, incidents of lawbreaking provoke calls for more effective law enforcement, not the abolition of the law itself. For example, during the 1980s, there was an average of more than twenty thousand persons murdered annually in the United States; yet, in slightly less than half of those cases was there a conviction.[131] There are tens of thousands of vehicular homicides, rapes, robberies, and burglaries each year.[132] It is never suggested that any of these crimes should be legalized because the law is broken or because so many crimes go unpunished. As Professor John Hart Ely wrote in reaction to the *Roe* decision, with considerable understatement, "it is a strange argument for the unconstitutionality of a law that those who evade it suffer."[133] Even Justice Blackmun, in his majority opinion in *Roe v. Wade*, noted that "[t]he prevalence of high mortality rates at illegal 'abortion mills' strengthens, rather than weakens, the State's interest in regulating the conditions under which abortions are performed."[134] Opponents of abortion law usually ignored any benefit of the law in protecting the unborn, and required that abortion law justify its own utility by demonstrating its general prevention effect to a *higher* degree than that required for any other area of criminal law, or by requiring the complete *elimination* of the crime.[135] In other words, it was claimed that abortion laws were ineffective because the laws were broken. This type of reasoning, of course, is usually not applied by Policy makers to other areas of law enforcement, and for good reason.

> Some may argue that the only appropriate level of crime is no crime at all. But
> while it may be technically possible to eradicate crime, the cost of such a pol-
> icy would most likely be exorbitant, especially in view of the multitude of
> other demands on public coffers. If there is not an unending supply of public
> funds and if there are more demands on public coffers than there are funds to
> satisfy these demands, then the public sector is faced with economic problems
> of choice and scarcity.[136]

Certain areas of criminal law—like laws against rape—continue to operate
without regard to proof of general prevention and despite claims that the incidence of the crime is increasing undeterred.[137]

> The disagreement over the importance of general prevention is of course
> largely due to the fact that its effectiveness cannot be measured. We do not
> know the true extent of crime. In certain areas of crime there is reason to be-
> lieve that the figures available for offenses which are prosecuted and punished
> corresponds roughly to the true incidence of crime. In other areas recorded
> crimes represent only a small fraction of the true incidence. We know still less
> about how many people *would* have committed crimes if there had been no
> threat of punishment.[138]

It was rarely recognized that general deterrence of abortion in a state could be
accomplished by one successful, well-publicized prosecution.[139]

Another common argument against abortion laws was that abortion laws
"discriminated" against the poor because rich women could "always" procure
abortions.[140] This argument, of course, betrays the underlying presumption that
abortion is a virtue and not a vice. It ignores the common understanding that society does not repeal criminal laws simply because the rich, unlike the poor, can
afford the higher cost of vices caused by criminalization itself (as with narcotics
and prostitution, for example).

Illegal Abortions

Much has been written about quantitative studies on numerous aspects of the
abortion issue.[141] Concerning much of abortion data, there are considerable problems. Judith Leavitt has summarized analogous problems with statistics on
childbirth:

> We simply do not know how often women in the past found themselves preg-
> nant or even how frequently women labored to give birth. It is only in the
> twentieth century that the recording of births (live and still) began to be noted
> reliably by local and state health departments, and even today we cannot cal-

culate precisely the risks women face each time they become pregnant. Because we can not be sure about the number of labors or pregnancies, our statistical conclusions have limited meaning.[142]

These same problems apply, at least in part, to abortion statistics before *Roe v. Wade*. Even since Roe, the availability and quality of data has been criticized.[143]

Throughout the twentieth century, social scientists have made widely varying estimates of the number of illegal abortions.[144] In the early part of this century, ambiguous estimates of the number of abortions were expressed by physicians and medical societies in their efforts to suppress illegal abortion. It was frequently stated that illegal abortion was widespread. But there were no data available, and no scientific efforts were made to estimate the numbers.[145] Anecdotal evidence was not evaluated for its representativeness—it was presumed to stand on its own—and to the extent that it came out of large cities, it was most unrepresentative.[146] The problem with all of these early estimates is that there were no hard data, and general labels such as "large" lacked the necessary context for comparison. In effect, the commentators—who seemed to invariably support the legalization of abortion—were often reduced to saying "We can only guess how many there are but it's a lot."[147]

At a 1942 national abortion conference, it was admitted by a number of physicians and statisticians that it was not possible to estimate reliably the number of illegal abortions, and, often, in making these estimates, distinctions were not drawn between spontaneous, therapeutic, or illegally induced abortions. They acknowledged that there was presently a lack of knowledge and "reliable figures are not available."[148]

A 1991 review by Professor Gerald Rosenberg listed more than twenty estimates of illegal abortions performed nationwide between 1936 and 1972. Another 1994 reviewer cited most of the same estimates.[149] Nearly all of these estimates were either by abortion advocates or by newspapers and magazines without original research. Rosenberg took them at face value despite a significant concession:

> while most students of illegal abortion agree that the number was substantial, they have differed markedly on the figures. By the mid-1960's, however, the range seemed to be settling around 1 million. For obvious reasons of partisanship and lack of hard data, these figures can only be taken as very rough estimates."[150]

The best critical analysis of these statistical claims is still Germain Grisez's 1968 review.[151]

Most estimates of illegal abortion begin with Frederick Taussig, the leading medical proponent of legalized abortion in the 1930s. His 1936 book on abortion first suggested a figure of 681,600 illegal abortions annually in the United States, and, because his estimate was novel and had the appearance of scientific objectivity, it was widely cited and relied upon.[152] As Grisez and Olasky point out, however, Taussig's figures were extrapolations based on speculations based on isolated figures that could not be demonstrated to be representative. Olasky writes:

> Basing his calculations on the records of a New York City birth control clinic, Taussig decided that one abortion took place for every 2.5 confinements [for delivery] in urban areas; he did not note that visits to still-controversial birth control clinics were hardly typical jaunts. He also postulated a rural total of one abortion for every five confinements throughout the United States; his evidence for that were estimates by some physicians in "the rural districts of Iowa." Dubious techniques yielded totals of 403,200 abortions in urban areas and 278,400 in rural areas, for a nationwide annual total of 681,600.[153]

In fact, it is rarely pointed out that Taussig subsequently repudiated his 1936 figure and adopted a lower estimate at a 1942 conference:

> I would like . . . to apologize for the very meager information contained in my book, which was published in 1935, on the actual number of abortions and abortion deaths. We had, at that time, the wildest estimates as to the number of abortions and the number of abortion deaths both in Europe and in this country, and I thought the numbers were conservative.
>
> Since 1936, I have reviewed the figures carefully. . . . They were trimmed down considerably, particularly as to the number of abortion deaths. . . . I think we can positively say there do not occur over 5,000 abortion deaths annually in this country, no matter how we try to cull the various brackets in the mortality statistics.[154]

J. E. Bates also questioned Taussig's 1936 estimate.[155]

Three other studies—by Marie Kopp, Regine Stix, and Alfred Kinsey—are also often cited.[156] Taussig relied on Kopp for his 1936 estimate, but recognized that Kopp's study was unrepresentative. At the 1942 Conference, Dunn was critical of both Kopp and Taussig.[157] Stix acknowledged her own earlier sample to be unrepresentative.[158] The Kinsey study is perhaps the most important because it is the only basis for the 1.2 million "upper limit" suggested by the 1955 Planned Parenthood Conference and the major authority for the standard "1 million" claim in the 1960s. The Kinsey study was based on a sample that was projected for the entire country, but the statistics committee for the 1955 conference doubted the representativeness of the study.[159] Others, like Robert G. Potter, also doubted the reliability of the Kinsey study.[160] Nevertheless, from 1960-1995, abortion advocates have continued to rely on Taussig, Kopp, Stix, or Kinsey without acknowledging their admitted weaknesses.[161]

The widely quoted 1955 Planned Parenthood Conference figure of 200,000-1,200,000 illegal abortions annually was based on meager data and was substantially contradicted by the conference participants themselves. The figure is taken from the statistics committee for the conference, which, in arriving at the figure, significantly qualified its foundation in fact: "There is no objective basis for the selection of a particular figure between these two estimates as an approximation of the actual frequency."[162] Indeed, the committee provided no authority for any "objective basis" for any figure *lower* or *higher* than those estimates. In addition, individual conference participants indicated that there were no reliable figures on illegal abortions.[163]

Despite the lack of factual basis for enormous estimates, they were allowed to be taken as common wisdom without verification. For example, a 1962 law review article cited a figure of "more than 1 million" illegal abortions annually based on "the mounting evidence that one out of every five pregnancies in this country terminates in illegal abortion."[164] This was "based upon a conservative estimate of illegal abortions per year, contrasted with the known birth rate" (which begs the question), and then four studies are cited, three of which were published no later than 1936. As late as 1964, J. E. Bates and Edward Zawadzki cited a figure of 1 million abortions annually. They based this figure on four sources: Taussig's 1936 figures, the figures by Kopp that Taussig relied on in 1936,[165] Stix's 1935 figures,[166] and Kinsey/Gebhard's.[167] Still, the figure of 1 million annually was said by Planned Parenthood's statistician, Christopher Tietze, to have become widely accepted in the 1960s.[168]

Other contradictory claims by abortion advocates refute the notion of hundreds of thousands of illegal abortions. Zad Leavy and Jerome M. Kummer cited the Planned Parenthood conference in 1955 for the proposition that "an extremely small number of physicians are believed to be engaged in the performance of illegal abortions" and they cited the conference for the proposition that "most of them [physicians] scrupulously refuse even to discuss abortion with their patients."[169] At the same time, Mary Calderone, the medical director of Planned Parenthood who edited the papers of that conference, stated that "90 per cent of all illegal abortions are presently being done by physicians."[170] These two facts together would make it impossible for there to be hundreds of thousands of illegal abortions annually, because it would be impossible for those "extremely small number of physicians" to perform large numbers. High volume has been achieved only since nationwide legalization of abortion by *Roe v. Wade* in 1973.

Another claim is that *Roe v. Wade* did not significantly increase the number of abortions because a high percentage would have occurred anyway. For example, Rosenberg cites figures by abortion rights activists that 70 percent of abortions performed after *Roe* merely *replaced* illegal abortions before *Roe*.[171] A 1974 study suggested that "between two-thirds and three fourths—of all legal abortions in the United States in 1971 were replacements for illegal abortions."[172] The replacement argument, of course, cannot verify pre-*Roe* estimates because it assumes accurate statistics of pre-*Roe* abortions as the denominator in the equation.

In addition to the unreliability of the pre-*Roe* estimates, there are significant reasons now to believe—twenty years after abortion was legalized nationwide—that the claims of even hundreds of thousands of illegal abortions annually in the United States before *Roe v. Wade* were much exaggerated. In light of the conceded lack of data and the widely varying estimates, the most compelling data on the actual number of illegal abortions before *Roe v. Wade* are the data from states which loosened their abortion laws between 1966 and 1973 and the actual increase in the number of legal abortions that were reported after abortion was legalized. If hundreds of thousands of illegal abortions were performed annually in the United States before legalization, there is no reason why these *illegal* abortions would not be reflected in figures on *legal* abortions after legalization. States which legalized abortion between 1967 and 1973 did not report a significant number of abortions in the initial years. For example, California reported only five thousand legal abortions in 1968, the first full year of legalized abortion after the new law became effective in November, 1967.[173] If there were one hundred thousand illegal abortions annually in California before 1967, why were there only five thousand reported abortions in the first full year of legalization? As a whole, the most dramatic rise in reported abortions came between 1966 and 1972, as nineteen states loosened their laws, not after *Roe*. The numbers grew as legalization grew. The rise in the number of abortions nationally between 1972 (the last year abortion was illegal in most states) and 1974 (the second year after abortion was legalized) was small.[174] Not until 1975—two years after abortion was legalized on demand nationwide and eight years after the states began to loosen their laws—did the number of induced abortions reach one million.

The great rise in the number of abortions *after* abortion was legalized is confirmed by the rise in the *repeat* abortion rate after legalization. The percentage of repeat abortions (the second or third abortion for the woman aborting) has almost tripled since 1973.[175] This, too, shows that legalization dramatically increased the availability of induced abortions.

Maternal Mortality Before *Roe v. Wade*

The fact that some women died from illegal abortions can be reliably determined from abortion prosecutions in the nineteenth and twentieth centuries.[176] The significance of that tragic fact for defining a sound public policy, however, can only be understood by evaluating a number of other factors, including the increase in the number of abortions since legalization and the loss of unborn lives, the threat of injury and death to women from *legal* abortion every year since abortion was legalized, and broader qualitative factors affecting women's health.

Tales of pain and fear from illegal abortion were the common currency of the abortion reform movement of the 1960s.[177] The constant refrain was that restrictive abortion laws prevented abortions from being performed "under proper conditions and by proper persons."[178] Typical of this genre is Pat Miller's 1993 book, *The Worst of Times* and Rickie Solinger's 1994 book, *The Abortionist*, which recasts Portland abortionist, Ruth Barnett, as an unsung hero. Miller's book is a series of undocumented vignettes. Solinger's book is long on claims and self-justifications but short on facts and documentation. Solinger tries to make out the grossly unrepresentative (by her own account) case of Ruth Barnett to be typical. Conveniently enough, Ruth Barnett died twenty five years ago. The book contains not one footnote citing authorities, references or sources, nor any index, and only a sparse bibliography.

Solinger's overriding themes are belied by the the book's numerous contradictions. For example, Solinger claims that Oregon's law was "tolerant," but the careful reader finds that it treated abortion as manslaughter if either the mother or unborn child was killed. Ruth Barnett supposedly operated undisturbed in Portland between 1930 and 1951, indicating "tolerance," but her boyfriend was a captain in the Police Department.[179] Portland society "tolerated" the abortion trade, but Ruth and her daughter were social pariahs. Public officials "tolerated" abortion, but the "young, politically ambitious" district attorney elected in 1950 was "the sort of official Ruth Barnett had always associated with abortion prosecutions."[180] Ruth was a caring hero who didn't do abortions for the money, but she made (by her own account) $17 million doing abortions and was financially pressured to maintain her lavish life-style and that of her profligate daughter who could not support herself.[181] Abortion was "tolerated" in the 1930s, but a large West Coast abortion operator, Reginald Rankin, was prosecuted in Los Angeles in 1936 and Rankin went to considerable lengths to avoid the law, including successfully bribing an employee of the California State Board of Medical Examiners to dispose of evidence in at least two abortion prosecutions.[182] Abortion was "tolerated" and abortion laws were ineffective, but Barnett was prosecuted numerous times between 1951 and 1968, hindered from performing abortions, under "persistent danger of arrest and imprisonment that dogged her for years," and finally imprisoned as an elderly woman in the late 1960s.[183] Barnett was revered and admired, but her sister and her cousins did not "like what Ruth did for a living one bit," and Ruth carried on a "war against Portland society" for many years.[184] Everyone in Portland knew what she was doing and tolerated it, but law enforcement "experts never considered the possibility of an abortionist like Ruth. . . ."[185] Even the slick book jacket, with the picture of a beautiful, youthful Ruth in expensive clothes, is belied by the reality of a profligate life-style, a family life in shambles, and a daughter who was married nine times, was an abortion patient of her mother's several times,[186] and could not support herself.[187] The irony is entirely lost on Solinger.

A review of maternal deaths from illegal abortion must begin with a statement by Mary Calderone, the medical director of Planned Parenthood, before the campaign for abortion rights in the 1960s got underway. Calderone said:

> Abortion is no longer a dangerous procedure. This applies not just to therapeutic abortions as performed in hospitals but also to so-called illegal abortions as done by physicians. In 1957 there were *only 260 deaths in the whole country attributed to abortions of any kind.* . . . Two corollary factors must be mentioned here: first, chemotherapy and antibiotics have come in, benefiting all surgical procedures as well as abortion. Second, and even more important, the [1955 Planned Parenthood] conference estimated that *90 percent of all illegal abortions are presently done by physicians.* Call them what you will, abortionists or anything else, they are still physicians, trained as such; and many of them are in good standing in their communities. They must do a pretty good job if the death rate is as low as it is. Whatever trouble arises usually comes after self-induced abortions, which comprise approximately 8 per cent, or with *the very small percentage that go to some kind of nonmedical abortionist.* Another corollary fact: physicians of impeccable standing are referring their patients for these illegal abortions to the colleagues whom they know are willing to perform them, or they are sending their patients to certain sources outside of this country where abortion is performed. . . . So remember fact number three: abortion, whether therapeutic or illegal, is in the main no longer dangerous, because it is being done well by physicians.[188]

This general sentiment was also expressed the year before by Dr. Alan Guttmacher—a participant in the 1955 Conference—in his 1959 book.[189]

Three key medical developments before *Roe v. Wade* must be emphasized. First, because of advances in medicine, cases of maternal mortality from *all* types of causes declined dramatically throughout the first half of the twentieth century.[190] Ironically, as professional support for abortion laws seemingly weakened, the medical need for therapeutic abortions was declining: As Dr. Ewen Cameron wrote in the foreword to Harold Rosen's 1954 book, *Therapeutic Abortion*:

> The progress of medicine is rendering therapeutic abortion less and less important, and less and less frequent. The rachitic pelvis is disappearing. The safety of Caesarian section has been immeasurably increased. Tuberculosis is a vanishing disease; and we are by no means so positive as we once were that the offspring of the mentally-deficient woman will be similarly afflicted.[191]

Doctors were increasingly able to treat pregnant mothers and sustain the pregnancy, and the medical reasons (indications) for therapeutic abortion were consistently decreasing.[192] As early as 1954, Alan Guttmacher said that "[t]he truly legal abortions, in which the procedure is *absolutely essential* to preserve a woman's life are relatively few."[193] Mary Calderone reached the same conclusion in 1960: "Medically speaking, that is, from the point of view of diseases of the various systems, cardiac, genitourinary, and so on, *it is hardly ever necessary today* to consider the life of the mother as threatened by a pregnancy."[194] Likewise, Leavy & Kummer wrote in 1962: "The advance of medical science has made rare the situation where illness in a pregnant woman cannot be treated so that her life is not immediately endangered by the pregnancy."[195] By the 1960s, it was widely acknowledged that, with advances in medical science, it was hardly ever necessary to perform an abortion to preserve the life of the mother.[196]

Second, owing to the same advances in medicine and the use of antibiotics occurring after World War II, deaths from illegal abortion (the primary reason being infection) were declining because infection was increasingly capable of being treated with medicine.[197] As Dr. Robert Nelson stated at the 1955 conference, "Since that time [1940-43] the deaths from septic abortions [in the District of Columbia] have ranged between five and none."[198] Likewise, Milton Halpern, the Chief Medical Examiner of New York City, stated at the 1955 conference that "annual incidence figures for abortion deaths in New York City . . . show a progressive drop" from one hundred forty four in 1921 to fifteen in 1951.[199] Consequently, as one scholar wrote, "By 1967, the year the [*New York Times*] was declaring 4,000 women dead annually from abortion, there were 133 such deaths on record. The *New York Times* had allowed itself an editorial adjustment of slightly more than 3,000 percent."[200] Dr. Bernard Nathanson, a founder of NARAL and a former abortionist who managed a clinic that performed tens of thousands of abortions in the early 1970s, wrote in retrospect:

> How many deaths were we talking about when abortion was illegal? In N.A.R.A.L. we generally emphasized the drama of the individual case, not the mass statistics, but when we spoke of the latter it was always "5,000 to 10,000 deaths a year." I confess that I knew the figures were totally false, and I suppose the others did too if they stopped to think of it. But in the "morality" of our revolution, it was a *useful* figure, widely accepted, so why go out of our way to correct it with honest statistics? The overriding concern was to get the laws eliminated, and anything within reason that had to be done was permissible.[201]

Even abortion proponents occasionally recognize the dramatic drop in maternal deaths due to antibiotics.[202]

Third, abortion technology improved up to the time of *Roe v. Wade* and after. These three aspects mean that maternal mortality, both generally and from abortion specifically, declined dramatically in the years *preceding Roe v. Wade*. They also mean that even if elective abortion is again criminalized, maternal mortality would continue to be at least as low as it was on the eve of *Roe v. Wade*, if not still lower.

Despite the unreliability of pre-World War II figures and the 1957 figure of 260 maternal deaths from abortions of all kinds, the common claim in the 1960s was that five thousand to ten thousand women died every year from illegal abortion,[203] and that claim is still made in 1994.[204] No author citing a figure of five thousand abortion deaths a year relied on any scientific, official, or government study. The common currency was anecdotes from coroners, or doctors, usually from unrepresentative locations such as public hospitals in the largest cities in the country.[205] But even these anecdotes fall far short of supporting the notion that maternal deaths were numerous. For example, Patricia Miller cites an autopsy technician working at a hospital in a large Pennsylvania city from the middle 1950s until 1966 (i.e., the year legalization of abortion started in nineteen states): "At the coroner's office, we would see 3 or 4 deaths a year from illegal abortion."[206] These anecdotes never explain how it was medically known that the cause of death was abortion. Nevertheless, based on such anecdotes, the common logic was to speculate, with absolutely no evidence, about "the tip of the iceberg."

In light of Calderone's comment that there were only 260 deaths nationwide in 1957 "attributable to abortions of any kind," what is the five thousand figure based on? That figure was derived from the large estimates of the 1930s, like Taussig's, that preceded World War II and the medical developments that brought about the dramatic decrease in general maternal mortality as well as abortion mortality in the decades after World War II. Even Robert Hall, a leading proponent of legalized abortion in the 1960s, repudiated the claim of five thousand to ten thousand maternal deaths.[207]

The official figures for maternal deaths from illegal abortion dropped still further in the fifteen years leading up to *Roe v. Wade*. Consequently, in 1972—the last year before *Roe v. Wade,* by which time nineteen states had loosened their laws—the Federal Centers for Disease Control (CDC) reported thirty nine deaths from illegal abortion and twenty four deaths from legal abortion.[208] This must be compared with the current figure of at least fifteen deaths per year from legal abortion.[209]

The Impact on Women's Health

Another major indication of the impact of the enforcement of abortion law is more qualitative. How has legalized abortion affected the overall health and well-being of women compared to the conditions that would prevail if abortion were illegal?[210]

One factor is the danger from *legal* abortion. The argument that death and injury from illegal abortion before *Roe* were directly attributable to abortion laws is based on individual, dramatic stories, not on reliable data. Yet, each pre-*Roe* anecdotal account of abortion deaths and injuries can be matched with a similar account from a legal abortion between 1973 and 1995. Each account of a fearful woman suffering before *Roe* can be matched by another fearful woman after *Roe.* Today, many abortions are done on a cash basis, most counseling is group counseling by nonphysicians, women never meet the abortionist until they are gowned and in stirrups, the abortion takes eight minutes, and the woman never sees the abortionist again.[211]

The common claim is that *illegal* abortion is invariably unsafe and *legal* abortion in invariably safe. Yet, the safety of abortion (for the woman) depends on technology, medicine, and the experience of the abortionist. The technology has reached a significant level, and that same technology would exist even if elective abortion were prohibited. Most of the pre-*Roe* maternal deaths—from *all* causes—were due to infection, and when antibiotics were introduced widely in the 1940s, maternal deaths declined precipitously. Again, as Mary Calderone wrote in 1960, there were only 260 maternal deaths from all causes in 1957.[212] Yet, some of the most experienced physician-abortionists still cause the death of women through abortion.[213] Legal proscriptions on abortion would not change these developments in medicine and technology.

In addition, twenty one years of legalized abortion has done little to shed abortion of its negative social and medical stigma, which is directly caused by consciously taking human life. That stigma still dissuades most ethical and competent physicians from getting into the business, and, consequently, it means that many abortionists lack high standards of skill and medical ethics.[214]

In fact, hundreds of women have died from legal abortion since 1973.[215] For each anecdote of a maternal death before *Roe*, there is an incident of maternal death from legal abortion since *Roe*. Take the case of thirteen-year-old Dawn Ravenell, who died after an abortion in New York City in January, 1985;[216] or twenty one-year-old Angelica Duarte, who bled to death from a perforated uterus after an abortion at the Women's Place Clinic in Las Vegas in October, 1991; or seventeen-year-old Latachie Veal, who died in Houston in November 1991 after an abortion at the West Loop Clinic; or thirteen-year-old Deanna Bell, who died in Chicago in September, 1992 after an abortion at the Albany Medical Surgical Center; or Guadalupe Negron, the thirty three-year-old mother of four who died in July 1993 in New York City from a punctured uterus and resulting blood loss; or Pamela Colson, who died from a perforated uterus, lacerated uterine artery, and loss of blood after an abortion in June 1994 at Women's Medical Services in Pensacola, Florida;[217] or Magdalena Ortega Rodriguez, a twenty three-year-old who died from a perforated uterus in December 1994 after an abortion in San Ysidro, California.[218] Numerous abortion malpractice are suits filed in local courts around the country every year for injuries short of death. Today, the "back alley" is on Michigan Avenue.

Besides the evidence of mortality and morbidity from legal abortion is additional evidence about the broader impact of legalized abortion on women's health. One indication of the impact on women's health is the repeat abortion rate, which had climbed to at least 42 percent of all abortions by 1988.[219] Numerous studies indicate that many women suffer psychological pain from abortion. Although "unwanted children" was a common reason cited for the need for legal abortion before *Roe v. Wade*, the illegitimacy rate has only increased since 1973.[220] Abortion has not solved "child unwantedness;" on the contrary, reported cases of child abuse have dramatically increased in the past twenty years.[221] Female deaths from AIDS have increased dramatically over the past decade.[222] There has been a a five-fold increase in hospitalizations for ectopic pregnancies over the past twenty years.[223] Recently, researchers with the National Cancer Institute reported that women may face a higher risk of breast cancer after abortion.[224] Many of these negative health trends for women are associated with sexual behavior patterns as well as with the legalization of abortion, and, as such, they impact on the merits of legal abortion.

CONCLUSION

Abortion laws can be successfully enforced, and abortion can be contained. This is demonstrated by the enforcement of abortion laws in the nineteenth and twentieth centuries as medical science developed more effective means of determining pregnancy, proving abortion, and reducing the medical indications for therapeutic abortion.

But the history of abortion law enforcement teaches us that attention must be given to several considerations. First, complete reliance for curtailing abortion should not be placed on criminal abortion laws. They are a necessary part of containing abortion, but the surrounding cultural and sociological conditions that create the demand for abortion must be understood and counteracted in concert with the enforcement of criminal prohibitions. Second, public opinion must be respected and cultivated. We must remember that print and electronic media can either assist or undermine abortion law enforcement. Third, abortion should be recognized as a business, and the market conditions that sustain it must be understood and inhibited. By understanding the market conditions that make abortion thrive, and by inhibiting them, reliance on criminal prohibitions can be reduced. Fourth, progress in medical science that allows fetal therapy, treatment, and surgery in utero clearly demonstrate the full humanity of the unborn child, and can be utilized to prove the *corpus delicti* of the crime with increasing sophistication. Finally, consideration must be given to the desperation with which some women seek abortion, and compassionate public or private social services must be increased and improved to support and complement the successful enforcement of abortion law.

A number of general conditions have marked the conduct of the abortion industry since nationwide legalization of abortion on demand by *Roe v. Wade*. Attention to these conditions will be necessary to successfully suppress the market after *Roe* is overturned. Legalization under *Roe* is virtually absolute and characterized by a significant lack of regulation, except for the requirement that the abortionist be a licensed physician. State and municipal health departments do very little to regulate clinics, and when they do, the courts often issue injunctions.[225] Within five years after the *Roe* decision, it became clear that the social stigma against doctors for performing elective abortion was not going to disappear, and that abortions were not going to be performed generally by the medical profession. Nor were hospitals going to get into the business of providing a high volume of elective abortions. The notion that abortion was "between a woman and her physician" quickly became a myth. Few women sought abortions from their family or personal physician; most sought abortions from high volume abortionists whom they had never seen before. As a result, the abortion business became limited to a relatively small number of abortionists practicing in about eight hundred assembly-line specialty clinics. By limiting the business to a small number of abortionists in assembly-line clinics, the abortion industry became dependent on high volume operation—a situation which requires physicians, if they wish to stay in business, to spend very little time with their patients, provide little counseling, and operate on an outpatient basis. Thus, it would seem that reducing high volume by itself would make abortion unprofitable.

The criminal law has played an essential role in the enforcement of abortion law for centuries. It has played a teaching role, emphasizing that abortion is the taking of human life. It has also inhibited the performance of abortions, and it has resulted in criminal convictions. But the best evidence indicates that the effectiveness of the criminal law in inhibiting abortion and protecting women and children from abortion has gone through an ebb and flow over the decades. It has not been entirely successful in stopping abortion. When the mixed record of effectiveness of other criminal laws is considered, this fact is unsurprising. The historical evidence indicates that supplementary enforcement schemes and nonlegal mechanisms are needed to bolster the effectiveness of the criminal law. The criminal law is a relatively blunt instrument in inhibiting abortion. Other steps must be taken to relieve the burden of reducing abortion from the criminal law, these include: significantly reducing unplanned pregnancies and the desperate pressure that induces women to consider abortion; encouraging men to assume responsibility and support for women they have impregnated; offering realistic, practicable alternatives for women in crisis pregnancies. These difficult but essential measures will not only ease the burden from the criminal law, but thereby make the criminal law more effective in protecting human life. This is asking no more than society asks of other aspects of criminal law, all of which depend on general deterrence along with the habits and character of the populace.

Support for such broader efforts has been ongoing throughout the United States. Public and private services exist throughout the country. There are thousands of private pregnancy care centers. But, as yet, these public and private services have been unsuccessful in stemming the tide of abortions, a tide that swelled to the rate of 1.6 million per year in the 1980s.

The overruling of *Roe v. Wade* will provide an essential first step in producing the climate in which a more meaningful balance can be achieved, with public and private services, between the rights of women to full civil, economic, and political equality of opportunity and those of the unborn child. *Roe*'s policy of abortion on demand clearly increased the number of abortions dramatically, fostered the widest possible advertising of abortion, crippled the states from inhibiting the abortion industry, and eliminated the economic attractiveness of any alternatives to abortion on demand. By raising the cost of abortion, other alternatives can be made more attractive. New coordination and publicity about available public and private services are needed to make them more attractive to women, and to help women avoid the tragic and deadly choice of abortion.

NOTES

1. Alan Keyes, in a speech given to the New Hampshire Republican State Committee, 19 February 1995.

2. John T. Noonan, Jr. *A Private Choice* (New York: Free Press, 1979), p. 192.

3. I am grateful for comments on an earlier draft by Joseph Dellapenna, Marvin Olasky, Paul Linton, Paige Cunningham, Lynn Murphy and Brian Clowes, for the research assistance of Kirsten Hildebrand (J.D. expected, University of Wisconsin, 1996) and John Little (J.D. Jones College of Law, expected 1996), and for the technical assistance of Margee Connolly and Roger Lewis. *(Since this essay is researched and written in the manner of a legal review, the notation style is different from the other chapters in this book—Ed.).*

4. 410 U.S. 113 (1973).

5. See e.g., Rickie Solinger, *The Abortionist: A Woman Against the Law* (New York: Free Press, 1994); Patricia G. Miller, *The Worst of Times* (New York: Harper-Collins, 1993); Ellen Messer and Kathryn E. May, *Back Rooms: Voices from the Illegal Abortion Era* (Buffalo, N. Y.: Prometheus Books, 1988); Mark A. Graber, "The Ghost of Abortion Past: Pre-Roe Abortion Law in Action," 1 *Va. J. Soc. Pol. and Law* 309 (1994); Rickie Solinger, "A Complete Disaster: Abortion and the Politics of Hospital Abortion Committees, 1950–1970," 19 *Feminist Studies* 241 (Summer 1993); Carole Joffe, "Portraits of Three Physicians of Conscience: Abortion Before Legalization in the United States," 2 *J. Hist. Sexuality* 46 (July 1991); Leslie J. Reagan, "About to Meet Her Maker: Women, Doctors, Dying Declarations, and the State's Investigation of Abortion, Chicago, 1867–1940," 77 *J. Amer. Hist.* 1240 (March 1991); Samuel W. Buell, "Criminal Abortion Revisited," 66 *N.Y.U.L. Rev.* 1774 (1991).

6. James Davison Hunter, *Before the Shooting Begins: Searching for Democracy in America's Culture Wars* 95 (New York: Free Press, 1994), (reporting that one-half of those surveyed in a 1990 Gallup Poll said that "the right to be born outweighs the right to choose at the instant of conception," Ibid at 95, and that 47 percent of those self-identified as "pro-choice" "favor a restriction of abortions after the third month of pregnancy unless it is required to save a woman's life." Ibid at 101).

7. 112 S.Ct. 2792 (1992).

8. See generally, Joseph W. Dellapenna, "The History of Abortion: Technology, Morality and Law," 40 *U. Pitt. L. Rev.* 359 (1979); Clarke D. Forsythe, "Homicide of the Unborn Child: The Born Alive Rule and Other Legal Anachronisms," 21 *Val. U.L. Rev.* 563 (1987).

9. See generally, *The Fetus As A Patient '87: Proceedings of the Third Inter'l Symposium* held in Matsue, Japan, 20–23 July 1987, (Kazuo Maeda ed., New York: Elsevier Science Publications, 1987); *The Fetus As A Patient, Proceedings of the First Inter'l Symposium* held in Sveti Stefan, Yugoslavia, 4–7 June 1984, (Asim Kurjak ed., New York: Elsevier Science Publications, 1985); M. Harrison et al., *The Unborn Patient: Prenatal Diagnosis and Treatment* (Orlando, Florida: Grune and Stratton, 1984); E. Volpe, *Patient in the Womb* (Macon, Georgia: Mercer, 1984); Michael R. Harrison, et al., "Successful Repair in Utero of a Fetal Diaphragmatic Hernia after Removal of Herniated Viscera from the Left Thorax," 322 *N. Eng. J. Med.* 1582 (1990).

10. Joseph D. Schulman, "Treatment of the Embryo and the Fetus in the First Trimester," 35 *Am. J. Med. Genetics* 197 (1990).

11. See generally, Forsythe, supra note 8.

12. Carl J. Pauerstein, ed., *Clinical Obstetrics* 110–114 (New York: John Wiley & Sons, 1987); Miller, *The Worst of Times*, 19.

13. See generally, Forsythe, supra note 8. As one mid-nineteenth century treatise stated:

The signs of abortion, as obtained by an examination of the female, are not very certain in their character. It is seldom, indeed, that an examination of the living female is had, and especially at a period early enough to afford any valuable indications. When abortion occurs in the early months, it leaves but slight and evanescent traces behind it.

James C. Mohr, *Abortion in America: The Origins and Evolution of National Policy, 1800–1900* 72 (New York: Oxford University Press, 1980) (quoting Francis Wharton and Moreton Stille, *Treatise on Medical Jurisprudence* 277 (Philadelphia, 1855)).

14. As late as the first decade of the twentieth-century, medical conferences of the American Medical Association recorded expressions of frustration by physicians that the public still held to the notion that the life of the child began with quickening and that the truth that human life began with conception was not widely understood. See, e.g., Walter Dorsett, M.D., "Criminal Abortion in its Broadest Sense," 51 *J. Amer. Med. Assoc.* 957 (19 Sept. 1908) (statement during discussion by R.W. Holmes, M.D. of Chicago: "The fact should be taught that life begins with conception and not with quickening..Many now make themselves believe that there is no life until the movements are felt.); Ibid. at 961 ("If our statutes are to accomplish the results they should we must first educate the public mind and morals to the belief that conception means human life, and that the interruption or destruction of that conception means murder just as much as if the child had been murdered with a bludgeon after it had been delivered into the world.") (Statement of Dr. Florus F. Lawrence).

15. See generally, Forsythe, supra note 8.

16. Ibid.

17. See generally, Forsythe, supra note 8.

18. See Joseph Dellapenna, *Dispelling the Myths of Abortion History*, Part XV, at 1–3 (unpublished manuscript) (hereafter Dellapenna, *Dispelling*).

Thereafter, English courts prosecuted abortions fairly routinely under the early Stuarts, Cromwell's Commonwealth and the Restoration. With the exception of Sir Matthew Hale's holding that the death of a mother from an abortion was a felony homicide, these later seventeenth-century cases produced convictions only for misdemeanors, lending credence to Coke's conclusion that abortion before quickening was only a misdemeanor. All important later commentators on the criminal law followed Coke's dictum in describing the law relating to abortions. By the opening of the eighteenth century, then, the criminality of abortion under the common law was well-established: courts had rendered clear holdings that abortion was a crime, no decision indicated that any form of abortion was lawful, and secondary authorities similarly uniformly supported the criminality of abortion.

See also Philip A. Rafferty, *Roe v. Wade: The Birth of a Constitutional Right* (Ann Arbor: U. M. I. dissertation services, 1992).

19. See, e.g., Glanville Williams, *The Sanctity of Life and the Criminal Law* 152 (New York: Knopf, 1957) ("Abortion before quickening was no crime."); Zad Leavy, "Criminal Abortion: Facing the Facts," *Los Angeles B. Bull.* 355 n.1 (Oct. 1959) (citing Williams, supra).

20. Cf. 1 William Blackstone, *Commentaries on the Laws of England* 125 (Chicago: U. Chi. Press edition, 1979), (concluding that "[l]ife is the immediate gift of God, a right inherent by nature in every individual; and it begins in contemplation of law as soon as an infant is able to stir in the mother's womb")(on the "Rights of Persons") with 4 Blackstone 198 ("To kill a child in it's [sic] mother's womb, is now no murder, but a great misprision: but if the child be born alive, and dieth by reason of the potion or bruises it received in the womb, it is murder in such as administered or gave them.").

21. See generally, John Keown, *Abortion, Doctors and the Law: Some Aspects of the Legal Regulation of Abortion in England from 1803 to 1982* (New York: Cambridge University Press, 1988); Joseph W. Dellapenna, "The History of Abortion: Technology, Morality and Law," 40 *U. Pitts. L. Rev.* 359 (1979); Joseph Dellapenna, "Brief of the American Academy of Medical Ethics as Amicus Curiae in Support of Defendants-Appellants, Hope v. Perales," 83 N.Y.2d 563, 634 N.E.2d 183, 611 N.Y.S.2d 811 (1994) [hereinafter Brief of AAME]; Joseph W. Dellapenna, "The Historical Case Against Abortion," 13 *Continuity* 59 (1989).

22. Cyril C. Means, "The Law of New York Concerning Abortion and the Status of the Foetus, 1664–1968: A Case of Cessation of Constitutionality," 14 *N.Y. Law Forum* 411 (1968); Cyril C. Means, "The Phoenix of Abortional Freedom: Is a Penumbral or Ninth-Amendment Right About to Arise from the Nineteenth Century Legislative Ashes of a Fourteenth Century Common-Law Liberty?," 17 *N.Y. Law Forum* 335

(1971). NARAL was first the National Association for the Repeal of Abortion Law, then the National Abortion Rights Action League, now the National Abortion and Reproductive Rights Action League. See also Rafferty, *Roe v. Wade: The Birth of a Constitutional Right*.

23. Rex v. de Bourton (The Twinslayer's Case), Y.B. Mich. 1 Edw. 3, f. 23, pl. 28 (K.B. 1327); Rex v. Anonymous (The Abortionist's Case), in Sir Anthony Fitzherbert, Graunde Abridgement tit. Corone, f. 268, pl. 263 (1st ed. 1516)[K.B. 1348]. Although Means implies that he discovered these cases, they were known by several judges and authorities before 1900, and no one before Means had ever suggested that the cases established any abortion "liberty." Justice Holmes cited them in his opinion for the Massachusetts Supreme Judicial Court in Dietrich v. Northampton, 138 Mass. 14 (1884). See Clarke D. Forsythe, "The Legacy of Oliver Wendell Holmes," 69 *U. Det. Mercy L. Rev.* 677, 685–689 (1992).

24. Dellapenna, *Dispelling*, supra note 18; Robert A. Destro, "Abortion and the Constitution: The Need for a Life-Protective Amendment," 63 *Cal. L. Rev.* 1250 (1975); Robert M. Byrn, "An American Tragedy: The Supreme Court on Abortion," 41 *Fordham L. Rev.* 807 (1973).

25. At least fifteen cases for abortion have been discovered, dating back to 1256. Dellapenna, Brief for the American Academy of Medical Ethics (AAME), supra note 21, at 13 n.18 (citing R. v. Haule, JUST 1/547A, m.20d (London Eyre 1321); R. v. Kultavenan, Calendar of Justiciary Roles or Proc. in the Ct. of the Justiciar of Ireland I to VII Years of Edward II, at 193 (Dublin Stationary Off., n.d.) (Cork, Ireland 1311); R.v. Code, JUST 1/789, m.1. (Hampshire Eyre 1281) [see Appendix B, at B-3]; R. v. Ragoun, JUST 1/547A, m.55d (London Eyre 1310); R. v. Eppinge, JUST 1/547A. m.46 (ms. dated 1321) (London Eyre 1304); R. v. Hervy, JUST 1/547A, m. 40d (1300, ms. dated 1321); R. v. Hokkestere, JUST 1/547A., m.3. (London Eyre 1298, ms. date 1321); R. v. Scot, JUST 1/547A, m.22 (1291, ms. dated 1321); R. v. Dada, JUST 1/547A, m.19d (1290, ms. dated 1321); R. v. Cliston, JUST 1/1011, m.62 (Wiltshire Eyre 1288); R. v. Mercer, JUST 1/710, m.45 (Oxford Eyre 1285) [see Appendix B, at B-4]; R. v. Brente, JUST 1/186, m.30 Devon Eyre 1281); R. v. Code, supra; R. v. Scharp, The London Eyre of 1276, at 23 (no. 76) (London Rec. Soc'y 1976); Juliana's Appeal (1256?) Somerset Pleas (Civ. and Crim.) from the Rolls of the Itinerant Justices 321 (no. 1243) (1897) [see Appendix B, at B-3]; Erneburga's Appeal, JUST 1/175, m.38 (1249). See also R. v. Haunsard, JUST 1/548, m.4. (London Eyre 1329) (defendant convicted of causing an abortion in the course of extorting money); R. v. Clouet, (1304), Cal. Ch. Warrants in the Pub. Rec. Off. Prepared under the Superintendence of the Deputy Keeper of the Rec., A.D. 1244–1326, at 232 (London 1927) (pardon; Island of Guernsey); R. v. Cheney, JUST 1/323, m.47d (Hertfordshire Eyre 1278) (defendant amerced in trespass for an accidental abortion caused by defendant's horse); R. v. Cordwaner, The London Eyre of 1276, at 18 (no. 62) (London Rec. Soc'y 1976) (defendant outlawed for causing the birth of a child; unclear whether the child died). There is stronger evidence, beginning in the 1500s, that elective abortion was treated as a crime. Ibid. at 14 (citing R. v. Lichefeld, K.B. 27/974, Rex. m.4 (1505)). In two other cases, a man was indicted for encouraging a woman to take an abortifacient and a woman was sentenced to death for

performing an abortion by "witchcraft." Ibid. (citing R. v. Wodlake, K.B. 9/513/m.23, K.B. 9/513/j.23d (1530), K.B. 29/162/m.11d (1531); R. v. Turnour, Assize 35/23/29 (Essex 1581)).

In 1732, there was a misdemeanor conviction for a prequickening abortion. Rex v. Beare, 2 *The Gentleman's Magazine* 931 (Aug. 1732). See also 2 *The Newgate Calender* 315–16 (Andrew Knapp and William Baldwin eds. 1825). See also Rafferty, *Roe v. Wade: The Birth of a Constitutional Right.*

    26. See, e.g., Norma McCorvey, *I Am Roe: My Life, Roe v. Wade, and Freedom of Choice* 8 (New York: HarperCollins, 1994) ("English law...held that abortion was legal up until the moment a fetus 'quickened'....In England, an abortion after quickening became a crime in 1803."); See also generally Solinger, *The Abortionist*, supra note 5; Reagan, supra note 5, at 1241.

    27. State v. Cooper, 22 N.J. (2 Zabr.) 52 (1849); Commonwealth v. Parker, 50 Mass. (9 Met.) 263 (1845).

    28. Eggart v. State, 40 Fla. 527, 25 So. 144, 145 (Fla. 1898) (dictum in case decided under statute abolishing quickening distinction); Arnold v. Gaylord, 16 R.I. 573, 576, 18 A. 177, 178–79 (R.I. 1889) (dictum in loss of services case); People v. Sessions, 58 Mich. 594 (1886); State v. Emerick, 13 Mo.App. 492, 495–98 (1883) (dictum in case decided under statute), aff'd, 87 Mo. 110 (1885); Mitchell v. Commonwealth, 78 Ky. 204, 205–10 (1879) (reversing conviction where indictment failed to allege that "the woman was quick with child"); Evans v. People, 49 N.Y. 86, 88 (1872) (dictum in case reversing conviction under manslaughter statute); Smith v. Gaffard, 31 Ala. 45 (1857) (dictum in slander case); Abrams v. Foshee, 3 Iowa 273 (1856) (dictum in slander case); Smith v. State, 33 Me. 48 (1851); Commonwealth v. Parker, 50 Mass. (9 Met.) 263 (1845); State v. Cooper, 22 N.J.L. 52 (1849) (dictum in case upholding indictment charging defendant with assault); Commonwealth v. Bangs, 9 Mass. 387, 387–88 (1812) (arresting judgment where indictment failed to allege that "the woman was quick with child").

    29. It was recognized that:

[A]s the life of an infant was not supposed to begin until it stirred in the mother's womb, it was not regarded as a criminal offense to commit an abortion in the early stages of pregnancy. A considerable change in the law has taken place in many jurisdictions by the silent and steady progress of judicial opinion; and it has been frequently held by Courts of high character that abortion is a crime at common law without regard to the stage of pregnancy.

Lamb v. State, 67 Md. 524, 533, 10 A. 208 (Md. 1887). See also, State v. Reed, 45 Ark. 333, 334 (1885); State v. Slagle, 82 N.C. 630, 632 (1880); Mills v. Commonwealth, 13 Pa. 630, 632–33 (1850); Marmaduke v. People, 45 Colo. 357, 361–62, 101 P. 337, 338 (Colo. 1909).

    30. Bishop, Statutory Crimes § 744, at 447 (2d ed. 1883); F. Wharton, American Criminal Law § 1220–30, at 210–18 (6th rev. ed. 1868). In the 20th century, Burdick said that these two authors were "the two most frequently cited American writers" on the criminal law." W. Burdick, *Law of Crime* v (foreword) (New York: M. Bender and

Co., 1946).

31. Julia Cherry Spruill refers to the case of Captain Mitchell in Maryland in 1652, who "was accused of a number of crimes, among which was attempted abortion." J. Spruill, *Women's Life and Work in the Southern Colonies* 325–26 (New York: Russell & Russell, 1938). She also refers to the seventeenth-century case of Elizabeth Robins, who was accused of "taking medicine to destroy her child." Ibid. at 325–26. A Rhode Island case of 1683 has also been discovered. There, a Deborah Allen was convicted and punished for "indeavoringe the dithuchion of the Child in her womb." L. Koehler, *A Search for Power: The "Weaker Sex" in Seventeenth-Century New England* 329 and n. 132 (Urbana: University of Illinois Press, 1980).

There are few reported cases and this may be because there were few abortions. At least historian Catherine Scholten has concluded that "few [women] tried to limit their pregnancies by birth control or abortion." C. Scholten, *Childbearing in American Society 1650–1850* 9 (New York: New York University Press, 1985).

32. Paul Linton, "Planned Parenthood v. Casey: The Flight From Reason in the Supreme Court," 13 *St. Louis Pub. L. Rev.* 15, 109–113 (1994) (Appendix A).

33. Dellapenna, *Dispelling*, supra note 18, at Part VIII; Mohr, supra note 13, at 276 n.15 ("[t]he nineteenth century had no preparations capable of directly producing abortion, though contemporary physicians and the public believed otherwise").

34. Marvin Olasky, *Abortion Rites: A Social History of Abortion in America* 43–59 (Wheaton, Ill.: Crossway Books, 1992).

35. Dellapenna, *Dispelling*, supra note 18, at Part IX, p. 38.

36. See Dennis J. Horan and Thomas J. Marzen, "Abortion and Midwifery: A Footnote in Legal History," in *New Perspectives on Human Abortion* 199 (Thomas W. Hilgers, et al., eds., Frederick, Md.: University Publications of America, 1981) (citing 3 Minutes of the Common Council of the City of New York 121 (1712–1729)); S. Massengill, *A Sketch of Medicine and Pharmacy* 294 (Bristol, Tenn.: S. E. Massengill Co., 2d ed. 1942).

37. Otto Pollak, *The Criminality of Women* 45–46 (Philadelphia: U. Penn. Press 1950, Perpetua paper ed. 1961)

The best illustration of the degree to which the criminal behavior of the abortee herself is disregarded by our law-enforcing agencies can be found in the proceedings against the Pacific Coast Abortion Ring...in the thirties. Not one of the women who had engaged the services of this organization seems to have been prosecuted, however.

See also, Reagan, supra note 5, at 1243–44 ("women were not arrested, prosecuted, or incarcerated for having abortions...."); Paul Linton, "Enforcement of State Abortion Statutes after Roe: A State-By-State Analysis," 67 *U. Det. Mercy L. Rev.* 157, 163–64 and n. 31 (1990).

38. Dellapenna, *Dispelling*, supra note 18, Part VIII at 25 and n.78.

39. Cf. Pollak, supra note 37, at 2 ("being an accessory to statutory rape is hardly ever charged to a woman").

40. See, e.g., People v. Reinard, 33 Cal.Rptr. 908, 912, 220 Cal.App.2d 720, 724 (Cal. Dist. Ct. App. 1963) ("The abortee is considered the victim of the crime."); Basoff v. State, 208 Md. 643, 654, 118 A.2d 917, 923 (1956) ("regarded by the law as a victim of the crime, rather than as a participant in it."); Thompson v. United States, 30 App.D.C. 352, 363 (1908) ("She is regarded as his victim, rather than an accomplice."); People v. Dunn (NY).

41. See, e.g., Petition of Vickers, 371 Mich. 114, 115, 123 N.W.2d 253, 254 (Mich. 1963) ("The majority view is that not only may she not be held for abortion upon herself but neither as an accomplice.").

42. Paul D. Wohlers, *Women and Abortion: Prospects of Criminal Charges* 1 (Washington D. C.: The American Center for Bioethics, undated).

43. See, e.g., State v. Barnett, 249 Or. 226, 228, 437 P.2d 821, 822 (Or. 1968); Zutz v. State, 52 Del. 492, 160 A.2d 727 (Del. 1967); People v. Kutz, 9 Cal.Rptr. 626, 187 Cal.App.2d 431 (Cal. Dist. Ct. App. 1961) (not an accomplice); State v. Miller, 364 Mo. 320, 261 S.W.2d 103 (Mo. 1953); People v. Stone, 89 Cal.App.2d 853, 202 P.2d 333 (Cal. Dist. Ct. App. 1949); People v. Clapp, 24 Cal.2d 835, 151 P.2d 237 (Cal. 1944); Commonwealth v. Sierakowski, 154 Pa.Super.Ct. 321, 327, 35 A.2d 790, 793 (Pa. 1944) ("not an accomplice or particeps criminis."); People v. Blank, 283 N.Y. 526, 29 N.E.2d 73 (N.Y. 1940); State v. Burlingame, 47 S.D. 332, 337, 198 N.W. 824, 826 (S.D. 1924) (regarded as victim rather an accomplice or participant); State v. McCurtain, 52 Utah 63, 172 P. 481 (Utah 1918); Gray v. State, 77 Tex. Crim. 221, 229, 178 S.W. 337, 341 (Tex. Crim. App. 1915) (not an accomplice); Seifert v. State, 160 Ind. 464, 67 N.E. 100 (Ind. 1903); State v. Pearce, 56 Minn. 226, 230, 57 N.W. 652, 653 (Minn. 1894) ("She was the victim of a cruel act."); People v. McGonegal, 136 N.Y. 62, 32 N.E. 616 (N.Y. 1892); People v. Vedder, 98 N.Y. 630, 632 (1885).

The only apparent exception was Alabama. Trent v. State, 15 Ala.App. 485, 73 So. 834 (Ala. Ct. App. 1916). See also Dykes v. State, 30 Ala.App. 129, 1 So.2d 754 (Ala. Ct. App. 1941); Steed v. State, 27 Ala.App.263, 170 So. 489 (Ala. Ct. App. 1936). As in the other cases, the woman's guilt was not the issue but whether her status as an accomplice prevented the introduction of evidence without corroboration. The court concluded, however, that the woman should be considered an accomplice because the statute would otherwise lose its moral force. This rationale, however, never influenced other states.

44. Wohlers, supra note 42, at 2.

45. State v. Barnett, 249 Or. 226, 228, 437 P.2d 821, 822 (1968) ("The acts prohibited are those which are performed upon the mother rather than any action taken by her. She is the object of the acts prohibited rather than the actor.").

46. See generally, Linton, supra note 37, at 163–64 n.31.

47. Reagan, supra note 5, at 1244.

48. Cf. Wohlers, supra note 42, at 8–10 (citing Gaines v. Wolcott, 119 Ga.App. 313, 167 S.E.2d 366 (Ga. Ct. App. 1969), aff'd, 225 Ga. 373, 169 S.E.2d 165 (Ga. 1969) (woman can sue abortionist for negligence); Henrie v. Griffith, 395 P.2d 809 (Okla. 1965); Castronovo v. Murawsky, 3 Ill.App.2d 168, 120 N.E.2d 871 (Ill. App.

Ct. 1954) (woman cannot recover for negligence); True v. Older, 227 Minn. 154, 34 N.W.2d 200 (1948) (woman could recover); Nash v. Meyer, 54 Idaho 283, 31 P.2d 273 (Idaho 1934) (woman cannot recover for negligence); Martin v. Morris, 163 Tenn. 10, 42 S.W.2d 207 (Tenn. 1931) (woman cannot recover); Andrews v. Coulter, 163 Wash. 429, 1 P.2d 320 (Wash. 1931) (woman could not recover damages for abortion but could recover for negligent treatment after abortion); Martin v. Hardesty, 91 Ind.App. 239, 163 N.E. 610 (Ind. App. 1928) (estate could recover after abortion death); Szadiwicz v. Cantor, 257 Mass. 518, 154 N.E. 251 (Mass. 1926) (woman could not recover); Milliken v. Heddesheimer, 110 Ohio St. 381, 144 N.E. 264 (Ohio Ct. App. 1924) (woman's estate could recover); Hunter v. Wheate, 63 App.D.C. 206, 289 F. 604 (D.C. Cir. 1923) (woman could not recover even if she was not an accomplice); Lembo v. Donnell, 117 Me. 143, 103 A. 11 (1918) (woman could recover); Larocque v. Couneim, 87 N.Y.S. 625, 42 Misc. 613 (N.Y. Sup. Ct. 1904); Wells v. New England Mutual Life Ins. Co., 191 Pa. 207, 43 A. 126 (Pa. 1899) (estate cannot recover); Goldnamer v. O'Brien, 98 Ky. 569 (1896) (cannot recover from person urging her to have abortion); Miller v. Bayer, 94 Wis. 123, 68 N.W. 869 (Wis. 1896) (woman could recover).

49. Williams, supra note 19, at 153–54.

50. Dellapenna, *Dispelling*, supra note 18, at Part VIII, at 26–27.

51. Paul B. Linton and Kevin J. Todd, "Abortion Under the Illinois Constitution: The Framers Did Not Incorporate A Right to Abortion," 81 *Ill. Bar. J.* 31 (Jan. 1993); J.M. Sheean, "The Common and Statute Law of Illinois," 7 *Ill. Med. J.* 37, 38 (January 1905).

52. Ibid.

53. See generally, Olasky, supra note 34, at 83–105.

54. C.S. Bacon, "The Duty of the Medical Profession in Relation to Criminal Abortion," 7 *Ill. Med. J.* 18, 21 (January 1905).

55. John E. Traeger, "Criminal Abortion As It Comes Before the Coroner's Office," 7 *Ill. Med. J.* 35 (January 1905).

56. See generally, R. Perkins and R. Boyce, *Criminal Law and Procedure* 263–288 (5th ed. 1977); Jerome Hall, "Criminal Attempt: A Study of Foundations of Criminal Liability," 49 *Yale L.J.* 789 (1940).

57. 720 Ill. Compiled Statutes 5/8–4(a) (1992).

58. People v. Paluch, 78 Ill.App.2d 356, 222 N.E.2d 508 (1966).

59. Hyde v. United States, 225 U.S. 347, 387–88 (1911) (Holmes, J., dissenting).

60. 141 Cal.App.2d 193, 296 P.2d 610 (Cal. Dist. Ct. App. 1956).

61. See also, Jeffrey F. Ghert, "Annotation, Comment Note-Impossibility of Consummation of Substantive Crime As Defense in Criminal Prosecution for Conspiracy or Attempt to Commit Crime," 37 *A.L.R.* 3d 375 (1971 and Supp. 1994); Arnold N. Enker, "Impossibility in Criminal Attempts: Legality and the Legal Process," 53 *Minn. L. Rev.* 665 (1969).

62. Cal. Penal Code § 317 (1915) (advertising to produce miscarriage). Subsequently, the scope of the statute was judicially narrowed. See People v. McKean, 243 P. 898 (Cal. Dist. Ct. App. 1925).

63. See generally, Olasky, supra note 34, at 194–96 and n.96–102; Marvin Olasky, *The Press and Abortion, 1838–1988* (Hillsdale, N. J.: Lawrence Erlbaum Associates, 1988).

64. See generally, Paul Linton, "Enforcement of State Abortion Statutes After Roe: A State-by-State Analysis," 67 *U. Det. L. Rev.* 157 (1990).

65. Dellapenna, *Dispelling*, supra note 18, at Part IX, p. 42; Olasky, supra note 34.

66. Olasky, supra note 34, at 170.

67. Ibid., at 170–71.

68. Ibid.

69. Ibid.

70. Note, "A Functional Study of Existing Abortion Laws," 35 *Col. L. Rev.* 87, 91 n.17–18 (1935).

71. Samuel B. Burk, "The Development of the Law of Criminal Abortion," 57 *Medical Times* 153, 158 (June, 1929).

72. Olasky, *The Press and Abortion*, supra note 63, at 68.

73. Pollak, supra note 37, at 45.

74. See Olasky, *The Press and Abortion*, supra note 63, at 80 (citing *San Francisco Examiner*, 22 May 1946, p. 8; "Four Seized in Alleged Illegal Operation Raids," *Los Angeles Times*, 30 Sept. 1948, p. 2).

75. "Illegal Operation Nets M.D. Three Years," *N.Y. J.-Am.*, 5 May 1950; "Three Doctors and 4 others Plead Guilty of Abortion," *N.Y. Tribune*, 18 Feb. 1952; "Charges M.D., Hospitals Hush Abortion Cases," *N.Y. Post*, 10 Dec. 1953.

76. See In re Lurie, 263 App. Div. 660, 34 N.Y.S.2d 247 (N.Y. App. Div. 1942); In re Madden, 24 N.Y.S.2d 127 (N.Y. App. Div. 1940). See also J. Bennett and J. Amen, "A Presentment on the Suppression of Criminal Abortions, By the Grand Jury for the Extraordinary Special and Trial Term," (New York Supreme Court, 15 October 1941) (hereafter Amen Report); J.E. Bates, "The Abortion Mill: An Institutional Study," 45 *J. Crim. Law and Crimin.* 157, 163–66 (1954).

77. John Harlan Amen, "Some Obstacles to Effective Legal Control of Criminal Abortions," in "The Abortion Problem," Proceedings of the conference held under the auspices of the National Committee on Maternal Health, Inc., at the New York Academy of Medicine, 19 and 20 June 1944, Howard C. Taylor Jr., chairman. Proceedings published by Williams and Wilkins, Baltimore, 1944. [Hereinafter "The Abortion Problem"].

78. Ibid., at 135.

79. Ibid.

80. Ibid., at 135.

81. Ibid.

82. Ibid., at 136.

83. Ibid., at 136.

84. Ibid., at 136.

85. Dellapenna, *Dispelling*, supra note 18, at Part IX, p. 39, n.90, 40. See also People v. Candib, 129 N.Y.S.2d 176 (N.Y. Sup. Ct. 1954).

86. 1942 N.Y. Laws, ch. 791, §1.

87. Weinstein v. Board of Regents of Univ. of State of New York, 267 App. Div. 4, 44 N.Y.S.2d 917, 918 (N.Y. App. Div. 1943).

88. "The Abortion Problem," supra note 77, at 139.

89. See Epstein v. Board of Regents of University of New York, 267 A.D. 27, 44 N.Y.S.2d 921 (N.Y. App. Div. 1943), rev'd, 295 N.Y. 154, 65 N.E.2d 756 (N.Y. 1946); Weinstein v. Board of Regents of Univ. of State of New York, 267 A.D. 4, 44 N.Y.S.2d 917 (N.Y. App. Div. 1943), rev'd, 292 N.Y. 682, 56 N.E.2d 104 (N.Y. 1944); Rothenberg v. Board of Regents, 267 A.D. 24, 44 N.Y.S.2d 926 (N.Y. App. Div. 1943), appeal denied, 267 A.D. 852, 47 N.Y.S.2d 284 (N.Y. App. Div. 1944).

90. Epstein v. Board of Regents of University of New York, 295 N.Y. 154, 65 N.E.2d 756 (1946).

91. Miller, supra note 5, at 35.

92. Bates, supra note 76, at 166.

93. See generally Solinger, *The Abortionist*, supra note 5; Graber, supra note 5, at 325–28. Many if not most of Graber's sources consist of anecdotes by the most committed abortion rights supporters regurgitating claims made in the 1960s that were designed to undermine the laws.

94. See Note, supra note 70, at 91 n.18; Amen Report, supra note 76. The Amen investigation received much publicity. See Weinstein v. Board of Regents of Univ. of State of New York, 267 App. Div. 4, 44 N.Y.S.2d 917, 919 (N.Y. App. Div. 1943).

95. See generally Solinger, *The Abortionist*, supra note 5, esp. at 149–168.

96. Ibid.

97. Zimmerman v. Board of Regents, 31 A.D.2d 560, 294 N.Y.S.2d 435 (N.Y. App. Div. 1968).

98. See, e.g., Zimmerman v. Board of Regents, 31 A.D.2d 560, 294 N.Y.S.2d 435 (N.Y. App. Div. 1968); Sos v. Bd of Regents, 26 A.D.2d 741, 272 N.Y.S.2d 87 (N.Y. App. Div. 1966) (annulled Board's determination based on insufficient evidence), aff'd, 19 N.Y.2d 990, 281 N.Y.S.2d 831 (N.Y. 1967); Shapiro v. Bd of Regents, 22 A.D.2d 243, 254 N.Y.S.2d 906 (N.Y. App. Div. 1964), Walsh v. New York State Liquor Authority, 16 N.Y.2d 783, 209 N.E.2d 821, 262 N.Y.S.2d 503 (1965); Ciofalo v. Bd of Regents, 23 A.D.2d 926, 258 N.Y.S.2d 881 (N.Y. App. Div. 1965); Robinson v. Bd of Regents, 4 A.D.2d 359, 164 N.Y.S.2d 863 (N.Y. App. Div. 1957); Genova v. Board of Regents of University of N.Y., 272 A.D. 1085, 74 N.Y.S.2d 729 (N.Y. App. Div. 1947); Friedel v. Board of Regents of University of New York, 296 N.Y. 347, 73 N.E.2d 545 (1947); Jablon v. Board of Regents of University of State of New York, 296 N.Y. 1027, 73 N.E.2d 904 (1947); Jablon v. Board of Regents of University of State of N.Y., 271 A.D. 369, 66 N.Y.S.2d 340 (N.Y. App. Div. 1946); Newman v. Regents of University of State of N.Y., 270 A.D. 964, 61 N.Y.S.2d 841 (N.Y. App. Div. 1946); Neshamkin v. Board of Regents of University of New York, 295 N.Y. 755, 66 N.E.2d 124 (1946); Application of Neshamkin, 269 A.D. 891, 56 N.Y.S.2d 146 (N.Y. App. Div. 1945); Neshamkin v. Board of Regents of University of State of New York, 281 N.Y. 683, 23 N.E.2d 16 (N.Y. 1939); Epstein v. Board of Regents of University of New York, 267 A.D. 27, 44 N.Y.S.2d 921 (N.Y. App. Div. 1943), rev'd, 295 N.Y. 154, 65 N.E.2d 756 (1946); Weinstein v. Board of Regents of Univ. of State of New York, 267 A.D. 4, 44 N.Y.S.2d 917 (N.Y. App. Div. 1943),

rev'd, 292 N.Y. 682, 56 N.E.2d 104 (1944); Rothenberg v. Board of Regents, 267 A.D. 24, 44 N.Y.S.2d 926 (N.Y. App. Div. 1943), appeal denied, 267 A.D. 852, 47 N.Y.S.2d 284 (N.Y. App. Div. 1944); Kasha v. Board of Regents of University of State of New York, 290 N.Y. 630, 48 N.E.2d 712 (1943); Kahn v. Board of Regents of University of State of New York, 254 A.D. 798, 4 N.Y.S.2d 233 (N.Y. App. Div. 1938); Kahn v. Board of Regents of University of State of New York, 281 N.Y. 684, 23 N.E.2d 16 (1939); Reiner v. Board of Regents of the University of the State of New York, 254 A.D. 920, 6 N.Y.S.2d 356 (N.Y. App. Div. 1938); Minton v. Board of Regents of University of State of New York, 247 A.D. 838, 287 N.Y.S. 502 (N.Y. App. Div. 1936).

99. "The Abortion Problem," supra note 77, at 137–38.

100. See generally Lawrence Lader, *Abortion II: Making the Revolution* (Boston: Beacon Press, 1973).

101. Any determination by a sub-committee would only be reviewed by a full committee at its semi-annual meeting. Amen did not believe that the cases received careful attention, since the full committee primarily relied on the recommendation of the subcommittee and rarely reviewed the record. Furthermore, the finding of guilt by the subcommittee, and recommendation of punishment to the Board of Regents, had to be unanimous. The proceedings were voided if a member was absent or did not vote.

102. "The Abortion Problem," supra note 77, at 142.

103. See In re Abortion in Kings County, 206 Misc. 830, 135 N.Y.S. 2d 381 (1954); Application of Grand Jury of Kings County, 286 A.D. 270, 143 N.Y.S.2d 501 (1955).

104. See Williams, supra note 19, at 168.

105. Zad Leavy and Jerome M. Kummer, "Criminal Abortion: Human Hardship and Unyielding Laws," 35 S. *Cal. L. Rev.* 123, 128 and n.42 (1962).

106. Alan F. Guttmacher, "Therapeutic Abortion: The Doctor's Dilemma," 21 *J. Mt. Sinai Hosp.* at 111, 118 (1954). See also, Guttmacher, "The Law that Doctors Often Break," 63 *Redbook* 24 (Aug. 1959).

107. Ibid., (citing K.P. Russell, "Therapeutic Abortions in California in 1950," 60 *West. J. Surg. Ob. Gyn.* 497 (1952) (according to which the procedure was "the system of choice in 11 per cent of 61 hospitals in California in 1950")). See Stewart v. Long Island College Hospital, 58 Misc.2d 432, 296 N.Y.S.2d 41 (N.Y. Sup. Ct. 1968), affirmed as modified, 35 A.D.2d 531, 313 N.Y.S.2d 502 (N.Y. App. Div. 1970).

108. Miller, supra note 5, at 37; Peter Broeman and Jeannette Meier, "Therapeutic Abortion Practices in Chicago Hospitals—Vagueness, Variation, and Violation of the Law," 4 *Law and Soc. Order* 757 (1971).

109. Guttmacher, supra note 106, 21 *J. Mt. Sinai Hosp.* at 118.

110. Ibid.

111. Ibid. Guttmacher stated that "[u]nrestricted therapeutic abortion leads to loose medical thinking. Flouting the abortion law also acts as a springboard for unorthodox, borderline medical ethical practices." Ibid., at 119.

112. Herbert L. Packer and Ralph J. Gampell, "Therapeutic Abortion: A Problem in Law and Medicine," 11 *Stan. L. Rev.* 417 (1959).

113. Leavy and Kummer, supra note 105, at 128 (citing Russell, "Sterilization and Therapeutic Abortion," 1 *Clin. Obst. N.Y.* 967 (1958)).

114. See e.g., Graber, supra note 5.

115. See, e.g., State v. Millette, 112 N.H. 458, 299 A.2d 150 (1972); State v. Coleman, 17 N.C.App. 11, 193 S.E.2d 395 (1972); State v. Campbell, 263 La. 1058, 270 So.2d 506 (1972).

116. See, e.g., Solinger, *The Abortionist*, supra note 5; *Time*, 12 March 1956, at 46.

117. State v. Barnett, 249 Or. 226, 437 P.2d 821 (1968).

118. Charles King, "Calling Jane: The Life and Death of a Women's Illegal Abortion Service," 20 *Women and Health* 75 (1993).

119. Commonwealth v. Kudish, 289 N.E.2d 856 (Mass. 1972).

120. Finding constitutional: Nelson v. Planned Parenthood, 19 Ariz.App. 142, 505 P.2d 580 (Ariz. Ct. App. 1973); Cheaney v. State, 259 Ind. 138, 285 N.E.2d 265 (Ind. 1972); State v. Abodeely, 179 N.W.2d 347 (Iowa 1970); Sasaki v. Commonwealth, 485 S.W.2d 897 (Ky. 1972); State v. Campbell, 263 La. 1058, 270 So.2d 506 (1972); State v. Moretti, 52 N.J. 182, 244 A.2d 499 (1968); State v. Kruze, (Ohio 1972), vacated and remanded, 410 U.S. 951 (1973); Spears v. State, 257 So.2d 876 (Miss. 1972); Rodgers v. Danforth, 486 S.W.2d 258 (Mo. 1972); Byrn v. New York City, 31 N.Y.2d 194, 286 N.E.2d 887 (1972); State v. Munson, 86 S.D. 663, 201 N.W.2d 123 (1972); Thompson v. State, 493 S.W.2d 913 (Tex. Crim. App. 1971); State v. Bartlett, 128 Vt. 618, 270 A.2d 168 (1970).

Finding unconstitutional: People v. Belous, 71 Cal.2d 954, 458 P.2d 194 (1969); State v. Barquet, 262 So.2d 431 (Fla. 1972); State v. Nixon, 42 Mich.App. 332, 201 N.W.2d 635 (1972); Beecham v. Leahy, 130 Vt. 164, 287 A.2d 836 (1972).

121. Miller, supra note 5, at 9.

122. Miller, supra note 5, at 32.

123. Solinger, *The Abortionist*, supra note 5, at 4.

124. Marian Faux, *Roe v. Wade: The Untold Story of the Landmark Supreme Court Decision that Made Abortion Legal* (New York: Macmillan, 1988); McCorvey, supra note 26 at 104–106.

125. Reagan, supra note 5.

126. See generally, R. Donnelly, et al., *Criminal Law* 252–523 (New York: Free Press of Glencoe, 1962).

127. Johs Andenaes, "General Prevention: Illusion or Reality?," 43 *J. Crim. L. Criminology and Pol. Sci.* 176, 180 (1952).

128. Ibid., at 179.

129. Ibid., at 180 (emphasis in original).

130. Cf. Gerald Gunther, *Learned Hand: The Man and the Judge* 451 (New York: Knopf, 1994). ("As an observer from the sidelines, Hand could and did criticize New Deal programs with regularity. But as a judge, Hand knew that his doubts about the effectiveness of these reforms could not legitimately affect the exercise of his official duties.").

131. David Savage, *Turning Right: The Making of the Rehnquist Supreme Court*

80 (New York: John Wiley & Sons, 1992).

132. Statistical Abstract of the United States 180 (112th ed. 1992) (Table No. 287) (83,000 forcible rapes in 1980; 102,600 in 1990), (23,000 murders in 1980, 23,400 in 1990), (566,000 robberies in 1980, 639,000 in 1990), (673,000 aggravated assaults in 1980, 1,055,000 in 1990).

133. John H. Ely, "The Wages of Crying Wolf: A Comment on Roe v. Wade," 82 *Yale L. J.* 920, 923 n.26 (1973).

134. 410 U.S. 113, 150 (1973).

135. See, e.g., Williams, supra note 19, at 212 ("The effect of the law is not to eliminate abortion but to drive it into the most undesirable channels."); Graber, supra note 5, at 321 (citing a number of general claims which rely on other unsubstantiated claims); Leavy and Kummer, supra note 105, at 126 and n.20 (1962) ("[f]or professional abortionists there exists a low rate of prosecution and an even lower rate of conviction").

136. Jeffrey Leigh Sedgwick, *Law Enforcement Planning: The Limits of An Economic Analysis* 42 (Westport, Conn.: Greenwood Press, 1984). ("The technique [for determining the optimal amount of crime in society] involved identifying the physical and psychic harm from crime, the costs of apprehension and conviction, the costs of wrongful conviction and punishment, and the social costs of punishing criminals." Ibid., at 56.).

137. Cf. Lawrence M. Friedman, *Crime and Punishment in American History* (New York: Basic Books, 1993), (arguing that crime has been a constant throughout American history and that criminals are never really deterred).

138. Andenaes, supra note 127, at 180 (emphasis in original).

139. See Olasky, supra note 34; Andenaes, supra note 127, at 179 ("General prevention may depend on the mere frightening or deterrent effect of punishment-the risk of discovery and punishment outweighs the temptation to commit crimes.").

140. See e.g., Graber, supra note 5, at 313.

141. A good overview is contained in Germaine Grisez, *Abortion: The Myths, the Realities, and the Arguments* 35–65 (New York: Corpus Books, 1970). See also Graber, supra note 5, at 315–16.

142. Judith Leavitt, *Brought to Bed: Childbearing in America, 1750–1950* 24 (New York: Oxford University Press, 1986). Another scholar has written: "The numerical base for the history of American prenuptial pregnancy and illegitimacy has serious gaps and limitations [beyond] the normal problems of data reliability." See Daniel Scott Smith, "The Long Cycle in American Illegitimacy and Prenuptial Pregnancy," in *Bastardy and Its Comparative History* (Peter Laslett, ed., Cambridge, Mass.: Harvard University Press, 1980).

143. Gerald Rosenberg, *The Hollow Hope: Can Courts Bring About Social Change?* 178 (Chicago: University of Chicago Press, 1991); Paige Cunningham and Clarke D. Forsythe, "Is Abortion the "First Right" for Women?," in *Abortion, Medicine, and the Law* 100 (J. Douglas Butler and David F. Walbert, eds., 4th ed., New York: Facts on File, 1992).

144. See generally, Rosenberg, supra note 143, at 353–55 (Appendix 6); Grisez, supra note 141, at 35–42; Pollak, supra note 37, at 45.

145. See Olasky, supra note 34.

146. For example, in 1903, a physician at the annual meeting of the Illinois Medical Society, stated that criminal abortion was "startlingly frequent." Others opined that "every physician" is, at one time or another, approached to perform elective abortion. In 1904, at a Chicago Medical Society symposium, a physician estimated that "probably 6,000 to 10,000 abortions [are] induced in Chicago every year." See Bacon, supra note 54, at 18. In 1921, a physician speaking at the 34th Annual meeting of the American Association of Obstetricians and Gynecologists and Abdominal Surgeons in St. Louis stated that it had been estimated that there were 80,000 criminal abortions annually in New York City. Others in 1921 suggested that criminal abortion was "practiced extensively."

147. See e.g., Graber, supra note 5; "The Abortion Problem," supra note 77, at 155 ("In the light of our present knowledge...we can only guess at the number of abortions that occur in the United States each year, since reliable figures are not available. We do know that their number is legion.") (statement of Herman N. Bundesen).

148. "The Abortion Problem," supra note 77, at 155 (Dr. Herman N. Bundesen).

149. See Graber, supra note 5.

150. Rosenberg, supra note 143, at 353–55 (Appendix 6). See also Solinger, *The Abortionist*, supra note 5, at ix; Graber, supra note 5, at 316 and n.28.

151. Grisez, supra note 141, at 35–42.

152. Frederick Taussig, Abortion, Spontaneous and Induced (1936). *Time* magazine blessed his book as "authoritative" and concluded that his calculations resulted from "careful figuring." *Time*, 6 March 1936, at 52.

153. Olasky, *The Press and Abortion*, supra note 63, at 70.

154. "The Abortion Problem," supra note 77, at 28.

155. J. E. Bates, supra note 76, at 8. Cf. Graber, supra note 5, at 322 (citing Taussig's 1936 estimate).

156. Marie E. Kopp, *Birth Control in Practice* (New York: R. M. McBride and Co., 1934); Regine Stix, "A Study of Pregnancy Wastage," 13 *Milbank Memorial Fund. Q.* 347 (1935); Paul Gebhard, et al., *Pregnancy, Birth and Abortion* (Westport, Conn. Greenwood Press 1958). The Kinsey study was published posthumously by Gebhard, et al. in 1958. Alfred Kinsey died in 1956.

157. "The Abortion Problem," supra note 77, at 5.

158. Regine K. Stix and Dorothy G. Wiehl, "Abortion and the Public Health," 28 *Am. J. Pub. Health* 621, 623 and fig. 1 (1938).

159. *Abortion in the United States* 179 (Mary Calderone, ed. New York: Hoeber-harper, 1958), (The Kinsey data "do not provide an adequate basis for reliable estimates of the incidence of induced abortion in the urban white population of the United States, much less in the total population."). *Abortion in the United States* consists of the papers of the 1955 conference sponsored by Planned Parenthood, which were edited and published by Mary Calderone, who was at that time the medical director of Planned Parenthood.

160. Robert G. Potter, Jr., "Abortion in the United States," 37 *Milbank Mem. Fund Q.* 92, 94 (January 1959) (Book Review) ("The lower estimate is based on a ratio

of 3.1 induced abortions per 100 pregnancies found by C. Kiser and P.K. Whelpton for their Indianapolis sample and also by D.G. Wiehl and K. Berry for a New York City sample. The upper limit is based on a ratio of 18.9 induced abortions per 100 pregnancies reported by the staff of the Institute of Sex Research [Kinsey] from their analysis of 5,293 women. The appropriateness of the upper limit is placed in doubt by an appendix in which Tietze analyzes the representativeness of the ISR respondents in relation to estimates of 1945 distributions for urban white women in the United States. Tietze concludes that the ISR respondents are usefully representative but his tables contradict this conclusion by showing not only gross differences with respect to age, education, and marital status, but also and more important, tangible differences with respect to age-specific marital fertility.").

161. See e.g., Graber, supra note 5, at 316 n.28 (citing Kopp).

162. *Abortion in the United States* 180 (Mary Calderone, ed. supra note 159), (hereafter Calderone). ("Taking into account the probable trend of the abortion ratio since the interwar period, a plausible estimate of the frequency of induced abortion in the United States could be as low as 200,000 and as high as 1,200,000 per year, depending upon the assumptions made as to the incidence of abortion in the total population as compared with the restricted group for which statistical data are available, and upon the assessment of the discretion and magnitude of bias inherent in each series of data. There is no objective basis for the selection of a particular figure between these two estimates as an approximation of the actual frequency." Ibid., at 180).

163. Calderone, supra note 159, at 37 ("Of course, we don't know what the total number of criminal abortions performed in the United States happens to be...") (Dr. Harold Rosen); Ibid., at 18 ("The incidence of criminal abortions is not better known in Norway than in the United States, the figures we have being mostly based on estimations or guesswork.") (Dr. Bard Brekke); Ibid. at 50 ("I think we have all been penalized in our thinking by lack of actual knowledge about illegal abortion...In the first place, there are no good figures that I know of that in any way depict the incidence. Taussig's book pulls out a nice round number, but when you try to analyze the formulae by which the number is derived, you could have substituted other values and gotten quite a different answer...we talk a lot about the practice of illegal abortion and how it is carried on—again without any factual data.") (Alan Guttmacher); Ibid., at 70 ("We have absolutely no hope of getting reports...of illegal induced abortions unless the woman requires subsequent hospital care, and...not even with all of these.") (Carl Erhardt, Director of Records and Statistics, Dept. of Health, NYC); Ibid. at 110 ("[T]he number of [illegal abortions] which we are aware of must be only a fraction of the problem, and it is doubtful if any combination of sources can give us reliable figures on this purposefully hidden area.") (Dr. Sophia Kleegman); See also Harold Rosen (ed.), 3–6 *Therapeutic Abortion: Medical, Psychiatric, Legal, Anthropological and Religious Considerations*, (New York: Julian Press, 1954) (330,000 illegal abortions, Dr. Russell Fisher). See also, Rosen, *Therapeutic Abortion*, at 180 ("There are no accurate figures on the number of spontaneous and induced abortions that occur annually in the United States.") (Dr. Manfred Guttmacher); Also, Joseph P. Kennedy, Jr. Foundation, *The Terrible Choice: The Abortion Dilemma* (R. Cooke, et al., eds., New York: Bantam Books, 1968), (figures on criminal abortion are "based on per-

sonal estimates"; "no way has yet been found of obtaining reliable statistics that would give an exact figure for the total population").

164. Leavy and Kummer, supra note 105, at 124.

165. Kopp, *Birth Control in Practice*. A number of subsequent researchers and historians have emphasized the probable bias of Kopp's sample. Pollak, supra note 37, at 47; "The Abortion Problem," supra note 77, at 5.

166. Regine Stix, "A Study of Pregnancy Wastage," 13 *Milbank Memorial Fund. Q.* 347 (1935); Stix and Wiehl, "Abortion and the Public Health," 28 *Am. J. Pub. Health* 623 (1938).

167. Paul H. Gebhard, et al., supra note 156, *Pregnancy, Birth and Abortion*.

168. Graber, supra note 5, at n.28 (citing Tietze).

169. Leavy and Kummer, supra note 105, at 125 (citing Calderone, supra note 159, *Abortion in the United States*).

170. M. Calderone, "Illegal Abortion as a Public Health Problem," 50 *Am. J. Pub. Health* 948, 949 (1960).

171. Rosenberg, supra note 143, at 355 (citing Christopher Tietze, "Two Years Experience with a Liberal Abortion Law: Its Impact on Fertility Trends in New York City," 5 *Fam. Plan. Perspect.* 36 (1973)). See Graber, supra note 5, at 316, 317 n.28.

172. June Sklar and Beth Berkov, "Abortion, Illegitimacy, and the American Birth Rate," 185 *Science* 909 (13 Sept. 1974).

173. Alan F. Guttmacher, "The Genesis of Liberalized Abortion in New York: A Personal Insight," in *Abortion, Medicine, and the Law* 246 n.16, ed. by J. Douglas Butler and David F. Walbert, supra note 143.

174. 745,000 in 1973 versus 586,800 in 1972. Statistical Abstract of the United States 70 (1989) (Tables No. 103 and 104).

175. Lynn D. Wardle, "Time Enough: Webster v. Reproductive Health Services and the Prudent Pace of Justice," 41 *Fla. L. Rev.* 881 (1989) (Appendix).

176. See e.g., State v. McMahan, 57 Idaho 240, 65 P.2d 156 (1937) (abortion homicide); Willis v. O'Brien, 151 W.Va. 628, 153 S.E.2d 178 (1967), cert. denied, 389 U.S. 848 (1969((abortion homicide). See also, Ernest F. Oakley, Jr., "Legal Aspect of Abortion," 3 *Am. J. Ob. Gyn.* 37 (Jan. 1922); Reagan, supra note 5.

177. See generally, Miller, supra note 5; Brian Clowes, "The Role of Maternal Deaths in the Abortion Debate," 13 *St. Louis U. Pub. L. Rev.* 327 (1993); Leavy and Kummer, supra note 105, at 124 and n.8 ("[T]he amount of human suffering at the hands of unskilled abortionists is inestimable.").

178. See e.g., Graber, supra note 5, at 319 (citing Glanville Williams).

179. He had to stop seeing Barnett after a new district attorney was elected who sought to vigorously enforce the law and his investigators discovered the relationship.

180. Solinger, *The Abortionist*, supra note 5, at 18.

181. Ibid., at 22, 37.

182. Ibid., at 65, 67, 69–72.

183. Ibid., at 53; State v. Barnett, 249 Or. 226, 437 P.2d 821 (1968).

184. Solinger, *The Abortionist*, supra note 5, at 26.

185. Ibid., at 36.

186. Ibid., at at 33.

187. Ibid., at 50–53.

188. Mary Calderone, supra note 170 at 948, 949 (July 1960) (emphasis added). See U.S. Dept. of Health, Education and Welfare, Public Health Service, Vital Statistics of the United States, 1957 cxxxix (1959) (Table CZ) (for 260 deaths attributed to abortions of all kind out of total 1,746 maternal deaths from all causes).

189. "The technique of the well-accredited criminal abortionist is usually good. They have to be good to stay in business, since otherwise they would be extremely vulnerable to police action." Alan Guttmacher, *Babies by Choice or by Chance* 216 (Garden City, N.Y.: Doubleday, 1959).

190. See Barbara J. Syska, et al., "An Objective Model for Estimating Criminal Abortions and Its Implications for Public Policy," in *New Perspectives on Human Abortion* 168 (Thomas W. Hilgers, ct al., eds. supra note 36), (citing National Center for Health Statistics data, showing drop in maternal deaths from 7,466 in 1940 to 2,697 in 1950, to 1,328 in 1960, to 684 in 1970 to 554 in 1972); See also Moore and Randall, "Trends in Therapeutic Abortion: A Review of 137 Cases," 63 *Am. J. Ob. Gyn.* 34 (1952).

191. Rosen, *Therapeutic Abortion*, supra note 163 at xvii. Rosen's book was republished in 1967 under the title *Abortion in America* (Boston, Beacon Press, 1967). In passing, it is important to note here that even as Dr. Cameron purports to address the "needs" for "therapeutic" abortion, his description sweeps well beyond the traditional definition of "therapeutic" as meaning "necessary to save the life of the mother."

192. See, e.g., Edwin M. Gold, "Therapeutic Abortions in New York City: A 20-Year-Review," 55 *Am. J. Pub. Health* 964, 969 (July 1965); Alan Guttmacher, "The Shrinking Non-Psychiatric Indications for Therapeutic Abortion," in Rosen, *Therapeutic Abortion*, supra note 163 at 12.

193. Guttmacher, supra note 106, at 119, emphasis added. Furthermore, he said, "Legitimate hospitals accept in addition some cases in a quasi-legal bracket, but only accept those of crying necessity. The greater the incidence of abortion in a given institution, the greater the proportion from the quasi-group, for the truly legal cases have a more or less constant incidence all over the country." Ibid. Guttmacher was once director of the obstetrical department at Mt. Sinai and a member of its therapeutic abortion committee.

Under the notion of abortion as a part of the constitutional right of privacy, the physician is viewed as a contractual agent of the patient who submits to her request to implement her constitutional right. Contrast this with Guttmacher's sentiment in 1954: "I do not feel that the obstetrician-gynecologist is simply the patient's agent who presents her request for interruption of pregnancy without himself evaluating it. I think he should pass this request on to the hospital authorities...only if he is convinced of the wisdom of the request. If he thinks the procedure unjustified, it behooves the physician consulted to discuss the matter in great detail with the patient and to attempt to persuade her to his viewpoint. If he fails to do this he has no further responsibility in the case." Ibid., at 119.

194. Calderone, supra note 170, at 948–49, emphasis added.

195. Leavy and Kummer, supra note 105, at 126 (citing Guttmacher, "The Shrinking Non-Psychiatric Indications for Therapeutic Abortion," in Rosen, *Therapeutic Abortion*, supra note 163).

196. See Daniel Callahan, "Abortion: Some Ethical Issues," in *Abortion, Society and the Law* 96 (David F. Walbert and J. Douglas Butler, eds., Cleveland: Press of Case Western Reserve University, 1973): "Except in the now-rare instances of a direct threat to a woman's life, an abortion cures no known disease and relieves no medically classifiable illness."); "Abortion: The Doctor's Dilemma," 35 *Modern Medicine* 12, 14–16 (24 April 1967) (quoting Dr. David Decker of Mayo Clinic based on poll of 40,000 American physicians in 1967: there were "few, if any, absolute medical indications for therapeutic abortion in the present state of medicine").

197. Miller, supra note 5, at 327.

198. Calderone, supra note 159, at 65.

199. Ibid., at 67–68.

200. James Burtchaell, *Rachel Weeping: And Other Essays on Abortion* 65 (Toronto: Life Cycle edition, 1990).

201. Bernard Nathanson, *Aborting America* 193 (Garden City, N.Y.: Doubleday, 1979).

202. Miller, supra note 5, at 327.

203. See, e.g., Leavy, 1959 *Los Angeles Bar Bull*, at 357 (between five and ten thousand annually) (citing 31 S. *Cal. L. Rev.* 181 (1958)).

204. Graber, supra note 5, at 318 n.33. Graber does not take notice of the dramatic decline in maternal deaths from all causes after World War II but relies on pre-World War II studies.

205. Lerner, "Death and Abortion," *N.Y. Post*, 9 April 1954 (claiming 5,000–6,000 maternal deaths per year).

206. Miller, supra note 5, at 13.

207. Robert E. Hall, "Commentary," in B. James George, et al., *Abortion and the Law* 228 (David T. Smith, ed., Cleveland: Press of Case Western Reserve University, 1967). Hall said:

I would quarrel with Niswander on only one point, namely, his perpetuation of Taussig's thirty-year-old claim that five thousand to ten thousand American women die every year as the result of criminal abortions. Whether this statistic was valid in 1936 I do not know, but it certainly is not now. There are in fact fewer than fifteen hundred total pregnancy deaths in this country per annum; very few others could go undetected and of these fifteen hundred probably no more than a third are the result of abortion. Even the 'unskilled' abortionist is evidently more skillful and/or more careful these days. Although criminal abortion is of course to be decried, the demand for its abolition cannot reasonably be based upon thirty-year-old mortality statistics.

208. U.S. Public Health Service, Centers for Disease Control, Abortion Surveillance, 61 (Nov. 1980).

209. See H.W. Lawson, et al., "Abortion Mortality, United States, 1972 through

1987," 171 *Am. J. Ob. Gyn.* 1365 (Nov. 1994).

210. See generally, Cunningham and Forsythe, supra note 143 at 100–158.

211. See, e.g., Cunningham and Forsythe, supra note 143, at 125–153; Dalton, "Doctor probed after abortion causes death," *San Diego Union*, 13 Dec. 1994, at B-1, B-3.

212. Calderone, supra note 170.

213. See, e.g., Moore, Estate of v. Bickham, 1993 WL 599846 (Cook Co. Cir. Ct.) ($2.05 million verdict for abortion death).

214. See, e.g., Signor, "Doctor's License Revoked," *St. Louis Post-Dispatch*, 15 Dec. 1993; (revocation of license of Dr. Bolivar M. Escobedo of St. Louis County because of botched 1986 abortion); Alexander, *N.Y. Newsday*, 16 Dec. 1993 (sentencing New York gynecologist Maxen Samuel to prison for performing abortions after his license was suspended); "Abortion Doctor Loses License," *Chicago Tribune*, 24 April 1994 (case of Mississippi doctor Thomas Tucker losing license in Mississippi and Alabama); *People Magazine*, 15 Aug. 1994 (abortionist Dr. Britton who was killed in Pensacola, FL in 1994 was investigated and disciplined by Florida medical authorities); Smothers, "Abortion Doctor Is Linked to Complaints in 5 States," *N.Y. Times*, 30 Sept. 1994, at A-19 (Dr. Steven Chase Brigham, who replaced Dr. Britton after killing in Pensacola, FL, had his medical license suspended in New York and Georgia and was investigated in New Jersey); Dalton, "Doctor probed after abortion causes death," *San Diego Union*, 13 Dec. 1994, at B-1, B-3 (case of San Ysidro abortionist Dr. Suresh Gandotra after death of Magdalena Ortega-Rodriquez, previously convicted of 17 felony and misdemeanor charges). See generally Cunningham and Forsythe, supra note 143, at 130–137.

215. H.W. Lawson, et al., "Abortion Mortality, United States, 1972 through 1987," 171 *Am. J. Ob. Gyn.* 1365 (Nov. 1994) (between 1972 and 1987, 240 women died as a result of legal induced abortions); Hani K. Atrash, et al., "Legal Abortion in the U.S.: trends and mortality," 35 *Contemp. Ob. Gyn.* 58 (1990) (213 legal abortion deaths 1973–1985); Hani K. Atrash, et al., "Legal abortion mortality and general anesthesia," 158 *Am. J. Ob. Gyn.* 420 (1988) (193 deaths 1972–1985); David A. Grimes, et al., "Fatal Hemorrhage from Legal Abortion in the United States," 157 *Surg. Gyn. and Ob.* 461 (Nov. 1983) (194 deaths 1972–1979); Scot A. LeBolt, et al., "Mortality from Abortion and Childbirth," 248 *J. Amer. Med. Assoc.* 188 (1982) (138 deaths 1972–1978); Willard Cates, Jr., et al., "Assessment of Surveillance and Vital Statistics Data for Monitoring Abortion Mortality, United States, 1972–1975," 108 *Am. J. Epidemiol.* 200 (1978) (204 deaths between 1972–1975, 104 from legal abortion).

These quantitative studies are sometimes flawed by their narrow definition of causation and by inadequate recordkeeping and reporting. The leading factors in death to due legal abortion include complications of anesthesia, hemorrhaging, infection, and anmiotic embolism. Deaths from complications of anesthesia are sometimes deleted from mortality statistics, though common sense would say that the deaths were due to the abortion procedure if but for undergoing the abortion, the woman would have lived.

CDC statistics relied on death certificates provided by states. One CDC official was reported as saying, "There have always been problems identifying deaths secondary to abortion. Death certificates are not the best source of death information, and we've always had concerns we're not getting all the deaths through the death certificate system." Price, "Statistics may be misleading on deaths caused by abortion," *Washington Times*, 4 June 1994, at A5. The official also stated that it is "likely" that many abortion-related deaths might not be reported. Ibid.

216. Ravenell, Estate of v. Eastern Women's Center, 1990 WL 467656 (N.Y.Sup.Ct.) ($1.2 million verdict).

217. *St. Petersburg Times*, 29 June 1994; *USA Today*, 30 June 1994. Police ended their investigation after one day, saying the abortion "was cared for by a licensed doctor in a licensed facility." "Woman Dies From Bleeding After Abortion," *Tallahassee Democrat*, 30 June 1994, at 1.

See generally, Cunningham and Forsythe, supra note 143, at 130–37. See also, Ruckman, Estate of v. Barrett, 1991 WL 444085 (Green Co., Mo. Cir. Ct.) ($25,000,000 verdict for abortion death); Redding v. Bramwell, 1990 WL 468158 (Cobb Co., Ga. Sup. Ct.) ($500,000 verdict for abortion death); Poteat, Estate of v. Dern, 1987 WL 232018 (Charleston Co. Com. Pl. Ct.) ($35,000 for abortion death).

218. The physician's lawyer was quoted as saying, "This is a standard risk of the procedure...We don't believe this was below the standard of care nor do we believe it is malpractice." Dalton, "Doctor probed after abortion causes death," *San Diego Union*, 13 December 1994, at B-1, B-3.

219. Wardle, supra note 175 (Appendix).

220. Statistical Abstract of the United States 67 (111th ed. 1991) (Table no. 92).

221. Statistical Abstract of the United States 182 (111th ed. 1991) (Tables No. 305 and 306).

222. Statistical Abstract of the United States 98 (111th Ed. 1994) (Table No. 130).

223. Centers for Disease Control, 44 Morbidity and Mortality Weekly Report No. 3, at 46 (January 27, 1995), ("The reported number of hospitalizations for ectopic pregnancy increased from 17,800 in 1970 to 88,400 in 1989.").

224. Janet R. Daling, et al., "Risk of Breast Cancer Among Young Women: Relationship to Induced Abortion," 86 *J. Nat'l Cancer Inst.* 1584 (1994).

225. Shortly after Roe was decided, the City of Chicago attempted to regulate Friendship Medical Center after a woman died at the clinic. The federal courts in Chicago prevented regulation. Friendship Medical Center v. Chicago Board of Health, 505 F.2d 1141 (7th Cir. 1974). Later, after the *Chicago Sun-Times* and the Better Government Association conducted an undercover investigation and published, in November 1978, a twelve part series on the unsafe conditions in Chicago abortion clinics, the department of health issued emergency regulations and the Illinois General Assembly passed additional legislation. But, seven years later, the federal courts, ignoring this history, enjoined against the regulations. Ragsdale v. Turnock, 841 F.2d. 1358 (7th Cir. 1988), appeal dismissed, 112 S.Ct. 1309 (1992).

Chapter 13

Supreme Court Jurisprudence and Prenatal Life

Tom Poundstone

[T]he question of when life begins is no longer a question for theological or philosophical dispute. It is an established scientific fact. . . . [T]heologians and philosophers may go on to debate the meaning of life or the purpose of life, but it is an established fact that all life, including human life, begins at the moment of conception.

—Dr. Hymie Gordon[1]

[Women] have literally been handed the right to slaughter their own children.
—Norma McCorvey, a.k.a. Jane Roe[2]

In the landmark case of *Roe v. Wade*, Justice Blackmun declares that the judiciary is not in a position to speculate as to when human life begins, nor need it resolve that difficult question.[3] Unhindered by his declaration of agnosticism, Blackmun then proceeds to perform a balancing test in which he weighs the respective interests of the pregnant woman against what he describes as the state's "important and legitimate interest in protecting the potentiality of human life."[4] That a woman in such a situation has significant and identifiable interests is beyond doubt. The questions for this chapter concern the other side of the scale. What are the state's "important and legitimate interests in protecting potential life," what value has the Supreme Court been giving the state's interests, and how did the Court establish the weight of that interest if, as Blackmun says, the Court may not and need not resolve the question of when human life begins?

After an introductory section which situates the debate in terms of constitutional law, this chapter reviews in four sections the Supreme Court's discussions on prenatal life. The first section looks at the description of the nature and status of the fetus in *Roe v. Wade*. The second section reviews the exchanges between the majority and dissenting justices on the state's interest in prenatal life during the nineteen years between *Roe* and *Planned Parenthood v. Casey*. The third section looks at the analysis of the state's interests presented by Justice Stevens in *Casey*. The final section notes the modifications which the justices in *Casey* made to the standard set in *Roe*.

THE CONSTITUTIONAL FRAMEWORK OF THE DISCUSSION

The major constitutional aspects of the abortion debate are centered in the meaning, scope, and intent of the Fourteenth Amendment. First and foremost, the Court has consistently held that the fetus is not a "person" within the meaning of the Amendment's declaration that "No state . . . shall deprive any person of life, liberty, or property, without due process of law." In the oral arguments heard by the Court in *Roe*, the attorneys arguing Jane Roe's case conceded that their case would collapse if the fetus's right to life were guaranteed by the Amendment. On the other hand, the State of Texas could not cite a case that held that the fetus was a person within the meaning of the Amendment. Indeed, no member of the Supreme Court has ever suggested that a fetus is a "person" within the context of that Amendment. If any of those in dissent on the abortion cases held that position, they would not recommend leaving the permissibility of terminating the life of the fetus to the will of state legislatures. Even Justice Scalia implicitly accepted this holding by characterizing the basic question as "a political issue." Furthermore, any compromise provision allowing for abortion in any situation except to save the life of the mother—such as incest, rape, or deformity—would be unconstitutional if the fetus were held to be a "person."

The Fourteenth Amendment's concept of personal liberty is also seen by the Court as the locus of the constitutional right to privacy. It is this right which Blackmun describes in *Roe* as "broad enough to encompass a woman's decision whether or not to terminate her pregnancy."[5] It is in this area that the initial dissent to *Roe* was made. The then Justice Rehnquist argued that Blackmun had found within the scope of the Fourteenth Amendment a right that was completely unknown to its drafters. Since thirty six states or territorial legislatures had enacted laws limiting abortion by the time the Amendment was adopted in 1868, and since there was no question concerning the validity of these laws at the time, Rehnquist argued that history would lead us to conclude that the drafters of the Amendment did not intend to take away the states' power to legislate with respect to this matter.[6]

These interpretations of the Constitution concerning the content of the term *person* and the existence and extent of a right to privacy raise profound questions for the abortion debate. If the fetus is not a rights-bearing "person," what interests can the state have in protecting the fetus's life that could ever become so compelling as to outweigh the constitutional rights of a pregnant woman? The state has no authority to overrule the Constitution by declaring that fetuses have rights competitive with the constitutional rights of pregnant women.[7] However, the state can legislate to protect those who are not "persons" just as it does to protect animals from unnecessary cruelty. Such laws which protect "nonpersons" are not rooted in the constitutional rights of these creatures but in deference to the rights of other persons. The state can also appeal to other compelling interests such as respecting the sanctity of life and protecting the community's sense that human life in any form has tremendous intrinsic value. The question is, can the State appeal to such interests to justify the abridgment of another person's constitutional rights, in this case a pregnant woman's right to control her own body?

Lastly, a procedural question underlying every abortion case heard by the Supreme Court is whether the right to abortion should be regarded as a "fundamental right" or a "liberty interest." If it is a fundamental right, the Court must pay strict scrutiny to any attempted restrictions of it, making sure that the statute's provisions are narrowly tailored to promote a compelling state interest. If it is only a liberty interest, the Court looks for no more than a reasonable relation between the means chosen by the state and a legitimate state interest. This later standard of review is extremely deferential to legislative bodies and can tolerate imperfect fits between means and ends. Once the Court decides that the traditional deferential review is appropriate, it is almost certain that the statute will be upheld. Conversely, if the court decides to apply strict scrutiny, it is almost invariable that the statute will be struck down. Thus, more important than the actual review of the statute is what standard of review the Court will employ.

Blackmun declared in *Roe* that abortion is a "fundamental right," thus calling for a strict scrutiny of all statutes regulating it. Most justices in dissent have maintained that abortion is not a fundamental right and that a more accommodating standard of review is called for. Until *Webster* (1989) and *Casey* (1992), justices supporting *Roe* have been in a majority. As a result, almost all restrictions on abortion were rejected from 1973 to 1989. What *Casey* adopted is neither a strict-scrutiny nor a rational-basis review, but a new standard of scrutiny described as an "undue burden" standard. The plurality of the Court did not apply strict scrutiny to the provisions of the Pennsylvania statute in question, and neither did they uphold them all. For the future, this new standard of review seems to indicate that state provisions which regulate the abortion process but do not present a substantial obstacle to it are much more likely to be sustained than they were prior to *Casey*.

THE NATURE AND STATUS OF THE FETUS IN *ROE V. WADE*

In this section I look closely at Justice Blackmun's opinion for the Court in *Roe v. Wade*, first tracing his analysis of when human life can be said to begin, then looking at how Blackmun sets up his balancing test, and finally noting

Blackmun's emphasis on viability as the decisive weight on the scales of justice.

Despite Blackmun's contention that the Court need not resolve the difficult question of when life begins, he proceeds to do just that, albeit in an indirect fashion. He first observes that the word "person" as used in the Constitution does not include the unborn. He briefly reviews the stance of tort law concerning recovery for prenatal injuries and the interests of the unborn in inheritance law. He concludes this section by observing that, apart from laws concerning abortion,

> [T]he law has been reluctant to endorse any theory that life, as we recognize it, begins before live birth or to accord legal rights to the unborn except in narrowly defined situations and except when the rights are contingent upon live birth. . . . [T]he fetus, at most, represents only the potentiality of life. . . . In short, the unborn have never been recognized in the law as persons in the whole sense.[8]

Note that in this passage Blackmun interchanges the term *life* with the term *person*. Blackmun wants to confine use of the term *person* to the narrow sense in which it is used in the Constitution. That can be granted him. To then treat "person" and "life" as interchangeable terms, however, is to smuggle in an answer to the question of when life begins. Without explicitly saying so, Blackmun has already answered the question as follows: human life begins when one is treated by the law as a person. Therefore, before that point the fetus may only be described as "potential human life." Blackmun has answered the very question which he not only said need not be resolved, but he has answered the question which he said, "[T]he judiciary, at this point in the development of man's knowledge, is not in a position to speculate as to the answer."[9]

Blackmun briefly notes that there is a wide diversity of thinking on the question of when life begins. He writes, "There has always been strong support for the view that life does not begin until live birth."[10] He then notes that others have placed significance on quickening and viability. He also observes that the Catholic Church, many non-Catholics, and many physicians believe that life should be recognized from the moment of conception. However, he immediately writes that substantial problems are posed to this last position by new embryological data that indicate that conception is a process over time rather than an event, by the "morning-after" pill, by artificial insemination, and by artificial wombs. What precise problems these matters pose and whether they may be responded to is not considered. No note is made of problems posed to the other marker events.[11]

His analysis complete, Blackmun writes, "In view of all this, we do not agree that, by adopting one theory of life, Texas may override the rights of the pregnant woman that are at stake."[12] Indeed, Texas did adopt one theory of when life begins, but so has Blackmun. In describing the fetus as "the potentiality of human life" rather than simply "human life," Blackmun has selected the lowest common denominator of the four theories which he considered: conception, quickening, viability, and birth.

Blackmun briefly acknowledges a difference between the claim that the fetus is a "human life" and the claim that it is merely "the potentiality of human life." He maintains that the state's legitimate interests in protecting prenatal life do not disappear if the belief that life begins at conception is not accepted. He writes, "[A]s long as at least *potential* life is involved, the State may assert interests beyond the protection of the pregnant woman alone."[13] Blackmun does not acknowledge, however, that the strength of the state's interests are determined by the nature of what it is protecting. If it is truly human life, the state has not merely an interest in protecting it; it is morally obliged to do so. Blackmun does not consider these nuances.

Before moving to the results of the balancing test, it is important to note that Blackmun does not place an unfettered right to privacy on the other side of the balance. Although Blackmun writes that the right of privacy "is broad enough to encompass a woman's decision whether or not to terminate her pregnancy,"[14] he is careful to note that the right to privacy as previously articulated by the Court does not encompass the claim that one has an unlimited right to do with one's body as one pleases.[15] Furthermore, he hints that the unique condition of pregnancy puts additional constraints on the right to privacy. "The pregnant woman," he writes, "cannot be isolated in her privacy." Since she carries an embryo and later a fetus, her situation is "inherently different" from the other situations in which the Court has acknowledged that a right of privacy exists. He concludes, "[I]t is reasonable and appropriate for a State to decide that at some point in time another interest, that of health of the mother or that of potential human life, becomes significantly involved."[16]

As Blackmun describes it, his balancing test is dynamic, not static. The state's interest in protecting maternal health and in protecting potential human life "grows in substantiality as the woman approaches term."[17] This interest becomes compelling at viability, the point at which the fetus is "potentially able to live outside the mother's womb, albeit with artificial aid."[18] Before that point, the pregnant woman's constitutional right of privacy permits her to choose abortion. After that point, the state may go so far as to proscribe abortion except when it is necessary to preserve the life or health of the mother.

Why does viability mark the transitional point for Blackmun? He writes, "This is so because the fetus then presumably has the capability of meaningful life outside the mother's womb. State regulation protective of fetal life after viability thus has both logical and biological justifications."[19]

That is the extent of Blackmun's argument. He does not supply a defense of his judgment; he simply repeats a definition of viability. In *Thornburgh*, Justice White remarks that Blackmun "mistakes a definition for a syllogism."[20] Blackmun makes no acknowledgment of the inherent problems in making "viability" at the constitutionally critical moment in pregnancy.

THE ABORTION CASES BETWEEN *ROE* AND *CASEY*

In this section, rather than attempt to survey the major abortion cases, I have chosen to trace the development of two themes in the Court's debate on abortion. First, I look at the debate on viability and the point at which the state's interests in protecting prenatal life become compelling. Second, I review the debate in *Akron v. Akron Center for Reproductive Health* (1983) and *Thornburgh v. American College of Obstetricians and Gynecologists* (1986) over whether the state can mandate that information concerning the nature of the developing fetus be shared with the pregnant woman seeking an abortion.

Viability and a Compelling State Interest

The appropriateness of selecting viability as the constitutionally significant moment in pregnancy has been a constant theme in the abortion cases. Justices White and O'Connor have questioned its significance. Justices Blackmun and Stevens have come to its defense.

In *Akron*, O'Connor wrote at length about the improvements in neonatology in the ten years since *Roe*. After citing recent studies which demonstrate increasingly earlier fetal viability, she concluded, "It is certainly reasonable to believe that fetal viability in the first trimester of pregnancy may be possible in the not too distant future."[21] Therefore, an assertion that a woman has a constitutional right to have an abortion up to the time of fetal viability might eventually mean that she has no right at all. As she put it, *"Roe* . . . is clearly on a collision course with itself."[22]

Blackmun responded directly to O'Connor in an extended footnote in *Webster*. Her critique, he said, had no medical foundation. He cites medical literature as conclusively demonstrating that there is an "anatomic threshold" for fetal viability of about 23-24 weeks gestation prior to which fetal organs are not sufficiently mature to provide self-sustaining functions. He writes, "[T]he threshold of fetal viability is, and will remain, no different from what it was at the time *Roe* was decided. Predictions to the contrary are pure science fiction."[23]

The more trenchant point lying behind this exchange asks what it is that viability indicates. Although Blackmun might be correct in writing that current science has reached an anatomic threshold, viability as he defines it still says more about available technology than it does about any inherent feature of the fetus. As Norman Fost, a pediatrician and medical ethicist, writes, "Fetuses of a particular gestational age and weight that were non-viable twenty years ago had all the intrinsic properties of similar fetuses today, which are in fact viable. Their change in status is entirely a result of the state of technology."[24] Justice

White echoes this theme in these remarks from his dissenting opinion in *Thornburgh*: "[T]he possibility of fetal survival is contingent on the state of medical practice and technology, factors that are in essence morally and constitutionally irrelevant."[25]

There is also something peculiar about an argument for abortion which turns upon viability, although no member of the Court has hinted at it. To determine whether an abortion is legal, one must first assess whether the fetus is "potentially able to live outside the mother's womb, albeit with artificial aid." If it is deemed capable, the Court declares that it may not be removed. Thus, a fetus that is capable of living independently of its mother is the only kind of fetus that has a constitutional right not to be forced to live independently of its mother.[26]

Closely related to the debate on viability is the discussion of when the state's interests in protecting prenatal life become compelling. In *Akron*, Justice O'Connor latches onto Blackmun's characterization of prenatal life as "potential" life. She takes that point to its logical conclusion in the following passage: "The difficulty with [the Court's] analysis is clear: *potential* life is no less potential in the first weeks of pregnancy than it is at viability or afterward. At any stage in pregnancy, there is the potential for human life. . . . Accordingly, I believe that the State's interest in protecting potential human life exists throughout the pregnancy."[27] O'Connor's conclusion is that the compelling nature of the state's interests does not depend on the trimester of pregnancy.

Similarly, Justice White writes that the character of the fetus worth protecting is present well before viability. From O'Connor's and White's perspectives, both the time that the state's interest in protecting the potentiality of this life becomes compelling, and the time that the state's interest in fostering a regard for human life in general becomes compelling, bear no discernible relationship to an assessment of when the fetus is viable. Thus, there is no reason to see the strength of the state's interest transformed at that point.

Justice Stevens directly responds to O'Connor's and White's contention that the state's interests in protecting prenatal life are compelling throughout pregnancy. Stevens argues that if a distinction may be made between the state's interest in protecting fetuses and its interest in protecting constitutional persons, then it is seems to him, "quite odd to argue that distinctions may not also be drawn between the state interest in protecting the freshly fertilized egg and the state interest in protecting the 9-month-gestated, fully sentient fetus on the eve of birth."[28]

Informed Consent Requirements

In *Thornburgh v. American College of Obstetricians and Gynecologists* (1986), the court considered sections of the Abortion Control Act in Pennsylvania which required that the pregnant woman be informed that literature was available from the state which describes the probable anatomical and physiological characteristics of the fetus at two-week gestational increments. As well, this literature lists public and private agencies willing to help the mother carry her child to term and to assist her after the child is born, whether she chooses to keep her child or to place her or him for adoption.

Justice Blackmun described these printed materials as "nothing less than an outright attempt to wedge the [state's] message discouraging abortion into the privacy of the informed-consent dialogue between the woman and her physician."[29] He writes that the description of the fetal characteristics at two-week intervals is information that "may serve only to confuse and punish her and to heighten her anxiety, contrary to accepted medical practice."[30] In a footnote, Blackmun further characterizes fetal-description requirements as having an "inflammatory impact."[31]

Blackmun writes that this information on fetal development and the requirement that the woman be advised that assistance may be available is irrelevant and inappropriate for some patients such as those with a life-threatening pregnancy. Therefore, since it is not always relevant information, it advances no legitimate state interest. The general tone of Blackmun's opinion, it should be clear, is that *Roe's* defenders on the Court disapprove of any attempt by states to legislate in this area. The Court was clearly straining to discover an unconstitutional element in these statutes.

In his dissenting opinion, Justice White describes the Court's opinion in *Thornburgh* as "linguistic nit-picking."[32] Whether the information will be irrelevant to some women is hardly a valid objection to the constitutionality of the law. Although it may upset some, in no way does it impair anyone's constitutionally protected interest to choose an abortion. It would seem that the more likely that information might influence a patient's choice, as long as it is accurate and nonmisleading, the more essential it is if her consent is to be truly informed.

O'Connor describes what the Court applies in *Thornburgh* as a "*per se* rule" meaning that "any regulation touching on abortion must be invalidated if it poses an unacceptable danger of deterring the exercise of that right."[33] In other words, the mere possibility that some women will be less likely to choose an abortion because of these laws is a sufficient reason to declare them constitutionally invalid.

In *Thornburgh*, Chief Justice Burger withdrew the support he had initially given *Roe* in 1973. In his concurring opinion in *Roe* he wrote, "Plainly, the court today rejects any claim that the constitution requires abortions on demand." That was simply a piece of wishful thinking on his part. *Roe's* trimester framework only allowed restrictions concerning the mother's health prior to fetal viability. In the 1977 case of *Maher v. Roe*, Burger wrote a concurring opinion maintaining that the Court's holdings in *Roe v. Wade* "simply require that a State not create an absolute barrier to a woman's decision to have an abortion."[34]

Again, that was Burger's wishful thinking. The stalwart supporters of *Roe* (Justices Blackmun, Brennan, Marshall, and Stevens in replacement of Douglas) all had a different conception of *Roe* than Burger.

In *Thornburgh*, Burger appears to recognize for the first time what he had unwittingly been supporting. He is astonished to find the Court in *Thornburgh* ruling against informed consent provisions based on the rationale "that such information might have the effect of 'discouraging abortion,' as though abortion is something to be advocated and encouraged."[35] Burger continues, "Can it possibly be that the Court is saying that the Constitution forbids the communication of such critical information to a woman? We have apparently passed the point at which abortion is available merely on demand. If the statute at issue here is to be invalidated, the 'demand' will not even have to be the result of an informed choice."[36] In response to the Court's rejection of the requirement of a second physician at postviability abortions to preserve the child's life, Burger described *Roe's* promise that the state's interests become compelling at viability as "mere shallow rhetoric."[37]

JUSTICE STEVENS'S UNDERSTANDING OF THE STATE'S INTERESTS

In *Planned Parenthood v. Casey*, Justice Stevens, the strongest supporter of abortion rights still on the Court, directly addresses the nature of the state's interests. He makes three basic observations: that the state's interests must have a secular basis; that the state's interests in protecting fetuses must be "indirect"; and that the most powerful of these indirect interests is the state's humanitarian concern.

First, the state's interest must have a secular basis. Stevens has consistently held that there is no secular basis for the view that human life begins at conception and that any such legislative proclamation is a violation of the Establishment Clause of the First Amendment.[38] Some try to escape Stevens's blanket statement by saying that a state's assertion that human life begins at conception is philosophical, not theological. Stevens would dismiss that basis as well. Note Stevens's equation of theological and philosophical speculation in this citation from his opinion in *Cruzan* concerning the State of Missouri's law on the withdrawal of nutrition and hydration. He held that the state had no "reasonable ground" for deciding that Nancy Cruzan had any personal interest in the perpetuation of her life. He defends his assertion by writing as follows: "[I]t would be possible to hypothesize such an interest on the basis of theological or philosophical conjecture. But even to posit such a basis for the State's action is to condemn it. It is not within the province of secular government to circumscribe the liberties of the people by regulations designed wholly for the purpose of establishing a sectarian definition of life."[39]

Nowhere does Stevens acknowledge that religious and state interests might merely coincide as they do, for example, in the prohibition of murder or in the decision to use the death penalty. It is simply inevitable that many of the state's positions will correspond to some religious beliefs and contradict others. Mere demonstration of similar conclusions does not demonstrate that the state's position is grounded in religious beliefs.[40]

Second, Stevens repeats his constant theme that the state's interest in protecting the fetus is not grounded in the Constitution because the fetus is not a "person" within the meaning of the Fourteenth Amendment.[41] Stevens puts it as follows: "[A]s a matter of federal constitutional law, a developing organism that is not yet a 'person' does not have what is sometimes described as a 'right to life.'"[42] Therefore, Stevens maintains that the state's interests in protecting potential life must be "indirect." By this he means they cannot refer to the rights of the fetus as such, but in stating the interests of the larger society, they might indirectly protect the fetus.

Third, Stevens lists two indirect interests of the state. The first he describes as a "humanitarian" concern since many citizens find abortions offensive. Stevens expresses it as follows: "Many of our citizens believe that any abortion reflects an unacceptable disrespect for potential human life and that the performance of more than a million abortions per year is intolerable; many find third-trimester abortions performed when the fetus is approaching personhood particularly offensive. The State has a legitimate interest in minimizing such offense."[43]

The second he describes as a "pragmatic" interest in expanding the population. Stevens expresses it as follows: "The state may also have a broader interest in expanding the population, believing society would benefit from the services of additional productive citizens—or that the potential human lives might include the occasional Mozart or Curie."[44]

In a footnote, Stevens observes that these two interests of the state are potentially in conflict. He uses the analogy of Haitian immigration to our country. Humanitarian concerns would support a policy allowing these people unrestricted entry. However, interests in population control support a policy of strict enforcement of immigration laws. As if he suddenly recognized the implications of his analogy, Stevens concludes his footnote by stating that the state's interest in population control would not be sufficient to require a woman to have an abortion.[45]

That concludes Stevens's analysis in *Casey* of the state's interests in protecting prenatal life. His final sentence—"These are the kinds of concerns that comprise the State's interest in potential human life"[46]—indicates that he does not view his list as exhaustive. However, his inability to list a more compelling state interest than the humanitarian desire to minimize the offense which abortion causes some in our society reveals that he thinks the state's interests in protecting prenatal life are hardly compelling enough to infringe upon a woman's decision to seek an abortion prior to fetal viability.

In earlier opinions, Stevens has referred to the fetus itself. In response to Justice White's claim in *Thronburgh* that the governmental interest in protecting fetal life is equally compelling from conception to birth, Stevens takes the *Roe* line of arguing for state interests which grow in tandem with the developing fetus. He writes,

> I should think it obvious that the State's interest in the protection of an embryo . . . increases progressively and dramatically as the organism's capacity to feel pain, to experience pleasure, to survive, and to react to its surroundings increases day by day. The development of a fetus — and pregnancy itself — are not static conditions, and the assertion that the government's interest is static simply ignores this reality.[47]

In *Webster* Stevens writes that the state has a valid interest in protecting a developed fetus from physical pain.[48] He is the only justice to make note of fetal sentience, a point which should have some significance for those advocating a developmental model.

Interestingly, Stevens's analysis of the state's interest in *Casey* makes no reference to this developing life of the fetus or the capacity of a third-trimester fetus to sense pain. Perhaps this omission, which could not be accidental, is a reflection of Stevens's understanding that, since the unborn have no constitutional rights, the only way that a pregnant woman's constitutional rights may be restricted is by deference to the rights of other citizens (such as the humanitarian concern of limiting the offense that late-term abortions cause to others) or for some other compelling state interest (the only one he could think of was that of population control, an example which he admits does not apply to our age). For the purposes of analyzing the state's interests, references to the fetus must somehow be subsumed by these other two categories, most likely that of humanitarian concern.

One point is worth noting about Stevens's coupling of the development of the state's interests in protecting prenatal life with the developing nature of the fetus. Such linking has tremendous implications for questions concerning the permissibility of experimentation on embryos. In *Webster* he writes as follows: "[A] State has no greater secular interest in protecting the potential life of an embryo that is still 'seed' than in protecting the potential life of a sperm or an unfertilized ovum." The idea of morally equating gametes and embryos demonstrates that Stevens is woefully out of touch with this century's advancements in genetics and embryology.

HOW AND WHY *CASEY* UPHELD *ROE*

There are three distinct voting blocs in *Casey*. The plurality opinion was written jointly by Justices O'Connor, Kennedy, and Souter. Such collaboration is quite rare; usually, an opinion is written by a single justice with others joining. They voted both to reaffirm what they called the central principle of *Roe v. Wade* and to allow state regulation which does not unduly burden a woman's freedom to choose to have an abortion. They were supported in their upholding of *Roe* by two justices, Blackmun and Stevens, who voted to uphold *Roe* completely and, hence, to reject all of the proposed regulations put forward by the State of Pennsylvania. Four justices—Chief Justice Rehnquist and Justices White, Scalia, and Thomas—voted to overturn *Roe* completely and to uphold all of the stipulations in the Pennsylvania law. In summary, the vote was 5-4 to uphold the core of *Roe* as a precedent, but 7-2 to allow states to regulate abortion more strictly than *Roe* and its progeny had allowed. The plurality's opinion commanded only three votes, far from a majority. The concurrence was in judgment, not in method.

The authors of the joint opinion candidly admit that in the cases subsequent to *Roe* the Court did not give proper consideration to the state's interests in potential life. They write, "[I]t must be remembered that *Roe v. Wade* speaks with clarity in establishing not only the woman's liberty but also the State's 'important and legitimate interest in potential life.' That portion of the decision in *Roe* has been given too little acknowledgment by the Court in its subsequent cases."[49] These justices maintain that *Roe's* trimester framework essentially precludes the state from expressing these interests prior to viability since it allows state involvement in second-trimester abortions only to protect the mother's health. The justices make this observation quite mildly: "[I]t *undervalues* the State's interest in potential life."[50]

In order to make *Roe's* declaration credible, the joint opinion in *Casey* discards the trimester system. They write that such measures as were taken by the state in *Akron* and *Thornburgh* to inform the pregnant woman of the developmental status of her fetus and of private and public assistance for alternatives to abortion did not necessarily present an undue burden to the abortion right recognized in *Roe*. Thus, they overturned the rulings in those cases. Now, even in the earliest stages of pregnancy, states may enact regulations designed to "encourage [the mother] to know that there are philosophic and social arguments of great weight that can be brought to bear in favor of continuing the pregnancy to full term."[51]

In keeping with the analysis so far, the point is not simply to look at what the justices write, but to analyze the justifications they give for writing it. For all the praise that *Casey* has received, its justifications are especially weak because they are rooted, not in principle, but in compromise. The most potent criticisms of *Casey* come from the pen of one of its co-authors. Justice

O'Connor has a lengthy paper trail of substantial criticisms of the very opinion she now jointly authors. I outline a few here, again focusing only on those passages that concern the protection of prenatal life.

In both *Akron*[52] and *Ashcroft*,[53] O'Connor writes that the state has a compelling interest in protecting and preserving fetal life throughout pregnancy. In the opinion for the Court in *Akron*, Justice Powell dedicated an extended footnote to O'Connor's position. He writes that she "rejects the basic premise of *Roe* and its progeny." He continues by saying that, "for all practical purposes," her reasoning would overrule *Roe*. Powell has no doubts about what O'Connor means when she writes that the state's interests are compelling throughout pregnancy. He writes that she "would uphold virtually any abortion-inhibiting regulation because of the State's interest in preserving potential human life." As proof of this he cites her argument that a 24-hour waiting period is justified in part because the abortion decision "has grave consequences for the fetus." Powell concludes: "This analysis is wholly incompatible with the existence of the fundamental right recognized in *Roe v. Wade*."[54] That O'Connor was not affected by Powell's critique is evidenced by her explicit remark three years later in *Thornburgh* that she had not changed her mind.[55]

In *Casey*, however, O'Connor and her collaborators downgrade the state's interests in the previable fetus from "compelling" to "substantial"[56] and "profound."[57] These words have little more significance in constitutional law than the words "legitimate" and "important" that Blackmun uses to describe the previability interests of the state. What caused O'Connor to abandon her earlier position? No clue is given. One assumes it was rooted in a spirit of compromise and not in a close examination of the interests involved. It was a sacrifice which had to be made, as the above-cited passage from Powell makes clear, if she was to participate in the joint opinion's reaffirmation of the central holding of *Roe*.

It might be suggested that what she meant by "compelling" in her earlier dissenting opinions was that the state's interest should be given some consideration prior to viability as it is now capable of receiving under *Casey*. But the word "compelling" has a distinct and clear meaning in the abortion cases, and to suggest that O'Connor might have used a word like "compelling" imprecisely over a period of years and in the face of direct attack by the pro-*Roe* justices would be to charge her with judicial recklessness. When Blackmun writes that the state's interests in protecting potential life increase throughout pregnancy and become compelling at viability, he means that from that point on they outweigh the woman's privacy interests and, unless her life or health are threatened, the state may proscribe abortion. For O'Connor to have written that the state's interests are compelling throughout pregnancy meant that she rejected the results of *Roe's* central balancing test.

Similarly, in *Akron* O'Connor describes *Roe's* focusing on viability as "no less arbitrary than choosing any point before viability or any point afterward."[58] However, in *Casey* she and her collaborators write, "Whenever it may occur, the attainment of viability may continue to serve as the critical fact, just as it has done since *Roe* was decided."[59] No argument is given to justify her acceptance of that which she had once explicitly rejected. In the next sentence, however, the joint opinion claims that this stance on viability is *Roe's* "central holding." To maintain her former position would be for her to call for *Roe* to be overruled. Again, it was a sacrifice which had to be made if she was to participate in the joint opinion's reaffirmation of the central holding of *Roe*.

Although they discard *Roe's* trimester framework, the authors of the joint opinion keep in place the result of *Roe's* balancing test without considering whether the interests were properly weighed when the test was first performed. Their only goal is to help *Roe* be true to itself by removing the trimester framework which devalued what *Roe* said were the State's important and legitimate interests.

Justice Scalia challenges the credibility of *Roe* on precisely this matter. Scalia describes the balancing test performed in *Roe* and in all of *Roe's* progeny as "begging the question . . . by assuming that the State is protecting the mere 'potentiality of human life.'"[60] He observes that, unless *Roe* is correct in its assessment of the fetus as "merely potentially human," then the result of its balancing test, which has since been applied in many cases, is wrong. As Scalia notes, the argument of most of those who oppose abortion focuses precisely on this begged question: that the fetus is not merely potentially human, but that it "*is a human life*."[61]

Consider the following passage in which the joint opinion lists those whose lives are affected by an abortion.

> Abortion is a unique act. It is an act fraught with consequences for others: (1) for the woman who must live with the implications of her decision; (2) for the persons who perform and assist in the procedure; (3) for the spouse, family, and society which must confront the knowledge that these procedures exist, procedures some deem nothing short of an act of violence against innocent human life; (4) and, depending on one's beliefs, for the life or potential life that is aborted.[62]

Although it is good to see that the Court is beginning to retreat from Blackmun's *de facto* decision that prenatal life is merely potential life, it is disheartening to see the fetus ranked fourth in terms of those who suffer the consequences of abortion. This description of the fetus's role in abortion is also a far cry from the bluntness with which O'Connor describes the consequences of abortion when she voted to uphold a 24-hour waiting period in *Akron*. She writes:

> The decision also has grave consequences for the fetus, whose life the State has a compelling interest to protect and preserve. No other medical procedure involves the purposeful termination of potential life. The waiting period is surely a small cost to impose to ensure that the woman's decision is well con-

sidered in light of its certain and irreparable consequences on fetal life, and the possible effects on her own.[63]

Most disturbing about *Casey* is that the joint opinion's authors themselves do not seem to believe that *Roe* was decided correctly. On at least five occasions, they strongly hint that *Roe's* standard is not what they would have endorsed had any of them been on the bench in 1973. They write, "[T]he reservations any of us have in reaffirming the central holding of *Roe* are outweighed by the explication of individual liberty we have given combined with the force of *stare decisis*."[64] After reviewing the doctrine of *stare decisis*, they repeat that sentiment, "[T]he stronger argument is for affirming *Roe's* central holding, with whatever degree of personal reluctance any of us may have, not for overruling it."[65] After further reviewing the obligation to follow precedent, the authors write: "a decision to overrule should rest on some special reason over and above the belief that a prior case was wrongly decided."[66] Similarly, they state: "A decision to overrule *Roe's* essential holding under the existing circumstances would address error, if error there was, at the cost of both profound and unnecessary damage to the Court's legitimacy, and to the Nation's commitment to the rule of law."[67] This series concludes with the final extended remark:

> We do not need to say whether each of us, had we been Members of the Court when the valuation of the State interest came before it as an original matter, would have concluded, as the *Roe* Court did, that its weight is insufficient to justify a ban on abortions prior to viability even when it is subject to certain exceptions. The matter is not before us in the first instance, and coming as it does after nearly twenty years of litigation in *Roe's* wake we are satisfied that the immediate question is not the soundness of *Roe's* resolution of the issue, but the precedential force that must be accorded to its holding.[68]

It appears that the revisions they make in the *Roe* standard are attempts to shore up a ruling which quite possibly none of them would have voted for in its original form. We might now have stability in knowing that the basic holdings of the previous nineteen years will remain in place. What we also have is decreased confidence that *Roe* itself was decided well. One would hope to have stronger justifications than the rule of *stare decisis* for maintaining such a significant constitutional doctrine.

The authors of the joint opinion expressed the basis for their maintaining *Roe* in the opening sentence of their opinion: "Liberty finds no refuge in a jurisprudence of doubt."[69] I stand with Scalia's mocking retort, "Reason finds no refuge in this jurisprudence of confusion."[70]

NOTES

1. In expert testimony before the U.S. Congress, 23 April 1981, as quoted in J. P. Moreland and Norman L. Geisler, *The Life and Death Debate: Moral Issues of Our Time* (Westport, Conn.: Greenwood Press, 1990), pp. 34–35.

2. "'Jane Roe' joins Operation Rescue," *The Orange County Register* 11 August, 1995, p. News 3.

3. *Roe v. Wade*, 410 U.S. 113 at 159 (1973).

4. Ibid., p. 162.

5. Ibid., p. 153.

6. Ibid., p. 177.

7. Ronald Dworkin makes this observation in "Unenumerated Rights: Whether and How 'Roe' Should be Overruled," *University of Chicago Law Review* 59 (1992): 401. Dworkin parallels this possible abridgment of a pregnant woman's rights with the following theoretical example: if the state could declare trees to be persons, the state could prohibit publishing newspapers in spite of the First Amendment's guarantee of free speech since that amendment does not grant a license to kill. This part of Dworkin's article is cited by Justice Stevens in *Planned Parenthood v. Casey*, 112 S.Ct. 2791 at 2839, n. 2 (1992).

8. *Roe*, pp. 161f.

9. Ibid., p. 159. In *Doe v. Bolton*, the companion case to *Roe v. Wade*, Justice Douglas wrote a concurring opinion which echoes this theme. He writes, "When life is present is a question we do not try to resolve. While basically a question for medical experts,...it is, of course, caught up in matters of religion and morality" (*Doe v. Bolton*, 410 U.S. 179 at 220). Note the equivocal meaning Douglas gives the term *life*. There is no doubt that the developing fetus is alive, a matter which medical experts can confirm and that Douglas' later references to such things as "embryonic life" belies. Douglas, however, is using the term in a value-oriented sense which is beyond the province of medical expertise to define. Justice Stevens is not at all hesitant to state his position on the disputed question of when life begins. He writes, "[U]nless the religious view that a fetus is a person is adopted ...there is a fundamental and well-recognized difference between a fetus and a human being" (Thornburgh, 476 U.S. 747 at 779). Note that "human" and the constitutional sense of "person" are equated without any justifying argument.

10. *Roe*, p. 160.

11. Ibid., p. 161.

12. Ibid., p. 162.

13. Ibid., p. 150. Italics in the original.

14. Ibid., p. 153.

15. Ibid., p. 154.

16. Ibid., p. 159.

17. Ibid., pp. 162f.

18. Ibid., p. 160.

19. Ibid., p. 163. In *Doe v. Bolton*, Douglas writes that society is rightfully concerned with the "life of the fetus after quickening" (*Doe v. Bolton*, 410 U.S. 179 at 215). Douglas treats "quickening" as the functional equivalent of Blackmun's "viability." However, quickening not only occurs four to seven weeks earlier than the earliest date which Blackmun gave for viability, but also as a marker event it tells us little about fetal development. The fetus has already been independently moving for quite some time. Quickening only denotes when the mother becomes aware of that movement.

20. *Thornburgh v. American College of Obstetricians and Gynecologists*, 476 U.S. 747 at 795, citing John Hart Ely, "The Wages of Crying Wolf: A Comment on 'Roe v. Wade'," *Yale Law Journal* 82 (1973): 924.

21. *Akron v. Akron Center for Reproductive Health*, 462 U.S. 416 at 457 (1983).

22. Ibid., p. 458.

23. *Webster v. Reproductive Health Services*, 492 U.S. 490 at 554 n. 9 (1989).

24. Norman Fost, David Chudwin, and Daniel Wikler, "The Limited Moral Significance of Fetal Viability," *Hastings Center Report* 10 (December 1980): 11.

25. *Thornburgh*, p. 795.

26. Fost, Chudwin, and Wikler, "The Limited Moral Significance of Fetal Viability," pp. 12f.

27. *Akron*, p. 461. Citations omitted. Emphasis in the original.

28. *Thornburgh*, p. 779.

29. Ibid., p. 762.

30. Ibid.

31. Ibid., p. 762, n. 10.

32. Ibid., p. 807.

33. Ibid., p. 829.

34. *Maher v Roe*, 432 U.S. 464, 484 (1977). Burger appears to be advocating what *Casey* would later describe as an "undue burden" standard which allows the state to express its interests in protecting prenatal life before viability.

35. *Thornburgh*, p. 783, n. *.

36. Ibid., p. 783f.

37. Ibid., p. 784.

38. Cf. *Thornburgh*, p. 778 (1986) and *Webster*, pp. 563–572 (1989).

39. *Cruzan v. Director, Missouri Department of Health*, 110 S.Ct. 2841 at 2888 (1990).

40. Cf. Justice White's dissent in *Thornburgh*, p. 795, n. 4.

41. *Thornburgh*, p. 779, n. 8; *Webster*, p. 568, n. 13; *Casey*, pp. 2839f.

42. *Planned Parenthood v. Casey*, 112 S.Ct. 2791 at 2839.

43. Ibid., p. 2840.

44. Ibid. When Stevens first wrote of this state interest in *Webster*, he quickly dismissed it as inapplicable to our historical age. Cf. *Webster*, p. 569 (1989).

45. *Casey*, p. 2840, n. 3.

46. Ibid.

47. *Thornburgh*, p. 778.

48. *Webster*, p. 490.

49. *Casey*, p. 2817.
50. Ibid., p. 2818. Emphasis added.
51. Ibid., p. 2818.
52. *Akron*, p. 461.
53. *Planned Parenthood v. Ashcroft*, 462 U.S. 476 at 505 (1983).
54. *Akron*, pp. 420f. n. 1.
55. *Thornburgh*, p. 828.
56. *Casey*, p. 2820.
57. Ibid., p. 2821.
58. *Akron*, p. 461.
59. *Casey*, pp. 2811f.
60. Ibid., p. 2875.
61. Ibid. Italics in the original.
62. *Casey*, p. 2807. Numbers added.
63. *Akron*, p. 474. Citations omitted.
64. *Casey*, p. 2808.
65. Ibid., p. 2812.
66. Ibid., p. 2814.
67. Ibid., p. 2816
68. Ibid., p. 2817.
69. Ibid., p. 2803.
70. Ibid., p. 2880.

Selected Bibliography

Adler, Mortimer. *Haves Without Have-Nots.* New York: Macmillan, 1991.

Alcorn, Randy. *Is Rescuing Right?* Downers Grove, Ill.: InterVarsity Press, 1990.

_____ . *Pro-Life Answers to Pro-Choice Arguments.* Sisters, Oreg.: Multnomah Books, 1992.

Anderson, John O. *Cry of the Innocents: Abortion and the Race Towards Judgment.* South Plainfield, N.J.: Bridge Publications, 1984.

Andrusko, Dave, ed. *To Rescue the Future.* Toronto and Harrison, N.Y.: Life Cycle Books, 1983.

Ankerberg, John, and John Weldon. *When Does Life Begin?* Brentwood, Tenn.: Wolgemuth and Hyatt, 1989.

Baird, Robert M., and Stuart E. Rosenbaum, eds. *The Ethics of Abortion: Pro-Life vs. Pro-Choice.* Buffalo, N.Y.: Prometheus Books, 1989.

Bajema, Clifford E. *Abortion and the Meaning of Personhood.* Grand Rapids: Baker Book House, 1974.

Baker, Don. *Beyond Choice: The Abortion Story No One is Telling.* Portland, Oreg.: Multnomah Books, 1985.

Batchelor, Edward Jr., ed. *Abortion: The Moral Issues.* New York: Pilgrim Press, 1982.

Beck, F., D. B. Moffat, and D.P. Davies. *Human Embryology.* Oxford: Blackwell, 1985.

Beckwith, Francis J. *Politically-Correct Death: Answering the Arguments for Abortion Rights.* Grand Rapids: Baker Book House, 1993.

Beckwith, Francis J., and Louis P. Pojman, eds. *The Abortion Controversy: A Reader.* Boston: Jones and Bartlett, 1994.

Beckwith, Francis J., and Norman L. Geisler. *Matters of Life and Death.* Grand Rapids: Baker Book House, 1991.

Belz, Mark. *Suffer the Little Children.* Westchester, Ill.: Crossway Books, 1989.

Blank, Robert H. *Fetal Protection in the Workplace: Women's Rights, Business Interests, and the Unborn.* New York: Columbia University Press, 1993.

Bonavoglia, Angela ed. *The Choices We Made: 25 Women and Men Speak Out About*

Abortion. New York: Random House, 1992.

Bopp, James Jr., ed. *Restoring the Right to Life: The Human Life Amendment.* Provo,Utah: Brigham Young University Press, 1984.

Boston Women's Health Collective. *Our Bodies, Ourselves.* New York: Simon and Schuster, 1973.

Bowers, James R. *Pro-Choice and Anti-Abortion: Constitutional Theory and Public Policy.* Westport, Conn.: Praeger Publishers, 1994.

Brennan, William. *The Abortion Holocaust: Today's Final Solution.* St. Louis: Landmark Press, 1983.

Brody, Brauch. *Abortion and the Sanctity of Human Life.* Cambridge, Mass: M.I.T. Press, 1975.

Browder, Clifford. *The Wickedest Woman in New York: Madame Restell, The Abortionist.* Hamden, Conn.: Archon Books, 1988.

Brown, Harold O.J. *Death Before Birth.* Nashville, Tenn.: Thomas Nelson, 1977.

Brown, Judie, Jerome LeJeune, and Robert G. Marshall. *RU-486: The Human Pesticide.* Stafford, Va.: American Life League, n.d.

Brown, Judy, and Paul Brown. *Choices in Matters of Life and Death.* Avon, N.J.: Magnificat Press, 1987.

Burtchaell, James Tunstead. *Rachel Weeping: The Case Against Abortion.* San Francisco: Harper and Row, 1982.

Butler , J. Douglas, and David F. Walbert, eds. *Abortion, Medicine, and the Law.* 4th edition revised. New York: Facts on File, 1992.

_____ . eds. *Abortion, Society and the Law.* Cleveland: Press of Case Western Reserve University, 1973.

Calderone, Mary, ed. *Abortion in the United States.* New York: Hoeber-Harper, 1958.

Callahan, Daniel. *Abortion: Law, Choice and Morality.* New York: Macmillan, 1970.

Callahan, Sidney, and Daniel Callahan, eds. *Abortion: Understanding Differences.* New York: Plenum Press, 1984.

Cameron, Nigel M. de S., and Pamela F. Sims. *Abortion: The Crisis in Morals and Medicine.* Leicester, England: InterVarsity Press, 1986.

Campbell, Robert, and Diane Collinson. *Ending Lives.* New York: Basil Blackwell, 1988.

Christian, Scott Rickly. *The Woodland Hills Tragedy.* Westchester, Ill.: Crossway Books, 1985.

Cochrane, Linda. *Women in Rama: A Postabortion Bible Study.* Falls Church, Va.: Christian Action Council, 1987.

Cohen, Marshall. *Rights and Wrongs of Abortion.* Princeton, N. J.: Princeton University Press, 1974.

Collins, Carol C., ed. *Abortion: The Continuing Controversy.* New York: Facts on File, 1984.

Collins, Vincent J, Steven R. Zielinsky, and Thomas J. Marzen. *Fetal Pain and Abortion: The Medical Evidence.* Chicago: Americans United For Life, 1984.

Condit, Celeste Michelle. *Decoding Abortion Rhetoric: Communicating Social Change.* Urbana and Chicago: University of Ilinois Press, 1990.

Connery, John. *Abortion: The Development of the Roman Catholic Perspective.* Chicago: Loyola University Press, 1977.

Davis, John Jefferson. *Abortion and the Christian.* Phillipsburg, N.J.: Presbyterian and Reformed, 1984.

Davis, Nanette J. *From Crime to Choice: The Transformation of Abortion in America.* New York: Greenwood Press, 1985.

Denes, Magda. *In Necessity and Sorrow: Life and Death in an Abortion Hospital.* New York: Basic Books, 1976.

Devereaux, George. *A Study of Abortion in Primitive Societies.* New York:Julian Press, 1955.

Doerr, Edd, and James W. Prescott, eds. *Abortion Rights and Fetal 'Personhood.'* Long Beach, Calif.: Centerline Press, 1989.

Drucker, Dan. *Abortion Decisions of the the Supreme Court, 1973 through 1989: A Comphrehensive Review with Historical Commentary.* Jefferson, N.C.: McFarland and Company, 1990.

Duden, Barbara. *Disembodying Women: Perspectives on Pregnancy and the Unborn.* Cambridge, Mass.: Harvard University Press, 1993.

Dworkin, Ronald M. *Life's Dominion : An Argument Abortion, Euthanasia and Inidividualism Freedom.* New York: Alfred A Knopf, 1993.

Eggebroten, Anne, ed. *Abortion: My Choice, God's Grace.* Pasadena, Calif: New Paradigm Books, 1994.

Everett, Carol. *The Scarlet Lady: Confessions of a Successful Abortionist.* Brentwood, Tenn.: Wolgemuth and Hyatt, 1991.

Feinberg, Joel, ed. *The Problem of Abortion.* Belmont, Calif.: Wadsworth, 1984.

Felix, Marilyn. *Ideology and Abortion Policy Politics.* New York: Praeger Publishers, 1983.

Fitzsimmons, Richard, and Joan P. Diana. *Pro-Choice/Pro-Life: An Annotated, Selected Bibliography.* New York: Greenwood Press, 1991.

Fleming, Anne Taylor. *Motherhood Deferred: A Woman's Journey.* New York: G. P. Putnam's Sons, 1994.

Ford, Norman. *When Did I Begin? Conception of the Human Individual in History, Philosophy and Science.* New York: Cambridge University Press, 1988.

Fowler, Paul. *Abortion: Toward and Evangelical Consensus.* Portland, Oreg.: Multnomah Books, 1987.

Franke, Linda Bird. *The Ambivalence of Abortion.* New York: Random House, 1978.

Frasier, Debra. *On the Day You Were Born.* San Diego: Harcourt Brace, 1991.

Frohock, Fred M. *Abortion: A Case Study in Law and Morals.* New York: Greenwood Press, 1983.

Gardner, R.F.R. *Abortion: The Personal Dilemma.* Grand Rapids: William B. Eerdmans Publishing Co., 1972.

Garfield Jay L., and Patricia Hennessey, eds. *Abortion: Moral and Legal Perspectives.* Amherst, Mass.: University of Massachusetts Press, 1984.

Garton, Jean. *Who Broke the Baby?* Minneapolis: Bethany House, 1979.

Gilligan, Carol. *In A Different Voice.* Cambridge, Mass.: Harvard University Press, 1982.

Ginsburg, Faye. *Contested Lives: The Abortion Debate in an American Community.* Berkeley: University of California Press, 1989.

Glenn, Evelyn Nakano, Grace Chang, and Linda Rennie Forcey, eds. *Mothering: Ideology, Experience, and Agency.* New York: Routledge, 1994.

Glendon, Mary Ann. *Abortion and Divorce in Western Law.* Cambridge, Mass.: Harvard University Press, 1987.

_____ . *Rights Talk*. New York: Free Press, 1991.

Glessner, Thomas. *Achieving and Abortion-Free America by 2001*. Portland, Oreg.: Multnomah Press, 1990.

Goldstein, Robert. *Mother-Love and Abortion*. Berkeley: Unversity of California Press, 1988.

Goodman, Michael F. ed. *What is a Person?* Clifton: N.J.: Humana Press, 1988.

Gorman, Michael J. *Abortion and the Early Church*. Downers Grove, Ill. InterVarsity Press, 1982.

Grant, George. *Grand Illusions: The Legacy of Planned Parenthood*. Brentwood, Tenn.: Wolgemuth and Hyatt, 1988.

_____ . *The Quick and the Dead: RU-486 and the New Chemical Warfare Against Your Family*. Westchester, Ill.: Crossway Books, 1991.

Grisez, Germain. *Abortion: the Myths, the Realities, and the Arguments*. New York: Corpus Books, 1970.

Harrison, Beverly Wildung. *Our Right To Choose: Toward a New Ethic of Abortion*. Boston: Beacon Press, 1983.

Hensley, Jeff Lane, ed. *The Zero People*. Ann Arbor: Servant Books, 1983.

Hentoff, Nat. *The Indivisible Fight for Life*. Chicago: Americans United for Life, 1987.

Hern, Warren M. *Abortion Practice*. Philadelphia: Lippincott, 1990.

Hilgers, Thomas, Dennis J. Horan, and David Mall, eds. *New Perspectives on Human Abortion*. Frederick, Md.: University Publications of America, 1981.

Hilgers, Thomas, and Dennis J. Horan, eds. *Abortion and Social Justice*. New York: Sheed and Ward, 1972.

Hinze, Sarah. *Life Before Birth*. Springville, Utah: Cedar Fort, 1993.

Hoffmeier, James, ed. *Abortion: A Christian Understanding and Response*. Grand Rapids: Baker Book House, 1987.

Horan, Dennis, Edward R. Grant, and Paige C. Cunninghan, eds. *Abortion and the Constitution: Reversing Roe v. Wade Through the Courts*. Washington, D.C.: Georgetown University Press, 1987.

Hunter, James Davison. *Before the Shooting Begins: Searching for Democracy in America's Culture Wars*. New York: Free Press, 1994.

Judges, Donald. *Hard Choices, Lost Voices*. Chicago: Ivan R. Dee Publishers, 1993.

Jung, Patricia Beattie, and Thomas A. Shannon, eds. *Abortion and Catholicism: The American Debate*. New York: Crossroad, 1988.

Kamm, F.M. *Creation and Abortion: A Study in Moral and Legal Philosophy*. New York: Oxford University Press, 1992.

Kennedy, D. James. *Abortion: Cry of Reality*. Fort Lauderdale, Fla.: Coral Ridge Ministries, 1989.

Kenny, Mary. *Abortion: The Whole Story*. London: Quartet Books Limited, 1986.

Koerbel, Pam. *Abortion's Second Victim*. Wheaton, Ill.: Victor Books, 1986.

Kolata, Gina. *The Baby Doctors: Probing the Limits of Fetal Medicine*. New York: Dell Publishing, 1990.

Koop, C. Everett. *The Right to Live: The Right to Die*. Old Tappan, N.J.: Revell, 1979.

Koop, C. Everett, and Francis A. Schaeffer. *Whatever Happened to the Human Race?*

Wheaton, Ill.: Tyndale House, 1976.

Krason, Stephen M. *Abortion: Politics, Morality and the Constitution*. Lanham, Md.: University Press of America, 1984.

Kreeft, Peter. *Making Choices*. Ann Arbor, Mich.: Servant Books, 1990.

_____ . *The Unaborted Socrates*. Downers Grove, Ill: InterVarsity Press, 1984.

Kuback, Michael M., and Carlo Valenti, ed. *Intrauterine Fetal Visualization*. Oxford: Excerpta Medica; New York: American Elsevier Publishing, 1976.

Kuhse, Helga and Peter Singer. *Should the Baby Live?* New York: Oxford Universtiy Press, 1985.

Lader, Lawrence. *Abortion*. Indianapolis: Bobbs-Merrill, 1966.

_____ . *Abortion II: Making the Revolution*. Boston: Beacon Press, 1973.

La Fleur, William R. *Liquid Life: Abortion and Buddhism in Japan*. Princeton, N. J.: Princeton University Press, 1992.

Leavitt, Judith Walzer. *Brought to Bed: Childbearing in America: 1750 to 1950*. New York: Oxford University Press, 1986.

Littlewood, Thomas B. *The Politics of Population Control*. Notre Dame: University of Notre Dame Press, 1977.

Lotstra, Hans. *Abortion: The Catholic Debate in America*. New York: Irvington, 1985.

Luker, Kristen. *Abortion and the Politics of Motherhood*. Berkeley and Los Angeles: University of California Press, 1984.

_____ . *Taking Chances: Abortion and the Decision Not to Contracept*. Berkeley: University of California Press, 1975.

Mall, David, and Walter F. Watts, eds. *The Psychological Aspects of Abortion*. Washington, D.C.: University Publications of America, 1979.

Mall, David. *In Good Conscience: Abortion and Moral Necessity*. Libertyville, Ill.: Kairos Books, 1982.

_____ . ed. *When Life and Choice Collide: Essays on Rhetoric and Abortion*. Vol. 1, *To Set the Dawn Free*, David Mall, ed. Libertyville, Ill.: Kairos Books, 1994.

Mannion, Michael. *Abortion and Healing*. Kansas City: Sheed and Ward, 1986.

Marsh, David, and Joanna Chambers. *Abortion Politics*. London: Junction Books, 1981.

Marshall, Robert, and Charles Donovan. *Blessed are the Barren: The Social Policy of Planned Parenthood*. San Francisco: Ignatius Press, 1991.

Martin, Walter R. *Abortion: Is it Always Murder?* Santa Ana, Calif.: Vision House, 1977.

Mathewes-Green, Frederica. *Real Choices: Offering Practical, Life-Affirming Alternatives to Abortion*. Sisters, Oreg.: Questar Publications, 1994.

Marx, Paul. *The Death Peddlers: War on the Unborn*. Collegeville, Minn.: St. John's University Press, 1971.

McCormick, Richard A. *How Brave A New World?* Garden City, N.Y.: Doubleday, 1981.

McDonnel, Kathleen. *Not an Easy Choice: A Feminist Reexamines Abortion*. Boston: South End Press, 1984.

McKeegan, Michele. *Abortion Politics*. New York: Free Press, 1992.

Merton, Andrew H. *Enemies of Choice: The Right to Life Movement and Its Threat to*

Abortion. Boston: Beacon Press, 1981.

Messer, Ellen, and Kathryn E. May. *Back Rooms: Voices from the Illegal Abortion Era*. Buffalo, N. Y.: Prometheus Books, 1994.

Michels, Nancy. *Helping Women Recover From Abortion*. Minneapolis: Bethany House, 1988.

Miller, Donald E., and Lorna Touryan. *Survivors: An Oral History of the Armenian Genocide*. Berkeley and Los Angeles: University of California Press, 1993.

Mohr, James. *Abortion in America: The Origins and Evolution of National Policy*. New York: Oxford University Press, 1978.

Montgomery, John Warwick. *Slaughter of the Innocents: Abortion, Birth Control, Divorce in Light of Science , Law and Theology*. Westchester, Ill.: Crossway Books, 1981.

Moore, Keith. *The Developing Human: Clinically Oriented Embryology*. Philadelphia: W. B. Saunders, 1977.

Moreland, J. P., and Norman L. Geisler. *The Life and Death Debate: Moral Issues of Our Time*. Westport, Conn.: Praeger Publishers, 1990.

Moreland, J. P., and David Ciocchi, eds. *Christian Perspectives on Being Human: An Integrative Approach*. Grand Rapids: Baker Book House, 1993.

Muldoon, Maureen. *The Abortion Debate in the United States and Canada: A Sourcebook*. New York: Garland Publishing, 1991.

Nathanielsz, Peter W. *Life Before Birth and A Time To Be Born*. Ithaca, N. Y.: Promethean Press, 1992.

Nathanson, Bernard. *Aborting America*. Garden City, N.Y.: Doubleday, 1979.

_____ . *The Abortion Papers: Inside the Abortion Mentality*. New York: Frederick Fell, 1983.

Nelson, Leonard, ed. *The Death Decision*. Ann Arbor, Mich.: Servant Books, 1984.

Neuhaus, Richard John. *America Against Itself*. Notre Dame: University of Notre Dame Press, 1992.

_____ . *The Naked Publid Square*. Grand Rapids: William B. Eerdmans Publishing, Co., 1984.

Nilsson, Lennart. *A Child is Born*. New York: Dell Publishing, 1977.

Noelle-Neumann, Elizabeth. *The Spiral of Silence*. Chicago: University of Chicago Press, 1984.

Noonan, John T. ed. *A Private Choice*. New York: Free Press, 1979.

_____ . *The Morality of Abortion: Legal and Historical Perspectives*. Cambridge, Mass.: Harvard University Press, 1970.

North, Gary. *Trespassing for Dear Life: What is Operation Rescue Up To?* Fort Worth, Tex.: Dominion, 1989.

Olasky, Marvin. *Abortion Rites*: A Social History of Abortion in America. Wheaton, Ill.: Crossway Books, 1992

_____ . *The Press and Abortion: 1838-1988*. Hillsdale, N.J.: Lawrence Erlbaum Associates, 1988.

Osofsky, Howard, and Joy , eds. *The Abortion Experience*. New York: Harper and Row, 1973.

Paige, Connie. *The Right-to-Lifers: Who They Are, How They Operate, Where They Get Their Money*. New York: Summit Books, 1983.

Peretti, Frank. *Tilly*. Westchester, Ill.: Crossway Books, 1988.

Petchesky, Rosalind. *Abortion and Woman's Choice: The State, Sexuality and Reproductive Freedom*. New York: Longman, 1984.

Pierson, Anne. *52 Simple Things You Can Do to Be Pro-Life*. Minneapolis: Bethany House, 1991.

Powell, John. *Abortion: A Christian Understanding and Response*. Grand Rapids: Baker Book House, 1987.

_____ . *Abortion: The Silent Holocaust*. Allen, Tex.: Argus, 1981.

Presser, Stephen B. *Recapturing the Constitution: Race, Religion, and Abortion Reconsidered*. Washington D. C.: Regnery Publishing, 1994.

Reagan, Ronald, and C. Everett Koop. *Abortion and the Conscience of the Nation*. Nashville, Tenn.: Thomas Nelson, 1984.

Reardon, David C. *Aborted Women, Silent No More*. Chicago: Loyola University Press, 1987.

_____ . *Abortion Malpractice*. Denton, Tex.: Life Dynamics, 1993.

_____ . *Give Us Love, Not Abortions: The Voices of Sexual Assault Victims and Their Children*. South Bend, Ind.: Fortress International, 1992.

_____ . *Life Stories*. Westchester, Ill.: Crossway Books, 1992.

Reed, James. *From Private Vice to Public Virtue*. New York: Basic Books, 1978.

Reisser, Teri and Paul. *Help for the Post-Abortion Woman*. Grand Rapids: Zondervan Publishing House, 1989.

Rice, Charles. *The Vanishing Right to Live: An Appeal for a Renewed Reverence for Life*. New York: Doubleday, 1969.

Rodman, Hyman et al. *The Abortion Question*. New York: Columbia University Press, 1987.

Rosen, Harold. *Therapeutic Abortion: Medical, Psychiatric, Legal, Anthropological and Religious Considerations*. New York: Julian Press, 1954.

Rubin, Eva R., ed. *The Abortion Controversy: A Documentary History*. Westport, Conn.: Greenwood Press, 1994.

Sachdev, Paul, ed. *Perspectives on Abortion*. Metuchen, N.J.: The Scarecrow Press, 1985.

Saltenberger, Ann. *Every Woman Has A Right to Know the Dangers of Legal Abortion*. Glassboro, N.J.: Air-Plus Enterprises, 1983.

Sanger, Margaret. *Woman and the New Race*. New York: Truth Publishing, 1920.

Sarvis, Betty, and Hyman Rodman. *The Abortion Controversy*. New York: Columbia Universtiy Press, 1973.

Sass, Lauren R., ed. *Abortion: Freedom of Choice and the Right to Life*. New York: Facts on File, 1978.

Schwarz, Stephen D. *The Moral Question of Abortion*. Chicago: Loyola University Press, 1990.

Selby, Terry. *The Mourning After*. Grand Rapids: Baker Book House, 1990.

Shettles, Landrum and David Rorvik. *Rites of Life: The Scientific Evidence for Life Before Birth*. Grand Rapids: Zondervan Publishing House, 1983.

Sider, Ron. *Completely Pro-Life: Building a Consistent Stance*. Downers Grove, Ill.: InterVarsity Press, 1987.

Smetana, Judith G. *Concepts of Self and Morality: Women's Reasoning About Abortion*. New York: Praeger Publishers, 1982.

Smith, F. LaGard. *When Choice Becomes God*. Eugene, Oreg.: Harvest House, 1990.

Solinger, Rickie. *The Abortionist*. New York: Free Press, 1994.

Sologub, Fedor. *The Kiss of the Unborn and Other Stories*. Translated by Murl G. Barker. Knoxville, Tenn.: University of Tennessee Press, 1977.

Sproul, R. C. *Abortion: A Rational Look at An Emotional Issue*. Colorado Springs, Col.: NavPress, 1990.

Steinbock, Bonnie. *Life Before Birth: The Moral and Legal Status of Embryos and Fetuses*. New York: Oxford University Press, 1992.

Swindoll, Charles. *Sanctity of Life*. Waco, Tex.: Word Publishing, 1990.

Szumski, Bonnie, ed. *Abortion: Opposing Viewpoints*. St. Paul, Minn.: Greenhaven, 1986.

Terry, Randall. *Accessories to Murder*. Brentwood, Tenn.: Wolgemuth and Hyatt, 1990.

_____ . *Operation Rescue*. Springdale, Penn.: Whitaker House, 1988.

Thomasma, David C. *Human Life in the Balance*. Louisville, Ken.: Westminster/John Knox Press, 1991.

Tickle, Phyllis, ed. *Confessing Conscience: Church Women on Abortion*. Nashville, Tenn.: Abingdon Press, 1990.

Tooley, Michael. *Abortion and Infanticide*. Oxford: Clarendon Press, 1986.

Tribe, Laurence. H. *Abortion: the Clash of Absolutes*. New York: W. W. Norton, 1990.

Trimble, Holly. *Healing Post Abortion Trauma*. Stafford, Va.: American Life League, 1989.

Vaux, Kenneth. *Birth Ethics: Religious and Cultural Values in the Generation of Life*. New York: Crossroad, 1989.

Wardle, Lynn, and Mary Anne Q. Wood. *A Lawyer Looks at Abortion*. Provo: Brigham Young University Press, 1982.

Wennberg, Robert. *Life in the Balance: Exploring the Abortion Controversy*. Grand Rapids: William B. Eerdmans Publishing Co., 1985.

Wilkie, John. *Abortion: Questions and Answers*. Cincinnati: Hayes Publishing Co., rev. ed., 1988.

_____ . *Abortion and Slavery: History Repeats*. Cincinnnati: Hayes Publishing Co., 1984.

Wilkie, John, and Barbara Wilkie, *Handbook on Abortion*. Cincinnati: Hayes Publishing Company, Inc., 1979.

Wittwer, Sherri Devashrayee. Gone Too Soon: The Life and Loss of Infants and Unborn Children. American Fork, Utah: Covenant Communications, 1994.

Young, Curt. *The Least of These: What Everyone Should Know About Abortion*. Chicago: Moody Press, 1984.

Zimmerman, Martha. *Should I Keep My Baby?* Minneapolis: Bethany House, 1983.

Zimmerman, Mary K. *Passage Through Abortion: The Personal and Social Reality of Women's Experiences*. New York: Praeger Publishers, 1977.

Index

Abortion: analogy to holocaust, xiii, 152–63, 164 n.9; argument for, 34–41, 47, 61, 63, 144, 242. *See also* pro-choice movement; counseling, 180; debate over, xi, xiv, xv, 1, 4–6, 15 n.39, 40, 66; ethical perversity of, 7–9, 40, 64, 73, 136, 138, 235; frequency of, 11 n.5, 47, 106, 108–10, 118, 125, 138, 159, 180, 183, 197, 199, 200, 202, 203, 205, 207, 222, nn.162, 163; grief over. *See* Grief from abortion; Women: as victims of abortion; guilt over. *See* Women: guilt over aborting; Women: as victims of abortion; law *see* Law and abortion; late in pregnancy, 8; license, xiii; maternal mortality and. *See* Women: as victims of abortion; media's attitude toward, 1, 9, 13 n.34; men and, 74, 121, 123, 139, 140, 158, 206, 207; methods, 8, 78–79, 97, 99. *See also* RU-486; moral deliberation about, 4, 6, 36–37, 39, 48, 74, 121, 136, 138–40; nature of, xii, 48, 124, 135, 137, 139, 141, 144, 153, 180, 204–7, 242; public opinion of , xiii, xiv, 2, 6, 7, 34, 34, 41

n.7, 97–98, 103–4, 108, 110, 136, 140, 180, 208 n.6; reasons for. *See* Women: reasons for aborting; rhetoric about, 4–5, 7, 43, 47, 140, 143–44, 158; right to. *See* Pro-choice movement; social consequences of, 10, 43, 45, 48–49, 56–58, 91, 110
The Abortionist, 201
Acquired Immune Deficiency Syndrome (AIDS). *See* Sexually transmitted disease
Akron v. Akron Center for Reproductive Health, 234–35, 240–42
Alan Guttmacher Institute, 11 n.5, 108, 140
Allen, William B., 61
The Ambivalence of Abortion, 140
Amen, John Harlan, 187–92
Amer, Margaret, 91–92, 109–10
American Civil Liberties Union (ACLU), 8
American College of Obstetricians and Gynecologists, 57
Apocalypticism, 156–58
Aquinas, Thomas, 19, 170
Archer, Anne, 72
Aristotle, 19, 23, 170
Augustus, 104

Babyfever, 119–20
Barnett, Ruth, 185, 194, 201, 223
    n.179
Bates, J. E., 198–99
Bauman, Michael, 4
Beauvoir, Simone de, 71, 123
Becker, Lawrence, 23–25
Bell, Deanna, 205
Benefit of the doubt argument, 36–39
Bentham, Jeremy, 85 n.12
Bernard, Viola, 159
Blackmun, Harry, 33, 35–36, 38,
    195, 229–36, 240, 241, 244 n.18
Blackstone, William, 182, 210 n.20
Blank, Robert H., 66
Boak, Arthur, 105
Bonhoeffer, Dietrich, 40
Boswell, John, 100
Brekke, Bard, 222 n.163
Brennan, William, 236
Brooks, Gwendolyn, 74
Bundesen, Herman N., 221 n.147
Burger, Warren, 236–37, 245 n.33
Butcher, Harry C., 164 n.6

Caesar, Julius, 104
Calderone, Mary, 199, 202, 204–5
Caldicott, Helen, 157
Callahan, Daniel, 140
Callahan, Sidney, 9, 14 n.35
Cameron, Ewen, 202, 224 n.191
Carroll, Mary Cate, 69
Casey, Robert, 3
Centers for Disease Control (CDC),
    204
"Choice," xi, 3–6, 9, 109, 140, 144,
    157
Christianity, 38, 100–1, 105, 152–
    54, 156–57, 160–63, 164 n.7,
    165 n.14, 169–75, 232
Christian Science, 38
Cicero, 104
Civil disobedience, 42 n.12, 154,
    162–63, 164 n.7
Clayburgh, Jill, 72–73
Clinton, Bill, 110

Colson, Pamela, 205
Conception (as beginning of human
    life), xii, 25–31, 34, 38, 43–46,
    118, 136–37, 144, 146, 152,
    169–75, 209 n.14, 229, 232
Constitution, 229–30, 237–38
Contraception, 65, 70–72, 86 n.24,
    103–4, 106, 109–10, 118
Couvade, 96
Crossing the Threshold of Hope, 121
*Cruzan v. Director, Missouri Depart-
    ment of Health*, 237
Culture, 6–7, 10, 15 n.38, 91–92,
    94, 97, 107, 110, 180; *see also
    Zeitgeist*; Abortion: debate over
Cuomo, Mario, 40
Curran, Charles, 22–23

Darley, John M., 161–62
Davis, Nathaniel, 43
Dellapenna, Joseph, 183–84
Denes, Magda, 143–44
Devereaux, George, 97
Dickinson, Peter, 77–78
Dobson, Shirley, 40
Doctors: 5, 8–9, 12 n.14, 54, 130,
    166 n.46, 202, 205, 206, 224
    n.193; as criminal abortionists,
    180–81, 184–85, 187–89, 191–
    92, 194, 199, 224 n.189; as deci-
    sion-makers, 51, 55–57, 159,
    192–93; legal liability and, 56–
    58, 193, 205
Doe v. Bolton, 244 nn.8, 18
Donohue, Michaela, 130–32
Douglas, William O., 236, 244 n.8
Downs, James F., 95
Dred Scott, xiii, 127
Duarte, Angelica, 205
Duden, Barbara, 117
Dworkin, Ronald, 244 n.6

Ecological consciousness, 46–47
Ehrlich, Paul, 156–57
Eisenhower, Dwight D., 164 n.3
Elders, Joycelyn, 1–2
Ely, John Hart, 195

Engelhardt, H. Tristam, Jr., 85 n.12
Ensoulment, 169–72
Erhardt, Carl, 222 n.163
Erikson, Erik, 46, 68
Evolution, 92–94

Family, 97, 101, 103–4, 106–8, 139
Fathers, 94–96
Faux, Marian, 194
Feinberg, Joel, 85 n.12
Feminism, 62, 65, 67, 71–73, 78–
    80, 84 n.6, 116–17, 120, 124,
    157
Feminists for Life of America, 84 n.6
Ferraro, Geraldine, 39
Fertility rate. See Infertility
Fetal experimentation and research,
    66–67, 85 n.19
Fetal life: xv, 1, 7–9, 44, 47, 49, 87
    n.32, 143, 181; agnosticism con-
    cerning status of, 33–36, 137,
    229, 232; obligations to, 10, 43–
    44, 48, 230; State's interests in,
    230–42; see also Personhood;
    Unborn human life
Fetus: 1–2, 9, 14, 28, 36, 43, 78, 86
    n.30, 87 n.43, 118, 136, 169–
    70, 181, 231–33, 236, 239, 242;
    as partially human, 14 n.35, 64,
    68, 137, 242; as threat, 65–67,
    73, 117, 157–58, 203; viability
    of, 26–27, 182, 232, 234–35,
    238; see also Unborn human life
Fleming, Anne Taylor, 70–71
Flesh, George, 9, 14 n.36
Fletcher, Joseph, 29
Fogel, Julius, 141–42, 147 n.18
Francke, Linda Bird, 139–40, 143–44
Frasier, Debra, 83
Freedom, 179
Friedan, Betty, 80
Frost, Norman, 234

Gebhard, Paul H., 199
Geisler, Norman L., 19
Gender hostility, 98–99
Genovese, Kitty, 160

Gillespie, Gary, 158
Goebbels, Joseph, 155
Goldberg, Whoopi, 40
Gordon, Hymie, 229
Graber, Mark A., 217 n.93
Green, Ronald, xii
Grief from abortion, 73–74, 77, 136,
    138–39, 144–46; see also
    Women: as victims of abortion
Griffin, Michael, 69
Grisez, Germain, 197–98

Hall, Robert E., 204, 225 n.207
Halpern, Milton, 203
Haskell, Martin, 8
Hawking, Steven, 64
Hentoff, Nat, 43
Hinckley, Thomas Kent, 78, 85 n.7
Hinduism, 38
Hinze, Sarah, 69
Hippocratic Oath, 51
Hogbin, Ian, 95
Holmes, Oliver Wendell, 187, 211
    n.23
Holmes, R. W., 209 n.14
Holocaust. See Abortion: analogy to
    holocaust
Human dignity, xiii, 10
Human Life Bill, 34–35
Human nature (essence), 20–25, 28,
    30–31, 33, 98
Hunter, James Davison, 1, 165 n.14,
    208 n.6
Hyatt, Abu, 8

Illegitimacy, 97–98, 107–8, 180,
    206
Implantation, 28–29, 171, 174
Infanticide, 99–101, 107
Infertility, 61, 84 n.4, 107–8, 160
Informed consent, 235–37
In Necessity and Sorrow, 143
Islam, 38, 100, 157

Jackson, Jesse, 10
Jelacic, Mary, 139–30

John Paul II, 121
Johnson, Jeffrey L., 12 n.14
Judaism, 152, 154–56, 163

Kali, 76, 82
Kant, Immanuel, 85 n.12
Kaplan, E. Ann, 65, 86 n.30
Kelly, Kevin, 173
Kennedy, Anthony, 239
Kerrison, Ray, 7
Keyes, Alan, 51, 179
Kidder, Margot, 73
Kindt, Anne, 12 n.18
Kinsey, Alfred, 198–99
Kleegman, Sophia, 222 n.163
Kopp, Marie, 198–99
Kristol, William, 123
Krupp, Charla, 120
Kuhse, Helga, 30, 32 n.21
Kummer, Jerome M., 199, 203, 223
     n.177

LaHaye, Beverly, 40
Laslett, Peter, 97
Latane, Bibb, 161–62
Law and abortion: 10 nn.3 and 4, 12
     n.14, 36, 167 n.65, 179–208,
     229–43; effects of enforcement of
     prohibitions, 195–206; enforce-
     ment of prohibitions, 180, 184–
     95; history of, 180–84, 206;
     problems associated with, 181–
     83, 185–86, 189, 192; recom-
     mendations for effective enforce-
     ment of prohibitions, 206–8; see
     also Doctors: as criminal abor-
     tionists
Lawrence, Florus F., 209 n.14
Leavitt, Judith, 196
Leavy, Zad, 199, 203, 223 n.177
Lehman, Herbert, 190, 192
Lejeune, Jerome, 33
Levi-Strauss, Claude, 102
Lewis, C. S., 160
Lindsey, Hal, 156
Littlehohn, Steven, 158
Livy, 104, 109

Lovejoy, C. Owen, 94
Lowinsky, Naomi Ruth, 76–77

Maher v. Roe, 236
Mahoney, John, 173–74, 175 n.5
Malinowski, Bronislaw, 91, 94, 110
Mann, Nancyjo, 135
Marriage, 105–7
Marshall, Thurgood, 236
Mathewes-Green, Frederica, 121, 135
McCormick, Richard, 174
McCorvey, Norma (a.k.a. Jane Roe),
     146 n.4, 194, 229
Means, Cyril, 182–83, 211 n.23
Michelman, Kate, 40, 61
Miscarriage, 28–29, 115, 117
Miller, Donald E., 154–55, 159, 163
Miller, James A., 108
Miller, Lorna T., 154–55, 159, 163
Miller, Patricia, 201, 204
Mohr, James C., 209 n.13, 213 n.33
Molech, 75, 77
Moore, R. I., 154–55
Moreland, J. P., 19, 29, 31 n.3
Mosher, Steven W., 98–99
Motherhood, 62, 67–71, 74, 80–83,
     85 n.10, 115–16, 118–21
Moynihan, Daniel Patrick, 107, 110
Muller, Steven, 66
Murder, 100–1, 182, 195, 238; see
     also Abortion; Infanticide
Murdock, George Peter, 91, 101, 107

Nagel, Thomas, 85 n.12
Najimy, Kathy, 73
Nathanson, Bernard, 203
Nathanson, Sue, 77
National Abortion Rights Action
     League (NARAL), 182–83, 203
National Institutes of Health (NIH),
     xii
Nature, 92, 102, 110, 179
Nazis, xiii, 152, 163 n.1, 164 n.3
Negron, Guadalupe, 205
Nelson, Robert, 203
Nineteen-sixties, 5, 106
Noelle-Neumann, Elizabeth, 11 n.6

Nominalism, 23, 31 n.9
Noonan, John T. Jr., 179

O'Connor, Sandra Day, 234–36,
    239–42
Olasky, Marvin, 183, 192, 198
Ontology, 19, 22
Operation Rescue, 40
Ottenberg, Perry, 159
Overpopulation, 156–57, 160–62

Packer, Herbert, 193
Papazoglou, Orania, 62
Patton, George S., 151, 163 n.2
Paul (St.), 64
Persecution, 153–60, 163
Personhood, xii, 19, 25–31, 32 n.32,
    35–36, 38–39, 44, 63, 157, 164
    n.8, 171, 174, 230, 232
Peters, Thomas P., 188
Pinnegar, Stefinee, 73, 87 n.44
Planned Parenthood, 6, 11 n.5, 117,
    198–99, 202
Planned Parenthood v. Ashcroft, 241
Planned Parenthood v. Casey, xiii,
    34, 64–65, 67, 180, 229, 231,
    237–41, 243
Political-correctness, 3–4, 7, 9, 11
    n.6, 160, 162
Pollitt, Katha, 116
Population Research Institute, 108
Postabortion syndrome, 138–46; *see
    also* Women: as victims of abor-
    tion
Potter, Robert G., 198
Powell, John, 164 n.5, 164 n.9
Powell, Lewis F., 241
Power, 46–48, 63, 67, 76–77, 83
Prager, Dennis, 19
Pregnancy: 52, 56, 64, 94, 116,
    120–21, 156, 162–63, 181, 206,
    233; as threat to woman's life,
    52–57, 63, 119, 202–3
Pregnancy care centers, 124–32, 207
Probabiliorism, 173
Pro-choice movement, xiii, xiv, 6,
    11 n.6, 33, 35–36, 39–41, 47–

48, 63, 65, 108, 140, 191, 193,
    197–98, 201, 203–4; *see also*
    Abortion: argument for
Procreation, 92–96, 101–2, 107
Pro-life movement: xiii, xiv, xvi, 1,
    6, 40–41, 108, 110; censored, 3;
    diversity of opinion in, xvi, 3, 42
    n.12, 84 n.6, 123, 132, 162,
    169–75, 206; inaction of, 152–
    63, 164 n.13; violence and, 13
    n.28, 69, 163
Properties, 19–25
Psychological sequelae to abortion.
    See Postabortion syndrome

Quickening, 27, 181–83, 209 n.14,
    232, 244 n.18

Rachel, 74–75, 77, 80
Rachels, James, 29
Rahner, Karl, 174
Rankin, Reginald, 201
Ravenell, Dawn, 205
Reagan, Leslie, 185, 194, 213 n37
Reardon, David C., 12 n.19
Redl, Fritz, 159
Rehnquist, William, 230, 240
Relativism, xii, xiii, 10, 47–48
Restell, Madame, 187
Rhode, Deborah L., 62, 64
Right to life, xiii, 10, 41, 230; *see
    also* Pro-life movement; Unborn
    human life
Rockefeller, Nelson, 194
Rodriguez, Ana, 8
Rodriguez, Magdalena Ortega, 205
Jane Roe. *See* Norma McCorvey
Roe v. Wade, xi–xiii, 12 n.19, 33–
    36, 56, 64, 124, 127, 129, 163,
    179–80, 182, 184–85, 187, 193–
    95, 197, 199–200, 202–8, 229–
    31, 236, 239–43
Rosen, Harold, 202, 222 n.163
Rosenberg, Gerald, 197, 199
RU-486, 14 n.35, 28, 78, 138, 157,
    232
Salamon, Julie, 120

Sargeant, Carolyn, 100
Scalia, Antonin, 230, 240, 242–43
Schindler's List, 152
Schlafley, Phyllis, 40
Schneider, David M., 103, 106
Scholten, Catherine, 213 n.31
Schumacher, E. F., 84 n.7
Science (and fertility), 72, 77–78; *see also* Infertility
Scrimshaw, Susan, 101
Sendak, Maurice, 80–81
Sentience, 27, 239. *See also* Fetal life; Fetus: viability of
Sex, 92–97, 105–9, 121, 126, 206
Sexton, Anne, 74
Sexually transmitted disease, 107–9, 206
Shepherd, Cybil, 40
Singer, Peter, 30, 32 n.21, 85 n.12
Sisterhood, 124-32
Skovgaard, Becky, 130–31
Smith, Walter Bedell, 152
Social change, 103–7
Social silence, sc, 2, 7, 9, 11 n.6
Solinger, Ricki, 201
Sologub, Fedor, 79
Sonogram. *See* Ultrasound
Souter, David, 239
Stare decisis, 243
Steinbock, Bonnie, 63–64, 85 n.19
Step-parents, 101
Stevens, John Paul, 229, 234–40, 244 nn.8, 18
Stigma, 109–10, 205, 207
Stix, Regine, 198–99
Substances, 19–25
Supreme Court of the United States, xiii, 33–34, 36, 229–43
Sutton, David
Szewczyk, Marilyn, 123–27, 129, 132
Tacitus, 104
Taney, Roger, 127
Taussig, Frederick, 197–99, 204
Thoday, J. M., 23
Thomas, Clarence, 240
Thomson, Judith Jarvis, 85 n.12, 157

Thornburgh v. American College of Obstetricians and Gynecologists, 233–38, 240–41
Thurer, Shari L., 117
Tietze, Christopher, 199, 222 n.160
Tiller, George, 8
Tolerance, 1, 39–41, 109
Tooley, Michael, 85 n.12
Tutiorism, 173
Twinning, 171, 174

Ultrasound, 69, 116–17, 120, 181
Unborn human life: 19, 25–31, 32 n.20, 61, 116, 167 n.63; as silent subject, xi, 1, 10, 69; children's literature and, 80–83; dehumanized, 2, 6–7, 10, 19, 30, 35, 43, 47, 63–67, 69, 116, 120, 139, 145, 158–59; knowledge of as human life, xii, 44, 72–73, 77–80, 115, 117–18, 124, 136–37, 139, 144; persecuted. *See* Persecution; poetry and, 73–77, 79, 89 n.73; significance of, 10, 43–46, 49, 51, 66, 68–71, 83; *see also* Fetal life; Fetus

Veal, Latachie, 205
Viability. *See* Fetus: viability of

Wagley, Charles, 102
Warren, Mary Ann, 29, 85 n.12, 157–58
Wattenberg, Ben, 107
Webster v. Reproductive Health Services, 231, 234, 239
Weigel, George, 115, 123
Wennberg, Robert, 37–38
White, Byron, 233–36, 238, 240
Wirthlin, Richard, 7
Women: 9, 61, 64–65, 68, 74, 82–83, 84 n.7, 87 n.44, 116–18, 121, 146; as victims of abortion, xiv, 3, 8, 12 n.19, 48, 115, 123, 132, 135, 138–39, 141–45, 180, 184–85, 200, 202–6, 226 n.215. *See also* Postabortion syndrome;

desire for children, 61–62, 70–72, 74–75, 80, 119–20, 138; guilt over aborting, 76, 79, 97, 138; reasons for aborting, 72–73, 75, 77, 96–98, 124, 136, 140–41, 205–6; supporting one another during pregnancy, 121, 124–32

Women's movement. *See* Feminism

Wood, Audrey, 81

Wood, Don, 81

Wordsworth, William, 68

World War II, 151–52, 155, 192, 203–4

The Worst of Times, 201

Wrongful birth, 57–58

Zawadzki, Edward, 199

Zeitgeist (contemporary), 3–6, 10

Zimmerman, Mary, 137

About the Editor and Contributors

Francis J. Beckwith, Ph. D. *Lecturer in Philosophy, University of Nevada, Las Vegas.; Senior Research Fellow, Nevada Policy Research Institute.* Dr. Beckwith is the author or editor of several books, including *The Abortion Controversy: A Reader* (Jones and Bartlett) and *Politically Correct Death: Answering the Arguments for Abortion Rights (*Baker). His articles have appeared in such publications as *International Philosophical Quarterly* and *Bibliotheca Sacra.*

Sidney Callahan, Ph. D. *Professor of Psychology, Mercy College.* Dr. Callahan is a regular contributor to *Commonweal* and *The Hastings Center Report.* Her many books include *With All Our Heart and Mind* (Crossroad) and *In Good Conscience: Reason and Emotion in Moral Decision Making* (HarperSanFrancisco).

Clarke D. Forsythe, J. D. *President, Americans United for Life.* Mr. Forsythe has written chapters in numerous books, including *Euthanasia and Other Controversies in the Care of the Dying Patient* and *Abortion, Medicine and the Law.* His articles have appeared in the *Notre Dame Law Review, Valparaiso University Law Review*, the *St. Louis University Public Law Review*, the *Brigham Young University Law Review* and *Issues in Law and Medicine.*

Thomas Murphy Goodwin, M. D. *Assistant Professor of Obstetrics and Gynecology, Division of Maternal-Fetal Medicine, University of Southern California School of Medicine; Director of Maternal-Fetal Medicine, Hospital of the Good Samaritan, Los Angeles, CA.* Dr. Goodwin has published articles on high risk pregnancy in *Obstetrics and Gynecology, The American Journal of Medical Genetics, The American Journal of Obstetrics and Gynecology*, and *The Journal of Clinical Endocrinology and Metabolism.*

Frederica Mathewes-Green, M. A. *Director of Communications, National Women's Coalition for Life.* Mrs. Mathewes-Green has published articles in *Policy Review*, the *Human Life Review*, *Crisis*, and *The World and I*. She currently writes a nationally syndicated column for Religion News Service, and is a national correspondent for *World* magazine. She is the author of *Real Choices: Offering Practical, Life-Affirming Alternatives to Abortion* (Questar).

Maria McFadden, B. A. *Executive Editor,* the *Human Life Review*. A regular contributor to the *Human Life Review*, Ms. McFadden writes frequently on American political trends and cultural aspects of the abortion debate. Her social commentary has appeared in *National Review* and other journals of opinion. She lives with her husband and son in New York City.

Michael McKenzie, Ph. D. *Adjunct Professor of Religion and Philosophy, Northwest College.* Dr. McKenzie has published articles in *The Simon Greenleaf Law Review*, *The Christian Research Journal* and the *Journal of the Evangelical Theological Society*, among other publications. He recently completed his dissertation on the ethics of theologian Paul Ramsey.

John A. Mitchell, M. A. A recent graduate of the Talbot School of Theology, Mr. Mitchell is currently a staff member with Campus Crusade for Christ at the University of Nevada, Las Vegas.

Richard John Neuhaus, *Editor in Chief, First Things; President, Institute on Religion and Public Life; Contributing Editor, National Review.* One of the nation's leading social analysts, Fr. Neuhaus writes the monthly column "The Public Square" in *First Things,* and regularly comments on social issues in other venues, including *The Wall Street Journal*. He is the author of over a dozen books, including *The Naked Public Square* (Eerdmans), *America Against Itself* (University of Notre Dame Press) and *Doing Well and Doing Good* (Doubleday).

Tom Poundstone, Ph. D. *Assistant Professor of Theology, Saint Mary's College.* Dr. Poundstone is presently at work on a second doctorate at the University of Notre Dame. He is a specialist in legal and medical ethics.

Scott B. Rae, Ph. D. *Associate Professor of Biblical Studies and Social Ethics, Talbot School of Theology, Biola University.* Dr. Rae has published in *The Christian Research Journal*, the *Linacre Quarterly* and other periodicals. His books include *An Introduction to Ethics* (Zondervan) and *The Ethics of Commercial Surrogate Motherhood: Brave New Families?* (Praeger).

David C. Reardon, Ph. D. *Director, The Elliot Institute; Editor, The Post-Abortion Review.* One of the nation's leading experts on the abortion experience of women, Dr. Reardon's books include *Abortion Malpractice* (Life Dynamics), *Aborted Women, Silent No More* (Loyola University Press), *Life Stories* (Crossway) and *Give Us Love, Not Abortions* (Fortress).

Brad Stetson, Ph. D. *Director, The David Institute.* Dr. Stetson is Director of Studies at The David Institute, a social research group. The permanent address of The David Institute is P. O. Box 1248, Tustin, CA 92681.

Olivia Vlahos, M. A. *Professor Emeritus of Social Science, Norwalk Community-Technical College.* Mrs.Vlahos is the author of several books, including *Body: The Ultimate Symbol* (Lipincott), and *Doing Business: The Anthropology of Striving, Thriving and Beating Out the Competition* (Franklin Watts). She has written for *First Things* and other journals of opinion.

Camille S. Williams, J. D. *Instructor in Philosophy, Brigham Young University.* Mrs. Williams has published essays and commentary in *First Things, The World and I, Deseret News, The Salt Lake Tribune*, and other periodicals. She has specialized in the study of American feminisms, and currently teaches--among other courses--a seminar in family law in BYU's Department of Family Sciences. She is the mother of five children.

ISBN 0-275-95032-8

90000>

EAN

9 780275 950323

HARDCOVER BAR CODE